Pearson Nursing Reviews & Rationales

Fluids, Electrolytes, & Acid–Base Balance

D0206679

Fourth Edition

SERIES EDITOR

MaryAnn Hogan, PhD(c), MSN, RN, CNE

Clinical Assistant Professor

College of Nursing

University of Massachusetts–Amherst

Amherst, Massachusetts

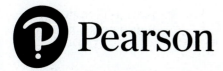

Vice President, Health Science and TED: Julie Levin Alexander
Portfolio Manager: Hilarie Surrena
Development Editor: Rachel Bedard
Portfolio Management Assistant: Taylor Scuglik
Vice President, Content Production and Digital Studio: Paul DeLuca
Managing Producer Health Science: Melissa Bashe
Content Producer: Michael Giacobbe
Vice President, Product Marketing: David Gesell

Executive Field Marketing Manager: Christopher Barry
Field Marketing Manager: Brittany Hammond
Managing Producer, Digital Studio, Health Science: Amy Peltier
Digital Producer: Jeff Henn
Full Service Vendor: SPi Global
Full-Service Project Management: Michelle Gardner, SPi Global
Cover Image: Andrew Brookes/Cultura/ Getty Images

Notice: Care has been taken to confirm the accuracy of the information presented in this book. The authors, editors, and the publisher, however, cannot accept any responsibility for errors or omissions or for the consequences for application of the information in this book and make no warranty, express or implied, with respect to its contents. The authors and the publisher have exerted every effort to ensure that drug selections and dosages set forth in this text are in accord with current recommendations and practice at time of publication. However, in view of ongoing research, changes in government regulations, and the constant flow of information relating to drug therapy and drug reactions, the reader is urged to check the package inserts of all drugs for any change in indications of dosage and for added warnings and precautions. This is particularly important when the recommended agent is a new and/or infrequently employed drug. The authors and publisher disclaim all responsibility for any liability, loss, injury, or damage incurred as a consequence, directly or indirectly, of the use and application of any of the contents of this volume.

Copyright © 2018 by Pearson Education, Inc. All rights reserved. Manufactured in the United States of America. This publication is protected by Copyright, and permission should be obtained from the publisher prior to any prohibited reproduction, storage in a retrieval system, or transmission in any form or by any means, electronic, mechanical, photocopying, recording, or likewise. For information regarding permissions, request forms and the appropriate contacts within the Pearson Education Global Rights & Permissions Department, please visit www.pearsoned.com/permissions/

Library of Congress Cataloging-in-Publication Data

Title: Fluids, electrolytes, & acid-base balance.
Other titles: Fluids, electrolytes, and acid base balance | Pearson nursing reviews & rationales series.
Description: Fourth edition. | Boston : Pearson, [2018] | Series: Pearson nursing reviews & rationales | Includes bibliographical references and index.
Identifiers: LCCN 2017034781| ISBN 9780134457710 | ISBN 0134457714
Subjects: | MESH: Water-Electrolyte Imbalance—nursing | Acid-Base Equilibrium | Acid-Base Imbalance—nursing | Water-Electrolyte Balance | Examination Questions
Classification: LCC RC630 | NLM WY 18.2 | DDC 616.3/992—dc23
LC record available at https://lccn.loc.gov/2017034781

1 17

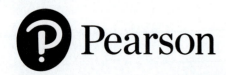

ISBN 10: 0-13-445771-4
ISBN 13: 978-0-13-445771-0

Contents

Welcome to the Pearson Nursing Reviews & Rationales Series!

This series has been specifically designed to provide a clear and concentrated review of important nursing knowledge and concepts in the following content areas:

- Nursing Fundamentals
- Fluids, Electrolytes, & Acid–Base Balance
- Medical–Surgical Nursing
- Pathophysiology
- Pharmacology
- Maternal–Newborn Nursing
- Child Health Nursing
- Mental Health Nursing

The books in this series are designed for use either by current nursing students as a study aid for nursing course work and NCLEX-RN® exam preparation, or by practicing nurses seeking a comprehensive yet concise review of a nursing specialty or subject area.

This series is truly unique. One key feature is that it has been developed and reviewed by a large team of nurse educators from the United States and Canada to ensure that each chapter is edited by a nurse expert in the content area under study. The series editor, Mary-Ann Hogan, designed the overall series in collaboration with a core Pearson team to take full advantage of Pearson's cutting edge technology. The consulting editors for each book, also experts in that specialty area, then reviewed all chapters and test questions submitted for comprehensiveness and accuracy. Finally, MaryAnn Hogan reviewed the chapters in each book and their corresponding questions for consistency, accuracy, and applicability to the latest NCLEX-RN® Test Plan.

All books in the series are identical in their overall design for your convenience. As an added value, each book comes with a comprehensive support package, including access to additional questions online and an appendix of valuable information for clinical reference and quick review.

What's New in this Edition

- Completely updated review material reflecting the 2016 NCLEX-RN® Test Plan

- Online access to Nursing Reviews and Rationales.com where students can complete quizzes on a computer or other device to practice for the NCLEX® experience.
- Hundreds of updated or brand-new NCLEX®-style practice test questions.
- Dozens of new alternate-item format questions
- The latest test prep advice from MaryAnn Hogan, trusted expert in what nursing students need to know.

Study Tips

Use of this book should help simplify your review. To make the most of your valuable study time, also follow these simple but important suggestions:

1. Use a weekly calendar to schedule study sessions.
   - Outline the time frames for all of your activities (home, school, appointments, etc.) on a weekly calendar.
   - Find the "holes" in your calendar, which are the times when you can plan to study. Add study sessions to the calendar at times when you can expect to be mentally alert and follow your plan!
2. Create the optimal study environment.
   - Eliminate external sources of distraction, such as online social media, smart phones, television, etc.
   - Eliminate internal sources of distraction, such as hunger, thirst, or dwelling on problems that you cannot work on at this time.
   - Take a break for 10 minutes or so after each hour of concentrated study, both as a reward and as a physical and mental break to reenergize you.
3. Use prereading strategies to increase comprehension of chapter material.
   - Skim the chapter headings (because they identify chapter content).

- Read the definitions of key terms to learn new words that will help you comprehend chapter information.
- Review all graphic aids (figures, tables, boxes) because they are often used to explain important points in the chapter.

4. Read the chapter thoroughly but at a reasonable speed.
   - Comprehension and retention are actually enhanced by not reading too slowly.
   - Do take the time to reread any section that is unclear to you.

5. Summarize what you have learned.
   - Use the accompanying online resource, NursingReviewsandRationales.com, to test yourself with hundreds of NCLEX-RN®-style practice questions.
   - Review again any sections that correspond to questions you answered incorrectly or incompletely.

Test-Taking Strategies

Test-taking strategies accompany the rationales for every question in the series. These strategies will assist you to select the correct answer by breaking down the question, even if you don't know the correct response. Use the following strategies to increase your success on nursing tests or examinations:

- Get sufficient sleep and have something to eat before taking a test. Eat carbohydrates that have a low glycemic index and a low-fat protein source to help maintain energy and focus. Avoid eating concentrated sweets (which have a high glycemic index) to prevent a rapid upward and then downward surge in your blood glucose. Also avoid high-fat foods that will make you sleepy.
- Take deep breaths periodically during the test. Remember, the brain requires oxygen to function well, not just calories.
- Read each question carefully, identifying the stem, all the options, and any critical words or phrases in either the stem or options:
  - Critical words in the stem such as *most important* indicate the need to set priorities, because more than one option is likely to contain a statement that is technically correct.
  - Remember that the presence of absolute words such as *never* or *only* in an answer

option is more likely to make that option incorrect.
- Determine who is the client in the question. Often this is the person with the health problem, but it may also be a significant other, relative, friend, or another nurse.
- Decide whether the stem is a true response stem or a false response stem. With a true response stem, the correct answer will be a true statement, and vice-versa.
- Determine what the question is really asking, sometimes known as the core issue of the question. Evaluate all answer options in relation to this issue, and not strictly to the "correctness" of the statement in each individual option.
- Use these strategies to answer questions in which only one option can be selected, such as standard multiple choice, exhibit, or graphic options questions:
  - Eliminate options that are obviously incorrect; then go back and reread the stem and any associated information. Evaluate those remaining options against the stem once more to make a final selection.
  - If two answers seem similar and correct, try to decide whether one is more global or comprehensive. If one option includes the alternative option within it, it is likely that the more global response is correct.
- When answering multiple response questions, which commonly contain the words "select all that apply," read each option and evaluate it as a true-false statement. If the wording of the question indicates the answers would be true/correct statements, select all of those that would represent appropriate nursing practice. If the question is wording negatively (with words such as "contraindicated, 'unsafe," etc.), select those that would not represent appropriate nursing practice. Remember that nurses need to practice safely but also must be able to identify threats to safe client care.

The NCLEX-RN® Licensing Examination

Upon graduation from a nursing program, you will need to pass the NCLEX-RN® licensing examination to begin professional nursing practice. The

NCLEX-RN® examination is a Computer Adaptive Test (CAT) that ranges in length from 75 to 265 individual (stand-alone) test items, depending on your performance during the examination. The blueprint for the exam is reviewed and revised every three years by the National Council of State Boards of Nursing using the results of a job analysis study of new graduate nurses practicing within the first six months after graduation. Each question on the exam is coded to a *Client Need* and an *Integrated Process*.

Client Needs Categories

There are eight *Client Needs* categories being tested on the licensing examination. Each exam will contain a minimum and maximum percent of questions from each of these categories. The percentages of questions from the *Client Needs* categories for the NCLEX-RN® Test Plan effective April 2016 are as follows:

- Safe Effective Care Environment
  - Management of Care (17–23%)
  - Safety and Infection Control (9–15%)
- Health Promotion and Maintenance (6–12%)
- Psychosocial Integrity (6–12%)
- Physiological Integrity
  - Basic Care and Comfort (6–12%)
  - Pharmacological and Parenteral Therapies (12–18%)
  - Reduction of Risk Potential (9–15%)
  - Physiological Adaptation (11–17%)

Integrated Processes

The integrated processes identified on the NCLEX-RN® Test Plan effective April 2016, with condensed definitions, are as follows:

- Nursing Process: a scientific and clinical reasoning approach to nursing practice that consists of assessment, analysis, planning, implementation, and evaluation.
- Caring: client–nurse interaction(s) characterized by mutual respect and trust and that are collaboratively directed toward achieving desired client outcomes.
- Communication and Documentation: verbal and/or nonverbal interactions between nurse and others (client, family, health care team); a written or electronic recording of activities or events during client care to demonstrate accountability and adherence to standards of care.
- Teaching/Learning: facilitating client's acquisition of knowledge, skills, and attitudes that lead to behavior change.
- Culture and Spirituality: interaction of nurse and client (individual, family, or identified group) which recognizes and considers the client-identified preferences for care as well as applicable standards and legal instructions.

More detailed information about this examination may be obtained by visiting the National Council of State Boards of Nursing website at http://www.ncsbn.org and viewing the *2016 NCLEX-RN® Detailed Test Plan*.[1]

[1]Reference: National Council of State Boards of Nursing, Inc. *2016 NCLEX-RN® Test Plan*. Effective April 1, 2016. Retrieved from https://www.ncsbn.org/testplans.htm

HOW TO GET THE MOST OUT OF THIS BOOK

Each chapter has the following elements to guide you during review and study:

Chapter Objectives describe what you will be able to know or do after learning the material covered in the chapter.

Objectives

➤ Review the basic physiology of acid–base balance.
➤ Identify potential acid–base imbalances.
➤ Identify priority nursing concerns for acid–base imbalances.
➤ Describe the therapeutic management of acid–base imbalances.

NCLEX-RN® Test Prep

Access the NEW Web-based app that provides students with additional practice questions in preparation for the NCLEX experience.

Review at a Glance contains a glossary of key terms used in the chapter, with definitions provided up-front and available at your fingertips, to help you stay focused and make the best use of your study time.

Review at a Glance

hyperkalemia serum potassium level above the laboratory normal value (usually 5.1 mEq/L)

hypokalemia serum level of potassium falls below 3.5 mEq/L

relative hyperkalemia movement of potassium from intracellular fluid to extracellular fluid, leading to elevated serum potassium levels without a true body increase of potassium, such as occurs with acidosis

relative hypokalemia movement of potassium from extracellular fluid to intracellular fluid, leading to lowered serum potassium levels without a true decrease of potassium in body, such as occurs with insulin therapy

sodium-potassium pump controls concentration of potassium by removing three sodium ions from cell for every two potassium ions that return to cell; fueled by breakdown of ATP and responsible for causing muscle cells to generate action potentials and transmit impulses

Pretest provides a 10-question quiz as a sample overview of the chapter material and helps you decide in what areas you need the most—or the least—review.

PRETEST

1 The nurse would expect a client to have a high serum level of magnesium after seeing which health problem listed in the medical history?

1. Malabsorption
2. Anemia
3. Overuse of laxatives
4. Excessive alcohol intake

Practice to Pass questions are open-ended, stimulate critical thinking, and reinforce mastery of the chapter information.

Practice to Pass

In caring for a client with hypernatremia, what should the nurse do to help ensure client safety?

NCLEX Alert identifies concepts that are likely to be tested on the NCLEX-RN® examination. Be sure to learn the information highlighted wherever you see this icon.

Case Study, found at the end of the chapter, provides an opportunity for you to use your critical thinking and clinical reasoning skills to "put it all together." It describes a true-to-life client case situation and asks you open-ended questions about how you would provide care for that client and/or family.

Case Study

A 69-year-old client with chronic obstructive pulmonary disease (COPD) is admitted with an acute respiratory infection. The client has a history of hypertension, diabetes mellitus, and mild renal insufficiency. You are the nurse assigned to the care of this client.

1. What would this client's ABGs look like based on the admitting diagnosis?

2. What will you do to help improve the client's respiratory status?

3. Why is this client's $PaCO_2$ different than a client who does not have COPD?

4. What teaching does this client require in order to prevent development of metabolic alkalosis?

5. Are there any other acid–base imbalances for which this client is at risk because of the client's medical history?

Posttest provides an additional 10-question quiz at the end of the chapter. It provides you with feedback about mastery of the chapter material after review and study. All pretest and posttest questions contain comprehensive rationales for the correct and incorrect answers, and are coded according to cognitive level of difficulty, NCLEX-RN® Test Plan category of Client Need, and Integrated Process. Each question also contains one or more suggested strategies for selecting answer(s).

POSTTEST

1 The nurse should identify which clients as being at risk for developing metabolic alkalosis? Select all that apply.

1. A client who has a nasogastric tube (NGT) to continuous suction
2. A client who has had diarrhea for 2 days
3. A client who is admitted with salicylate toxicity
4. A client who takes antacids frequently for heartburn
5. A client who is admitted with asthmatic bronchitis

NCLEX-RN® Test Prep: NursingReviewsandRationales.com

For those who want to prepare for the NCLEX-RN®, practicing online will help you become more familiar with the computer-based testing experience, especially for alternate item format questions. With this new edition, use the code printed inside the front cover of the book to access Nursing Reviews & Rationales, which offers hundreds of practice questions using a variety of NCLEX®-style formats. This includes the practice questions found in all chapters of the book as well as 30 additional questions per chapter. Nursing Reviews & Rationales allows you to choose two ways to prepare for the NCLEX-RN®. Both approaches personalize your practice experience according to where you are in your NCLEX® preparation.

Nursing Notes Appendix

This appendix provides a reference for frequently used facts and information. It is designed to provide quick and easy access to information for the NCLEX® licensing examination.

About the Fluids, Electrolytes, and Acid–Base Balance Book

Chapters in this book cover "need-to-know" information about principles of fluids, electrolytes, and acid–base balance, including focused assessments and how they affect entire body systems. Individual chapters focus on specific electrolytes (sodium, chloride, potassium, calcium, magnesium, and phosphorus), acid–base disturbances, and replacement therapies for common fluid and electrolyte imbalances. Each chapter includes definitions, etiologies, clinical manifestations, and therapeutic management of fluids, electrolytes, and acid–base problems in the context of the nursing process.

Acknowledgments

This book is a monumental effort of collaboration. Without the contributions of many individuals, this edition of *Fluids, Electrolytes, & Acid–Base Balance: Reviews & Rationales* would not have been possible. Thank you to the reviewers for this edition for their thoughtful comments, which were used in the preparation of this fourth edition. These reviewers are Kim Amer, PhD, RN, Depaul University, Chicago, IL; Charlene Gagliardi, RN, BSN, MSN, Mount Saint Mary's University, Emmitsburg, MD; Susan Growe, DNP, RN, Nevada State College, Henderson, NV; Sylvia Jones, MSN, RN, National University, San Diego, CA; Christine Kleckner, RN, Minneapolis Community Technical College, Minneapolis, MN; Rebecca Otten, EdD, RN, California State University, Fullerton, CA; Donna Volpe, RN-BC, MSN, Penn State University, State College, PA.

Thanks also to the contributors and reviewers for previous editions of this book: Margaret M. Gingrich, RN, MSN, Harrisburg Area Community College, Harrisburg, PA; Edward Nichols, RN, MSN, San Jacinto College Central, Houston, TX; Daryle Wane, APRN, BC, MS, Pasco-Hernando Community College, New Port Richey, FL; Faisal Aboul-Enein, DrPH, RN, NP, Texas Women's University, Houston, TX; Julie A. Adkins, RN, MSN, FNP, Family Nurse Practitioner, West Frankfort, IL; Patricia Boyle Egland, MSN, RN, CPNP-PC, The City University of New York, Borough of Manhattan Community College, New York, NY; Susan J. Brillhart, DNS(c), RN, PNP-BC, Borough of Manhattan Community College, New York, NY; Linda Wilson Covington, PhD, RN, Middle Tennessee State University, Murfreesboro, TN; June S. Goyne, RN, MSN, EdD(C), CEN, Columbus State University, Columbus, GA; Ann Putnam Johnson, EdD, RN, Western Carolina University, Cullowhee, NC; Kathy M. Ketchum, RN, PhD, Southern Illinois University Edwardsville, Edwardsville, IL; Andrea R. Mann, MSN, RN, CNE, Aria Health School of Nursing, Philadelphia, PA; Kristy A. Nielson, BSN, CCRN, BS, Western Wyoming Community College, Memorial Hospital of Sweetwater County, Rock Springs, WY; Mary Catherine Rawls, Castleton State College, Castleton, VT; Lynn Rhyne, MN, RN, Coastal Georgia Community College, Brunswick, GA; Bernadette VanDeusen, MSN, RN, Ohlone College, Fremont, CA; Karen Whitman, RN, MS CCPN, Walter Reed Army Medical Center, Washington DC. Their work will surely assist both students and licensed nurses alike to extend and/or freshen their knowledge of fluid, electrolyte, and acid–base balance and imbalances.

I owe a special debt of gratitude to the wonderful team at Pearson for their expertise and encouragement during development of this fourth edition. Hilarie Surrena, Nursing Portfolio Manager, oversaw this revision and fostered a culture of collaboration and teamwork. Rachel Bedard, Developmental Editor, shared her immense expertise with warmth and enthusiasm while coordinating different facets of this project. Her high standards and attention to detail contributed greatly to the final "look" of this book. Portfolio Management Assistant, Taylor Scuglik, helped to keep the project moving forward on a day-to-day basis, and I am grateful for her efforts as well. A very special thank you goes to the designers of the book and the production team, led by Michael Giacobbe, Managing Editor, who brought the ideas and manuscript into final form.

Thank you to the publishing team at SPi Global, led by Michelle Gardner and Karen Berry, Project Managers, for the detail-oriented work of creating this book. I greatly appreciate their diligence, attention to detail, and spirit of collaboration.

Finally, I would like to acknowledge and gratefully thank my children, Michael Jr., Kathryn, Kristen, and William, whose love and unending support enrich my life beyond words. I would also like to thank my nursing students, past and present, for continuing to inspire me daily with their quest for knowledge and passion for nursing. You are indeed the future of nursing!

–*MaryAnn Hogan*

Fluid Balance and Imbalances

1

Objectives

➤ Explain concepts related to fluid movement.

➤ Identify assessment data and diagnostic testing indicated to determine fluid volume deficit (dehydration) and fluid volume excess (overload).

➤ Identify clinical presentations of clients exhibiting fluid volume deficit or fluid volume excess.

➤ Identify priority nursing concerns for clients experiencing fluid imbalance.

➤ Describe the therapeutic management of clients exhibiting fluid volume deficit and fluid volume excess.

➤ Describe the management of nursing care for clients exhibiting fluid imbalances.

NCLEX-RN® Test Prep

Access the NEW Web-based app that provides students with additional practice questions in preparation for the NCLEX experience.

Review at a Glance

albumin a major plasma protein produced by the liver

aldosterone adrenal gland hormone that causes the kidneys to reabsorb sodium into the blood (causing more water to be reabsorbed by osmosis) and excrete potassium into urine, resulting in concentrated urine and lower urine output

anasarca generalized edema in the body

antidiuretic hormone (ADH) hormone produced by hypothalamus and stored/released by posterior pituitary that causes the kidneys to retain more water in the blood, thus increasing body water, resulting in concentrated urine and lower urine output

colloid osmotic pressure (COP) pulling force for water created by colloids in solution

colloid large solute particle, such as protein, in solution that exerts a pulling force for water

diffusion movement of particles in a solution from an area of higher concentration to an area of lower concentration in order to equalize the concentration

electrolyte a substance that, when dissolved in water, separates into charged particles (ions)

extracellular fluid (ECF) fluid space that lies outside of cells; composed of two spaces, the interstitial (tissue) spaces around cells and the vascular space inside blood vessels

filtration movement of fluid and solute through a semipermeable membrane due to hydrostatic and osmotic forces

free water a hypotonic solution that provides more water than electrolytes, diluting the ECF, making it hypotonic; water then shifts by osmosis from the ECF to the ICF until osmotic equilibrium is reached in both spaces; this rehydrates the ICF as well as the ECF

hemoconcentration condition in which the plasma is more concentrated

than normal (higher osmolality than normal)

hemodilution condition in which the plasma is more dilute than normal (lower osmolality than normal)

hydrostatic pressure pushing force of a fluid against the walls of the space it occupies

hypertonic having an osmolality higher than normal plasma

hypervolemia a state of fluid volume excess or overload in the bloodstream

hypotonic having an osmolality lower than normal plasma

hypovolemia a state of insufficient fluid volume circulating in the bloodstream

interstitial fluid fluid space that lies around the cells (cells "float" in interstitial fluid); the interstitial space and vascular space make up the extracellular fluid (ECF)

intracellular fluid (ICF) fluid space that lies inside of the cells

PRETEST

isotonic having the same osmolality as normal plasma

oncotic pressure pulling force a solution has for water due to its protein content

osmolality concentration of solute (particles) per kilogram of water, which creates the pulling power of that solution for water

osmolarity concentration of solute (particles) per liter of solution, which creates the pulling power of that solution for water

osmosis the pulling of water through a semipermeable membrane from an area of lower concentration (fewer particles, more water) to an area of higher concentration (more particles, less water) in order to equalize concentration on both sides

osmotic pressure pulling force a solution has for water; a solution's osmotic pressure is determined by its osmolality (concentration)—the higher the osmolality, the higher the osmotic pressure (force with which it will pull water in from other areas)

semipermeable membrane a membrane that allows some particles to pass through freely and not others (e.g., cell walls and capillary membranes)

specific gravity a measure of the concentration of a solution using solute–solvent ratio; specific gravity of water (no solute) is 1.000; urine specific gravity is normally 1.010–1.030, and is used to indirectly reflect serum osmolality

vascular space space within the blood vessels, usually discussed in terms of blood volume carrying capacity

PRETEST

1 The nurse determines that which client is at highest risk for developing a fluid volume deficit (FVD)?

1. A 76-year-old client who has a nasogastric (NG) tube attached to low suction following abdominal surgery
2. A thin 55-year-old client who smokes cigarettes and takes glucocorticoids for chronic lung disease
3. A 1-year-old child being treated in the clinic for a runny nose and an ear infection
4. A generally healthy 30-year-old client who is jogging in 45-degree weather

2 The nurse is assisting in a health fair at a senior citizen center. Which instruction should the nurse provide to an older adult when discussing guidelines about remaining hydrated in hot weather?

1. "If your urine is clear yellow, you are drinking adequate fluids."
2. "Drink only water to keep yourself properly hydrated."
3. "Popsicles, gelatin, and ice cream provide fluid intake as well as the liquids you drink."
4. "Use your thirst as a guide to the amount of fluid you should be drinking."

3 An adult client in the clinic reports a cough, fever, weakness, dizziness, and nausea and vomiting for 3 days. Examination reveals dry tongue and oral mucosa and concentrated urine. To assess the client's fluid status, the nurse checks which pertinent assessment parameters? Select all that apply.

1. Skin temperature
2. Heart rate
3. Presence of dyspnea
4. BP in lying and standing positions
5. Oxygen saturation at rest

4 The nurse evaluates the hydration status of a client who has been receiving intravenous (IV) fluids at 150 mL/hour. The nurse identifies that the client has fluid volume excess (FVE) after assessing which of the following? Select all that apply.

1. Neck veins are distended when head of the bed is elevated 45 degrees
2. Hand veins empty when hand is raised above the heart
3. Peripheral pulses are rapid and weak
4. Client becomes short of breath when ambulating
5. Pitting edema is present over tibia

5 A client hospitalized for gastrointestinal (GI) bleeding has a prescription for nasogastric tube (NGT) placement with irrigations until the returns are clear. Which prescribed solution should the nurse plan on using?

1. 10% dextrose in water ($D_{10}W$)
2. 5% dextrose in water (D_5W)
3. 0.9% sodium chloride (NaCl)
4. 0.45% sodium chloride (½ NaCl)

6 A 70-year-old client with a past medical history of hypertension and myocardial infarction is postoperative after stomach surgery. Vital signs have been stable with an IV of D_5½NS infusing at 100 mL/hour. The client now reports dyspnea, has a moist cough, and oxygen saturation has fallen to 92%. What action should the nurse take first?

1. Measure blood pressure (BP) and heart rate.
2. Assess legs and arms for pitting edema.
3. Notify the healthcare provider.
4. Slow the intravenous rate to 10–20 mL/hour.

7 A 45-year-old client with fluid volume excess (FVE) because of acute kidney dysfunction is placed on a 1000 mL fluid restriction per 24-hour period. The client asks the nurse, "Why is there such a severe fluid restriction when I already have dry lips and mouth?" Which response by the nurse is best?

1. "The healthcare provider prescribed the fluid restriction, so it is important to comply with the restriction."
2. "Your kidneys cannot eliminate extra fluid right now, so intake must be limited to protect your heart and lungs from being overloaded with fluid."
3. "You probably drank too much fluid before you got sick, so you can't compare your usual intake to your limitations now that your kidneys are not working."
4. "Too much fluid will cause your heart to fail and your lungs to fill with fluid, which could be dangerous."

8 A 45-year-old client is receiving a loop diuretic as treatment for edema caused by fluid overload. The nurse determines the client is experiencing an excessive response to the medication when the client demonstrates which assessment findings?

1. Blood urea nitrogen (BUN) 28 mg/dL, hematocrit (Hct) 45%, and a 3.6-kg (8-lb) weight loss in 24 hours
2. BUN 21 mg/dL, Hct 29%, and a 3.6-kg (8-lb) weight gain in 24 hours
3. BUN 16 mg/dL, Hct 31%, and a 3.6-kg (8-lb) weight loss in 24 hours
4. BUN 25 mg/dL, Hct 33%, and a 3.6-kg (8-lb) weight gain in 24 hours

9 During intershift report, the nurse is told that a client who experienced a stroke has now developed diabetes insipidus (DI). The nurse concludes this client is now at risk for which problem?

1. Severe fluid volume deficit because of excess urine output
2. Severe fluid volume overload because of inadequate urine output
3. Hyperglycemia and associated polyuria because of poor insulin production
4. Hypoglycemia from excess insulin production with uncertain effect on fluid volume

10 When caring for an adult receiving an intravenous (IV) infusion of 3% sodium chloride (NaCl), the nurse places priority on monitoring what client parameters to detect complications of therapy? Select all that apply.

1. Neurologic status
2. Urine specific gravity
3. Serum glucose levels
4. Lung sounds
5. Serum sodium level

➤ *See pages 28–29 for Answers and Rationales.*

I. OVERVIEW OF FLUID MOVEMENT

A. Fluid transport issues

    1. Body fluid spaces (see Figure 1-1)

        a. Intracellular fluid (ICF): fluid within body cells; two-thirds of body fluid is ICF

        b. Extracellular fluid (ECF): fluid outside body cells; consists of two components, the **interstitial fluid** (fluid surrounding cells) and fluid within the **vascular space** (blood vessels)

        c. Fluid constantly moves among the intracellular, interstitial, and vascular spaces to maintain body fluid balance

            1) ICF is most stable and is fairly resistant to major fluid shifts

            2) Vascular fluid is least stable; it is quickly lost or gained in response to fluid intake or losses

            3) Interstitial fluid is reserve fluid, replacing fluid either in blood vessels or cells, depending on need

    2. Osmosis (see Figure 1-2)

        a. Water moves through a **semipermeable membrane** (membrane that allows water and small particles, but not large particles, to easily pass through) from an area of lower concentration (fewer particles, more water) to an area of higher concentration (more particles, less water) until concentrations are equalized on both sides of the membrane

Figure 1-1	
Body fluid spaces	

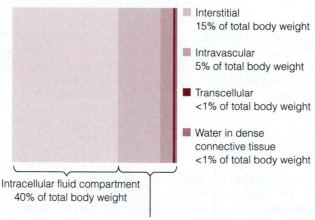

Total body fluids = 60% of body weight

    Interstitial
    15% of total body weight

    Intravascular
    5% of total body weight

    Transcellular
    <1% of total body weight

    Water in dense
    connective tissue
    <1% of total body weight

Intracellular fluid compartment
40% of total body weight

Extracellular fluid compartment
20% of total body weight

Figure 1-2	
Osmosis	

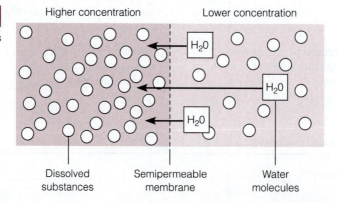

Higher concentration   Lower concentration

H_2O

H_2O

H_2O

Dissolved substances   Semipermeable membrane   Water molecules

b. Osmosis is a major force in body fluid movement and intravenous (IV) fluid therapy

    1) Cell membranes and capillary membranes are semipermeable

    2) Water moves into and out of cells and capillaries by osmosis

3. Osmolality and osmotic pressure

    a. *Osmolality* and *osmolarity* are both terms that refer to a solution's concentration, which creates its **osmotic pressure** (pulling power of a solution for water)

        1) **Osmolality** is the concentration of solute (particles) per kilogram of water, whereas **osmolarity** is the concentration of solute (particles) per liter of a solution (solvent does not have to be water)

        2) Because body fluid solvent is water and 1 liter of water weighs 1 kilogram, the terms can be used interchangeably in discussing human fluid physiology; the term *osmolality* is used here

        3) The higher the osmolality (concentration) of a solution, the greater its pulling power for water

    b. Serum osmolality is the concentration of particles (major particles are sodium and protein) in the plasma

        1) Normal serum osmolality is 275–295 milliosmoles/liter (mOsm/L)

        2) Serum osmolality can be estimated

            a) Sodium is the major solute in plasma contributing to its osmolality (estimated serum osmolality = 2 times the serum sodium level)

            b) Urea (BUN) and glucose are both large particles that increase serum osmolality when present in excess amounts in blood

            c) When either BUN or glucose or both are elevated, the serum osmolality will be higher than 2 times the sodium level, so the following formula will be more accurate:

$$\text{Serum osmolality} = 2 \times \text{serum sodium} + \frac{\text{BUN}}{3} + \frac{\text{glucose}}{18}$$

    c. The term ***isotonic*** is defined as having the same osmolality as normal plasma

        1) Isotonic IV fluids have the same osmolality as normal plasma; no osmotic pressure difference is created, so fluids remain primarily in the ECF

        2) Isotonic IV fluids are used to replace extracellular fluid and electrolyte losses and to expand vascular volume quickly

        3) Isotonic IV fluids (see Table 1-1)

            a) Normal saline (NS; 0.9% NaCl): sodium and chloride in water with same osmolality as normal plasma; NS provides no calories or **free water** (water without solute)

            b) Ringer's solution: contains sodium, potassium, and calcium in similar concentrations to plasma, but no dextrose, magnesium, or bicarbonate; Ringer's solution provides no calories or free water

            c) Lactated Ringer's (LR) solution: contains sodium, chloride, potassium, calcium, and lactate in concentrations similar to normal plasma; LR provides no dextrose, magnesium, or free water

    d. The term ***hypotonic*** is defined as having a lower osmolality than normal plasma

        1) Hypotonic IV fluids have a lower osmolality than normal plasma (<290 mOsm/L)

        2) Water is pulled out of blood vessels into cells, resulting in decreased vascular volume and increased cell water

        3) Hypotonic IV fluids are used to prevent and treat cellular dehydration by providing free water to cells or to restore renal functioning

Table 1-1	Hydrating Solutions	
Solution	**Uses**	**Nursing Implications**
Isotonic 0.9% sodium chloride (normal saline or NS) Lactated Ringer's (LR) 5% dextrose in water (D₅W)	Has same concentration of solutes as plasma, so it remains in vascular compartment, expanding vascular volume NS and LR are crystalloid solutions that ↑ fluid volume in both intravascular and interstitial spaces with minimal fluid volume expansion NS is the only solution to be administered with blood products D₅W is isotonic on initial administration but provides free water when metabolized, expanding intra- and extracellular fluid volumes	Assess for signs of hypervolemia • Bounding pulse • Shortness of breath • Distended neck veins Assess for signs of hypovolemia • Urine output <30 mL/hr • Weak, thready pulse • Subnormal temperature • Flat neck veins
Hypotonic 0.45% sodium chloride (½NS) 0.225% sodium chloride (¼NS)	Has lesser concentration of solutes than plasma, so treats cellular dehydration through fluid shifting out of blood vessels into cells; promotes elimination by kidneys	Do not administer to clients at risk for third-space fluid shift or fluid sequestration in a body space (results in circulating volume loss and ↑ risk for organ failure or ↑ intracranial pressure)
Hypertonic 5% dextrose in normal saline (D₅NS) 5% dextrose in 0.45% sodium chloride (D₅½NS) 5% dextrose in lactated Ringer's (D₅LR) 10% dextrose in water (D₁₀W) 20% dextrose in water (D₂₀W) 50% dextrose in water (D₅₀W)	Has higher concentration of solutes than plasma, thus causing fluid to shift from cells into vascular compartment, expanding vascular volume 10% dextrose—stand-by solution for clients receiving TPN 50% dextrose—used for hypoglycemia	Do not administer to clients with kidney or heart disease or clients who are dehydrated; monitor for signs of hypervolemia
Volume Expanders (colloid solutions) Albumin 5% Albumin 25% Dextran 40 Hetastarch Plasma protein fraction	Contain substances that cannot diffuse through capillary walls, resulting in ↑ plasma volume and ↑ osmotic pressure, causing fluids to move into vascular compartment; used to treat hypovolemic shock	Establish baseline vital signs, lung and heart sounds, and central venous pressure; repeat per agency protocols Administer with a large-gauge (18- to 19-gauge) needle Monitor intake and output Monitor for signs of hypervolemia
Nutrient 5% dextrose (D₅W) 5% dextrose in 0.45% sodium chloride (D₅½NS)	Contain some form of carbohydrate (e.g., dextrose, glucose) and water D₅W provides 170 calories per liter	Useful in preventing dehydration but does not provide sufficient calories to promote wound healing, weight gain, or normal growth in children
Electrolyte 0.9% sodium chloride (NS) Ringer's solution (has sodium, chloride, potassium, calcium) 5% dextrose in 0.45% sodium chloride (D₅½NS)	Saline and electrolytes restore vascular volume and replace electrolytes LR is also an alkalinizing solution that treats metabolic acidosis D₅½NS is an acidifying solution to treat metabolic alkalosis	Monitor fluid and electrolytes Monitor arterial blood gases Monitor intake and output

Source: Hogan, Mary Ann, *Pearson Reviews & Rationales: Comprehensive Review for NCLEX-RN*, 2nd Ed., © 2012. Reprinted and Electronically reproduced by permission of Pearson Education, Inc., New York, NY.

4) Clients requiring hypotonic IV fluids require frequent monitoring of vital signs, level of consciousness, and circulation to detect depletion of vascular volume and cerebral cellular edema

5) Hypotonic IV fluids are contraindicated in acute brain injuries because cerebral cells are very sensitive to free water, absorbing it rapidly and leading to cellular edema

6) Hypotonic intravenous fluids (see Table 1-1 again)
   a) 5% dextrose in water (D_5W): *although D_5W is isotonic in the IV bag, it has a hypotonic effect in the body*; the dextrose is quickly metabolized once infused, leaving free water that shifts by osmosis from vessels into cells; for each liter of D_5W, roughly ⅔ enters cells and ⅓ remains in extracellular space
   b) 0.45% saline (½NS) and 0.225 saline (¼NS): provide free water to cells as well as small amounts of sodium and chloride; approximately ½ of each liter infused moves into cells and ½ remains in extracellular space
   c) Maintenance fluids: saline mixed with dextrose and water
      i. 5% dextrose in 0.45 saline (D_5½NS) and 5% dextrose in 0.225% saline (D_5¼NS): both are hypertonic in the IV bag, but because of rapid dextrose metabolism, both also have a degree of hypotonic effect, providing some water to cells; provide calories and are often used as maintenance fluids; dextrose content does not meet daily nutritional caloric requirements, but does help prevent ketosis associated with starvation
      ii. 5% dextrose in 0.9% saline (D_5NS) is also hypertonic in the bag, but provides some free water and calories to cells; dextrose is mixed with NS and provides less free water and more extracellular water than D_5½NS or D_5¼NS

e. The term ***hypertonic*** is defined as having a higher osmolality than normal plasma
   1) Hypertonic IV fluids have a higher osmolality than normal plasma, causing water to be pulled from cells into blood vessels, resulting in increased vascular volume and decreased cell water
   2) Hypertonic solutions are used to treat very specific problems and are administered in carefully controlled, limited doses in order to avoid vascular volume overload and cellular dehydration; they are also used to pull excess fluid from cells and to promote osmotic diuresis
   3) Hypertonic IV solutions (see Table 1-1 again)
      a) Include saline solutions greater than 0.9% (3% saline and 5% saline); used infrequently
      b) Clinically indicated when serum sodium is dangerously low (115 mg/dL or less); given with great caution in carefully controlled, limited doses using an IV infusion pump
      c) *Note:* Clients receiving hypertonic saline solutions require frequent monitoring of vital signs, neurologic status, lung sounds, urine output (UO), and serum sodium levels to avoid hypernatremia and vascular volume overload
      d) Dextrose solutions greater than 5% (such as 10% dextrose and 50% dextrose) are also considered hypertonic; these are used on a limited basis to treat clients with hypoglycemia
      e) Hypertonic dextrose solutions are given in controlled settings by IV push or IV infusion pump; 50% dextrose is used as part of a hypoglycemic treatment protocol; a 10% dextrose solution is used to treat newborns as part of a hypoglycemic treatment protocol
      f) **Colloid** volume expanders (albumin, dextran)
         i. A colloid is a large solute particle, such as protein in solution, that normally does not pass through cell and capillary membranes (semipermeable membranes)
         ii. Colloid volume expanders have increased osmolality and pull fluid from tissue into blood vessels by osmosis, increasing vascular volume

Practice to Pass

A 16-year-old client is in the intensive care unit 12 hours after a bicycle collision in which the client, who was not wearing a helmet, landed head first on the pavement. CT scan is negative for bleeding, but the client remains unresponsive except to painful stimuli. What IV fluids would be dangerous for this client? Why?

Figure 1-3

Diffusion

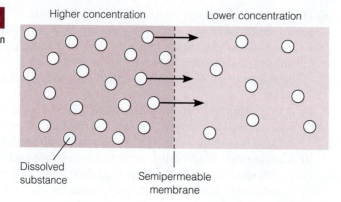

Higher concentration   Lower concentration

Dissolved
substance

Semipermeable
membrane

> g) Osmotic diuretics (such as mannitol) pull fluid from third spaces, tissues, and cells into blood vessels for elimination by kidneys

4. **Diffusion** (see Figure 1-3)
   a. Particles move from an area of higher concentration (more particles, less water) to an area of lower concentration (fewer particles, more water) until concentrations are equalized; some particles easily diffuse through semipermeable membranes and others do not
   b. **Electrolytes** (e.g., sodium, potassium, chloride, calcium, magnesium, and phosphate) are small particles that tend to move through semipermeable membranes easily
   c. Urea, glucose, and **albumin** (a plasma protein produced by liver) are large particles that do not pass through semipermeable membranes easily

B. **Capillary fluid movement** (see Figure 1-4)
   1. **Hydrostatic pressure**
      a. Hydrostatic pressure is the pushing force of a fluid against the walls of the space it occupies
      b. Hydrostatic pressure in blood vessels is generated by heart's pumping action and varies within the vascular system
   2. **Oncotic pressure**
      a. Oncotic pressure (also called **colloid osmotic pressure** or **COP**) is the pulling force exerted by colloids in a solution (pulling force of proteins within vascular space)
      b. Albumin is important in maintaining normal serum oncotic pressure (pulling force for water) and adequate vascular fluid volume
      c. Since plasma proteins do not normally cross blood vessel walls, plasma protein concentration remains the same in arteries, veins, and capillaries

Figure 1-4

Capillary filtration dynamics

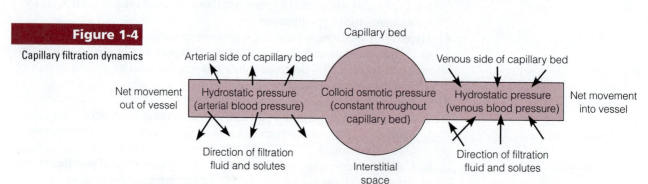

Capillary bed

Arterial side of capillary bed

Venous side of capillary bed

Net movement out of vessel

Hydrostatic pressure (arterial blood pressure)

Colloid osmotic pressure (constant throughout capillary bed)

Hydrostatic pressure (venous blood pressure)

Net movement into vessel

Direction of filtration fluid and solutes

Interstitial space

Direction of filtration fluid and solutes

3. Starling's Law of the Capillaries
   a. **Filtration** (net fluid movement into or out of capillary) is determined by the difference between the forces favoring filtration and those opposing it (like a tug of war—pushing and pulling)
   b. Interstitial hydrostatic pressure (pushing water into capillary) and interstitial oncotic pressure (pulling water out of capillary) are very low and are essentially equal, thus normally exert little influence on fluid movement into or out of capillaries
   c. Capillary hydrostatic pressure (pushing water out of capillary) and capillary oncotic pressure (pulling water into capillary) are not the same, and fluid movement is seen in the capillary bed
      1) At arterial end of capillary, hydrostatic pressure (pushing water out of capillary) exceeds oncotic pressure (pulling water into capillary), thus net fluid movement is from capillary into tissue, carrying nutrients with it
      2) At venous end of capillary, hydrostatic pressure (pushing water out of capillary) is less than capillary oncotic pressure (pulling water into capillary), thus net fluid movement is into capillary from tissue, carrying wastes with it

C. **Chemical regulation of fluid balance**
   1. **Antidiuretic hormone (ADH)** (see Figure 1-5)
      a. ADH is a hormone synthesized by hypothalamus and secreted by posterior pituitary gland, which regulates water by acting on distal tubules of kidneys
      b. ADH is released and inhibited in a feedback loop
         1) ADH release is triggered by a drop in BP or blood volume or by a rise in blood osmolality (increased concentration), causing kidneys to reabsorb more water (resulting in higher vascular volume and low output of concentrated urine)
         2) ADH release is inhibited by a rise in BP or blood volume or by a drop in blood osmolality (decreased concentration), causing kidneys to excrete more water in urine (resulting in lower vascular volume and high output of dilute urine)
   2. **Aldosterone** (see Figure 1-6)
      a. Aldosterone is an adrenal gland hormone that conserves sodium in body by causing kidneys to retain sodium and excrete potassium in its place
      b. Water follows sodium due to osmosis, thus aldosterone has an indirect effect on water
      c. Aldosterone is released and inhibited in a feedback loop as part of renin–angiotensin–aldosterone system (refer again to Figure 1-6)
         1) Aldosterone release is triggered by a drop in BP, blood volume, or serum sodium, or a rise in serum potassium
            a) Aldosterone causes kidneys to reabsorb more sodium into blood, increasing serum sodium levels; water follows sodium into blood by osmosis, raising vascular volume
            b) As more sodium is retained in blood, kidneys must excrete more potassium in urine to maintain a balance of positive ions in blood; this mechanism lowers serum potassium levels
         2) Aldosterone release is inhibited by a rise in BP, blood volume, or serum sodium, or a drop in serum potassium
            a) A decreasing aldosterone level causes kidneys to excrete more sodium in urine, decreasing serum sodium levels; water follows sodium, thereby lowering vascular volume
            b) As more sodium is excreted in urine, kidneys must retain more potassium in blood to maintain positive ion balance; this mechanism raises serum potassium levels

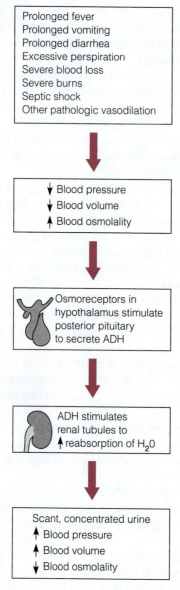

Figure 1-5

ADH regulation of water

Prolonged fever
Prolonged vomiting
Prolonged diarrhea
Excessive perspiration
Severe blood loss
Severe burns
Septic shock
Other pathologic vasodilation

↓ Blood pressure
↓ Blood volume
↑ Blood osmolality

Osmoreceptors in hypothalamus stimulate posterior pituitary to secrete ADH

ADH stimulates renal tubules to ↑ reabsorption of H_2O

Scant, concentrated urine
↑ Blood pressure
↑ Blood volume
↓ Blood osmolality

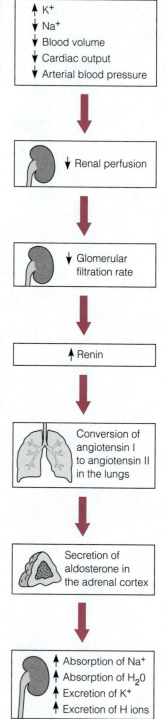

Figure 1-6

Aldosterone regulation of sodium and water

↑ K^+
↓ Na^+
↓ Blood volume
↓ Cardiac output
↓ Arterial blood pressure

↓ Renal perfusion

↓ Glomerular filtration rate

↑ Renin

Conversion of angiotensin I to angiotensin II in the lungs

Secretion of aldosterone in the adrenal cortex

↑ Absorption of Na^+
↑ Absorption of H_2O
↑ Excretion of K^+
↑ Excretion of H ions

3. Glucocorticoids (cortisol)
   a. Cortisol is a glucocorticoid hormone produced and released by adrenal gland cortex when body is stressed
   b. Glucocorticoids promote renal retention of sodium and water
4. Atrial natriuretic peptide (ANP)
   a. ANP is a cardiac hormone found in atria of heart that is released when atria are stretched by high blood volume or high BP

      b. ANP lowers blood volume and BP by the following:

        1) Causing vasodilation by direct effect on blood vessels and suppression of renin–angiotensin system

        2) Decreasing aldosterone release by adrenal glands, causing increased urinary excretion of sodium and water

        3) Decreasing ADH release by pituitary gland, causing increased urinary excretion of water

        4) Increasing glomerular filtration rate, increasing rate of urine production and water excretion

5. Brain natriuretic peptide (BNP)

      a. BNP is a cardiac hormone found within ventricles that is released when increased blood volume and pressure lead to ventricular stretching

      b. BNP works to decrease blood volume and pressure through these mechanisms:

        1) Vasodilates arteries and veins

        2) Decreases release of aldosterone

        3) Causes diuresis with excretion of both sodium and water

6. Thirst mechanism

      a. Thirst normally occurs with even small fluid losses or small increases in serum osmolality; it is stimulated by thirst receptors in hypothalamus, which can detect as little as 1 mOsm/L change in plasma concentration

      b. Thirst also stimulates ADH and aldosterone release, which promotes reabsorption of water

      c. Thirst mechanism is depressed in older adults (>age 60 years), including both healthy older adults and those living with debilitating illnesses

Practice to Pass

An adult client has 3% saline infusing intravenously. What nursing observations and measures should be implemented to protect client safety? Why?

II. FLUID VOLUME DEFICIT (FVD)

A. Etiology and pathophysiology

1. Isotonic fluid loss

      a. Fluid and solute are lost in proportional amounts, thus serum osmolality remains normal and no osmotic force is created

      b. Intracellular water is not disturbed and fluid losses are primarily ECF (especially vascular volume), which can quickly lead to shock

      c. Causes

        1) Hemorrhage results in loss of fluid, electrolytes, proteins, and blood cells in proportional amounts, often resulting in inadequate vascular volume (**hypovolemia**)

        2) Gastrointestinal losses (vomiting, continuous NG suction, diarrhea, drainage from tubes, fistulas, and ostomies) contain abundant electrolytes; thus GI fluid and electrolytes tend to be lost in fairly proportional amounts

        3) Large amounts of wound drainage or wound suctioning can lead to both fluid and electrolyte losses

        4) Fever, environmental heat, diaphoresis, and shock can result in profuse sweating, which causes water and sodium loss from skin in fairly equal proportions

        5) Burns (especially large burns) initially damage skin and capillary membranes, allowing fluid, electrolytes, and proteins to escape into burned tissue area, which often results in inadequate vascular volume

        6) Diuretics can cause excessive loss of fluid and electrolytes in fairly proportional amounts

        7) Third-space fluid shifts occur when fluid moves from vascular space into physiologically useless extracellular spaces (where it is unavailable as reserve fluid or to transport nutrients)

        d. Isotonic fluid loss is primarily an extracellular fluid loss that requires extracellular fluid replacement, with emphasis on vascular volume

  2. Hypertonic dehydration

        a. More water is lost than solute (primarily sodium), creating a fluid volume deficit and a relative solute excess

        b. Fluid loss is both extracellular and intracellular

        c. Solute (sodium or glucose more commonly) can also be gained in excess of water, creating a similar imbalance

        d. Serum osmolality is elevated, resulting in hypertonic extracellular fluid that pulls fluid into vessels from cells by osmosis and causes cells to shrink and become dehydrated

        e. Causes of hypertonic dehydration

            1) Inadequate fluid intake

                a) Clients who cannot respond to thirst independently (infants, older adults, those who are disabled or bedridden), who have nausea, anorexia, or dysphagia, or who are NPO (nothing by mouth) without IV fluid replacement are at risk to develop fluid volume deficit

                b) Decreased water intake results in increased ECF solute concentration, which leads to cellular dehydration

                c) A client can go several weeks to months without food, but only 2–3 days without water

            2) Severe or prolonged isotonic fluid losses

                a) May occur in conditions such as vomiting and diarrhea and eventually result in loss of more water than solute

                b) ECF becomes hypertonic as compensatory mechanisms are exhausted, and body has no more water to conserve via the kidneys

                c) The hypertonic ECF then begins to draw water from cells, dehydrating them as well

            3) Watery diarrhea causes loss of more water than electrolytes

            4) Diabetes insipidus (DI) is caused by insufficient ADH production or release, which leads to massive, uncontrolled diuresis of very dilute urine (as much as 30 liters per day) and can quickly lead to shock and death

                a) Brain injury that damages or puts pressure on hypothalamus or pituitary gland often causes DI

                b) Once acute DI develops, parenteral administration of vasopressin, a pharmacological form of ADH, is indicated to stop massive fluid loss

            5) Increased solute intake (e.g., salt, sugar, protein) without a proportional intake of water increases plasma osmolality, resulting in water being pulled from cells, increasing ECF, and causing cellular dehydration; increasing ECF is dangerous for clients with heart or kidney problems, and the resulting osmotic diuresis actually worsens cellular dehydration; conditions such as the following can lead to hypertonic dehydration:

                a) Highly concentrated enteral or parenteral feedings (increased glucose)

                b) Improperly prepared infant formulas (too concentrated)

                c) Hyperglycemia and/or diabetic ketoacidosis (excess glucose and ketones in the blood)

                d) Increased sodium ingestion (e.g., seawater ingestion, salt tablets)

                e) Excess osmotic diuretic use

  3. Third spacing

        a. Third spaces are extracellular body spaces in which fluid is not normally present in large amounts, but in which fluid can accumulate

      b. Fluid that accumulates in third spaces is physiologically useless because it is not available for use as reserve fluid or to transport nutrients

      c. Common locations for third-space fluid to accumulate include tissue spaces (edema), abdomen (ascites), pleural spaces (pleural effusion), and pericardial space (pericardial effusion)

      d. Causes of third spacing

        1) Injury or inflammation (e.g., massive trauma, crush injuries, burns, sepsis, cancer, intestinal obstruction, abdominal surgery) increase capillary permeability, allowing fluid, electrolytes, and proteins to leak from vessels

        2) Malnutrition or liver dysfunction (e.g., starvation, cirrhosis, chronic alcoholism)interfere with liver production of albumin, thus lowering capillary oncotic pressure

        3) High vascular hydrostatic pressure (e.g., heart failure, renal failure, or other forms of vascular fluid overload) pushes abnormal volumes of fluid from vessels

B. Dehydration concepts

    1. Isotonic dehydration involves equal losses of all fluid components and is the most commonly seen type of fluid volume deficit

    2. Hypotonic dehydration involves greater losses of electrolytes, leading to a decreased plasma osmolality; fluid shifting occurs as ECF volume decreases

    3. Hypertonic dehydration involves greater losses of ECF volume than electrolytes, leading to an increased plasma osmolality; fluid shifting occurs as body tries to compensate to restore balance

C. Assessment

    1. Clinical manifestations of dehydration (see Table 1-2)

    2. Acute weight loss (an important sign in infants and young children); see Table 1-3 for comparison of weight loss to degree of fluid deficit

      a. 1 L water = 1 kg (2.2 lb)

      b. Considered a more accurate reflection of fluid balance than intake and output (I&O) because of difficulty in keeping accurate records

      c. *Note:* Exception occurs in weight changes with significant third-space fluid shifts as weight gain is often seen; clients with third spacing may initially have signs/symptoms of **hypervolemia** but primary problem is fluid volume deficit

    3. Diagnostic and laboratory findings

      a. Normal or high hematocrit (Hct) and blood urea nitrogen (BUN) because of **hemoconcentration** (plasma is more concentrated than normal, with increased number of red blood cells [RBCs] and urea particles per liter of plasma); *variation:* if hemorrhage is causing fluid volume deficit, RBCs are being lost in proportion to plasma, thus Hct will be low

      b. High urine specific gravity (>1.030) as kidneys conserve water while continuing to excrete solute (unless cause is diabetes insipidus, in which specific gravity will be low [<1.010])

      c. Urine osmolality (measurement of particle numbers in solution and reflects ability of kidneys to concentrate urine; normal 500–800 mOsm/kg); is a more precise indicator of hydration

      d. In hypertonic dehydration, lab values will also reflect increased plasma concentration

        1) Serum osmolality elevated >300 mOsm/kg

        2) Serum sodium elevated (hypernatremia) >150 milliequivalents/liter (mEq/L)

        3) Serum glucose elevated (if that is the cause of the dehydration) >120 mg/dL

Table 1-2	Clinical Manifestations Consistent with Fluid Volume Deficit
Assessment Parameter	**Signs Consistent with Fluid Volume Deficit (Dehydration)**
Thirst	An early sign; slightly to greatly increased as state worsens; unreliable as indicator in older adults and those who cannot express needs
Urine	Normal to decreased volume as state worsens (<1 mL/kg/hr in children and <0.5 mL/kg/hr in adults); becoming concentrated, dark, increased **specific gravity** (>1.030) Variation: if diabetes insipidus is cause of dehydration, urine is pale, dilute, high in volume, with low specific gravity (<1.010)
Skin turgor	Normal to decreased with "tenting" as interstitial fluid loss progresses; not a reliable sign in infants (skin very elastic) and older adults (loss of skin elasticity with aging) Test skin of older adults on sternum, forehead, inner thigh, or top of hip bone rather than arms or legs; check tenting in infants over abdomen or inner thighs
Mucous membranes	Increasing dryness as state worsens; note that breathing and environmental conditions can cause dry lips when oral mucosa is actually moist; dry tongue with longitudinal furrows is a reliable sign in all age groups
Eyes	Normal to sunken eyeballs as state worsens; decreased tearing and dry conjunctiva
Fontanelles	Sunken or depressed fontanels in infants and children <18 months old; not applicable once fontanelles close
Vital signs	*Temperature:* normal to low-grade fever (higher fever can occur in severe dehydration) as body's perceived loss of fluid volume results in blood vessel constriction, which decreases heat loss *Heart rate:* normal to increased depending on severity of state *Respirations:* usual and regular rate, progressing to rapid rate (tachypnea, usually without shortness of breath or dyspnea); possible change in regularity *Blood pressure:* normal at first, then postural hypotension (rise in pulse rate >10–15 beats/min and/or fall in systolic BP >10–15 mm Hg after rising from lying to standing position) in older children, adolescents, and adults; frank hypotension even at rest (late sign)
Peripheral vascular	Normal pulse volume diminishing to weak and thready as state worsens; warm extremities progressing to cool; normal to delayed capillary refill as state worsens; poor peripheral vein filling; flat neck veins even when head of bed <45 degrees (adult sign only); possible lightheadedness, dizziness, and syncope (reduced circulation to brain)
Mental status	Mental status change is first sign noticed in older adults and first sign that causes alarm in caregivers of infants and small children Normal initially with progressive changes (e.g., irritability and restlessness progressing to lethargy, drowsiness, and finally coma); older adults may experience apprehension

Table 1-3	Correlation of Weight Change to Severity of Fluid Volume Deficit or Excess	
Weight Change	**Degree of Fluid Deficit**	**Degree of Fluid Excess**
2% body weight	Mild fluid deficit (may only see thirst; ~1–2 L fluid loss in adult)	Mild fluid excess
5% body weight	Moderate fluid deficit (signs and symptoms appear; ~3–5 L fluid loss in adult)	Moderate fluid excess
8% body weight	Severe fluid deficit (frank hypotension and delirium; ~5–10 L fluid loss in adult)	Severe fluid excess
>15% body weight	Very severe fluid deficit; can be fatal (anuria, coma; >10 L fluid loss in adult)	Very severe fluid excess

4. Identification of risk factors predisposing to fluid volume deficit
   a. Age, gender, and body fat
      1) Infants and young children
         a) Total body water percentage is higher (infant 80%, premature infant 90%, adult 60%); thus, infants require more water for size than older children and adults
         b) ECF, which is more easily lost, equals 40% of an infant's body water (compared to 20% of an adult's); infants may exchange 50% of their ECF daily, compared to 18% in an adult
         c) Kidneys are immature up to age 2 years, thus cannot conserve or excrete water or sodium as efficiently as adults, making them less able to handle large amounts of solute-free water or concentrated fluids
         d) Body surface area is relatively large, thus infants lose more fluid through skin for their size than adults
         e) Higher metabolic rate of infants requires more water for size than adults and produces more heat, which results in more water loss
         f) Fever tends to be higher and last longer in acute illnesses of infants and children, which increases fluid loss with acute illness
         g) Children 2–12 years of age have less stable regulatory responses to fluid imbalances than adults
      2) Older adults
         a) After age 60, only 45–50% of body weight is water (compared to 60% in younger adult), thus small water losses have a greater impact
         b) Skeletal muscle mass (which holds more water than fat) declines and percentage of body fat rises with aging
         c) Kidneys lose function and cannot concentrate or dilute urine as efficiently, thus cannot compensate as easily for imbalance or excrete heavy solute loads (such as those from tube feedings)
         d) Diminished thirst mechanism is seen with aging
         e) Decreased pancreatic function and glucose tolerance with aging increases risk of hyperglycemia and resulting osmotic diuresis
      3) Women and obese individuals have a higher percentage of body fat, which holds less water than muscle; thus, they have a lower percentage of body water for their weight
   b. Acute illness
      1) Surgery can result in blood and fluid loss
      2) Nasogastric suction and gastroenteritis causing nausea and vomiting and/or diarrhea lead to fluid and electrolyte loss
      3) Burns: the larger the burn surface area, the greater the fluid loss
      4) Brain injury from stroke, trauma, or tumor can cause cerebral edema, which can put pressure on hypothalamus and/or pituitary, altering ADH release and possibly leading to syndrome of inappropriate ADH secretion (SIADH) or more commonly, diabetes insipidus (DI)
      5) Large draining wounds and wound suctioning lead to fluid loss by interruption of skin barrier
   c. Chronic illness
      1) Liver disease reduces albumin production, which reduces ability to maintain adequate circulating vascular volume
      2) Renal disease limits ability to regulate fluid or electrolytes via UO
      3) Diabetes mellitus increases risk for hyperglycemia and hypertonic dehydration
      4) Cancer can predispose to fluid shifts; chemotherapy often causes nausea and vomiting with loss of fluid and lack of intake

    d. Environmental factors

       1) Vigorous exercise increases metabolism, ventilation, and sweating, causing both an increased demand for fluid as well as increased fluid losses

       2) Exposure to hot, humid environments can increase sweat production to as much as 2 L/hour; body fluid weight loss >7% is associated with failure of body cooling mechanisms, leading to heat injuries

    e. Diet and lifestyle

       1) Difficulty chewing or swallowing can lead to inadequate intake of oral fluids and food (which is also a major source of fluid intake)

       2) Malnutrition, starvation, and low protein intake will affect volume status

       3) Excess alcohol consumption causes liver damage and/or malnutrition, leading to altered volume status

    f. Medications

       1) Diuretics and laxatives can predispose client to excess fluid loss

       2) Chemotherapy can cause nausea and vomiting and poor oral intake

D. Priority nursing concerns

    1. Fluid volume deficit related to excessive fluid losses and/or decreased intake; possible shock if severe and untreated

    2. Possible client injury because of altered sensorium and/or dizziness

    3. Reduced client comfort associated with manifestations of fluid deficit

    4. Possible interruption of skin and mucous membranes because of dryness

    5. Inadequate client knowledge of risk factors and therapeutic interventions

E. Therapeutic management

    1. Oral replacement therapies

    a. Oral fluids are indicated if deficit is mild, thirst is intact, and client can drink

       1) Commercial oral rehydration solutions (ORSs) provide fluids, glucose, and electrolytes in a concentration that is quickly absorbed even if vomiting and diarrhea are present

       2) Infants and young children may only tolerate a few teaspoonfuls every few minutes, but over time intake should total 60–120 mL (if <10 kg weight) or 120–240 mL (if >10 kg weight) for each episode of vomiting or diarrhea with mild dehydration; moderate dehydration requires an additional 50–100 mL/kg every 3–4 hours

       3) For small children, freeze fluids into flavored ice pops, which are often better received than liquids; as fluids are replaced, begin alternating with low-sodium fluids such as water, breast milk, lactose-free formula, or half-strength lactose formula

       4) Adults should sip frequent, small amounts of ORS, progressing to a variety of oral fluids

    b. During initial rehydration, avoid sodas, fruit juice, and sports drinks because their high sugar content (hypertonic) can worsen diarrhea and promote fluid loss; avoid salty fluids that can make diarrhea worse; avoid caffeine (mild diuretic that may worsen fluid loss)

    c. Early reintroduction of regular diet has been shown to decrease the number of diarrhea stools and shorten the duration of gastroenteritis; BRAT diet (bananas, rice, applesauce, and toast) may be recommended by some providers in first 24 hours of acute illness, but provides inadequate fiber, protein, and fat

    2. Parenteral replacement therapies

    a. Parenteral therapy for isotonic fluid losses

       1) Initially, expand ECF volume with isotonic IV fluids until adequate circulating blood volume and renal perfusion are achieved

       a) Fluid challenges (large amounts of IV fluids infused rapidly, often in 30 minutes or less) may be used

Practice to Pass

A 23-year-old client is admitted to the emergency department with multiple fractures of the legs and pelvis. BP is 86/40, heart rate 120, respirations 30, skin is cool and pale, and peripheral pulses are weak and thready. What intravenous fluids should be given immediately? Why?

b) Infuse a 1–2 liter bolus of isotonic fluid (e.g., NS) for adults, with up to two or three additional boluses to achieve response to therapy (improving UO, BP, heart rate, and mental status)

c) Infuse a 20–30 mL/kg bolus of isotonic fluid (e.g., NS) for infants and young children, with up to two or three further boluses to achieve response to therapy (improving UO, heart rate, respiratory rate, and mental status)

d) Blood transfusion should be considered to replace lost RBCs for clients experiencing severe hypovolemia due to hemorrhage

2) Once initial parenteral rehydration is accomplished for mild to moderate fluid losses, oral rehydration can be continued at home

3) If dehydration is severe, IV rehydration may continue with maintenance IV fluids (usually saline and dextrose combination fluids such as $D_5\frac{1}{2}NS$ or D_5NS)

4) If third spacing is causing the fluid volume deficit, osmotic diuretics may mobilize some fluid; however, because of the nature of diseases that often cause third spacing, this is often a temporary measure; large third-space fluid collections may need to be physically removed (paracentesis for ascites; thoracentesis for pleural effusion) and the vascular space rehydrated with IV fluids

b. Parenteral therapy for hypertonic dehydration

1) If hypovolemia and impending shock are present, isotonic fluids are given first to achieve adequate circulation and renal perfusion

2) Cellular dehydration is corrected with hypotonic IV solutions (provide free water to cells); be alert—hypotonic fluids must be given slowly to prevent rehydrating brain cells too rapidly, which could result in cerebral edema and brain injury

3) If hypervolemia is present (as with excess sodium intake), a diuretic may be given with hypotonic fluid infusions (to provide free water to cells while preventing vascular volume overload)

3. Monitoring of client during therapy

a. Vital signs for changes in heart rate, BP, respiratory rate; breath sounds and mucous membranes

b. Mental status and behavior for improvement in mentation (less lethargic, more alert, less confused, appropriate behavior for situation); lack of improvement or worsening mental status could indicate too-rapid infusion of hypotonic fluids

c. Monitor UO and concentration for improvement; adequate UO of normal color and concentration (in healthy kidneys) is a good indicator of adequate vascular volume

d. Monitor IV infusion rate to avoid administration of excess fluid, especially in those with cardiac or renal dysfunction, older adults, infants, and young children (who are all at increased risk for fluid volume overload); use infusion pumps to prevent fluid overload

e. Monitor I&O and daily weights (same scale, same time of day, same clothing for consistency)

f. Auscultate breath sounds for crackles, which could indicate fluid accumulation in alveoli of lungs

F. Client-centered nursing care

1. Monitor specific assessment parameters related to management of FVD

2. Assist with rehydration and promote return to adequate oral intake

a. Provide indicated oral fluids in frequent, small amounts; keep fluids fresh and place within easy reach

b. Remind older adults to drink something each hour due to decreased thirst mechanism

    c. Chill, warm, or freeze indicated fluids to enhance intake based on client's preference

    d. Clients with reduced mobility may need assistance in drinking fluids

    e. Check IV infusion pump frequently to ensure fluid is delivered according to programmed settings

3. Provide comfort measures

    a. Provide oral hygiene frequently, including brushing teeth and rinsing mouth, to promote comfort

        1) A rinse of equal parts peroxide and water can help deodorize mouth

        2) Avoid glycerin and lemon or alcohol-based commercial mouthwash, which can be drying

        3) Avoid having client use hard candy or chewing gum with sugar, both of which can further dry oral mucous membranes

    b. Apply a lip moisturizer and/or skin moisturizer to dry skin to prevent cracking and breakdown

4. Provide measures to prevent fluid volume deficits and dehydration; provide additional plain water boluses periodically during enteral feedings

    a. *Note:* 1 mL of water is recommended for each kCal of formula

    b. If one can of formula has 380 kCal in 240 mL of fluid, an additional 140 mL of fluid is needed to achieve the recommended total fluid intake

    c. Excessive water boluses can lead to signs of water toxicity and hyponatremia; check serum sodium levels periodically

5. Implement measures to control nausea and vomiting, diarrhea, and high fever to prevent further fluid losses

6. Recognize acutely ill clients at risk for inadequate fluid intake and initiate measures to provide adequate fluids by the oral, enteral, or parenteral routes

G. Medication therapy

1. Antiemetics are used to prevent fluid losses due to nausea and vomiting (e.g., promethazine)

2. Antidiarrheals are used to prevent fluid losses from the GI tract (e.g., loperamide)

3. ADH: vasopressin is used to correct diabetes insipidus

4. Antipyretics are used to control fever and minimize fluid losses (e.g., acetaminophen or ibuprofen)

H. Client education

1. Awareness of predisposing factors

    a. Explain the nature of client's condition and relevant risk factors (e.g., age, gender, body size, physical activities, illnesses, medications, diet, and lifestyle)

    b. Explain early signs of impending fluid volume deficit and importance of initiating ORS in small, frequent amounts early to decrease nausea and replace electrolytes

    c. Explain importance of contacting a healthcare provider if illness lasts more than 24 hours, if client is an older adult or very young, or if client has a chronic illness (such as diabetes, heart disease, kidney disease, or liver problems)

2. Explain measures to help prevent fluid deficit and dehydration

    a. Older adults should drink a variety of fluids frequently during day even if not thirsty, especially in hot, humid weather, since thirst mechanism is diminished

    b. Foods that are liquid at room temperature provide fluid intake (frozen ice pops, ice cream, gelatin) for those at risk

    c. Drink cool water prior to and after exercise, and 5–6 oz every 15 minutes during exercise

        1) If exercise is prolonged (>1 hour for average person) or vigorous or if it occurs in a hot, humid climate, drink solutions for hydration that contain water, carbohydrates, and electrolytes (e.g., sports drinks)

Practice to Pass

An 80-year-old client is admitted to the hospital for treatment of urinary tract infection and dehydration. While in the emergency department, one liter of NS has infused and now $D_5\frac{1}{4}NS$ is infusing at 80 mL/hour. What monitoring is important during therapy and why?

2) Avoid highly salty fluids or salt tablets, which can raise sodium levels and draw fluid from cells, worsening dehydration

3. Provide dietary education
   a. Commercial oral rehydration solutions are recommended for vomiting and diarrhea, especially in children; they contain needed electrolytes but do not have large amounts of sugar that could worsen diarrhea and dehydration
   b. During diarrhea, avoid ingesting salty fluids (e.g., salty broth) and fluids high in sugar (gelatin, soda, and fruit juice) because the high solute content can worsen diarrhea and dehydration
   c. Avoid caffeine because it acts as a mild diuretic, increasing fluid loss
   d. Recommend early progression to a soft, easily digestible, regular diet; limiting intake to a BRAT diet has fallen out of favor, especially in acute diarrhea; recommend use of ORSs that are rich in electrolytes

I. Evaluation

1. Adequate fluid volume reflected by the following:
   a. Adequate UO and concentration
   b. Stable heart rate and BP (lying and standing) within individual norms
   c. Skin and mucous membranes moist with normal turgor and elasticity; fontanels soft
   d. Return to usual mental state and behavior
   e. Hct, BUN, serum osmolality, and serum electrolytes within normal range during first 48–72 hours

2. Free of injury
   a. No signs of injury from falls (e.g., bruises, abrasions, bumps)
   b. No reported episodes of falls with injury

3. Skin and mucous membranes intact
   a. Absence of cracks, fissures, or ulcers
   b. Mouth and oral mucosa moist

4. Verbalizes adequate knowledge of condition, therapeutic and preventive measures, and any indicated follow-up care

Practice to Pass

A young mother contacts the clinic and reports that her 8-month-old infant awakened about 6 hours ago with fever, vomiting, and diarrhea. She has stopped giving food and formula and has been giving him plain water to drink. What advice should you give her and why?

III. FLUID VOLUME EXCESS (FVE)

A. Etiology and pathophysiology

1. Isotonic fluid excess (hypervolemia and edema)
   a. Fluid and solute (primarily sodium) are gained or retained in proportional amounts, leading to an overall gain in extracellular fluid volume without a change in serum osmolality
   b. Excess vascular fluid volume leads to development of hypervolemia
   c. Excess tissue (interstitial) fluid volume leads to development of edema, which can occur throughout body or can be situated in specific body tissues or organs
   d. Causes of isotonic FVE (see Table 1-4)

2. Hypotonic fluid excess (water intoxication) (see Table 1-4)
   a. More fluid is gained than solute (primarily sodium), creating FVE and a relative deficit of sodium
   b. Serum osmolality falls, resulting in hypotonic ECF that gets pulled into cells by osmosis, causing cells to swell; cerebral cells absorb free water more readily than other cells, thus are very sensitive to hypotonic ECF

B. Mechanisms of edema formation

1. Increased capillary hydrostatic pressure disrupts normal filtration of fluid into and out of capillaries (refer back to Figure 1-4)

Table 1-4	Types of Fluid Volume Excess (FVE)	
Type	**Causes**	**Related Physiology**
Isotonic	1. Renal failure 2. Heart failure 3. Excess fluid intake 4. High corticosteroid levels due to therapy, stress, or disease 5. High aldosterone levels due to stress response, adrenal dysfunction, liver damage, or metabolic problems	1. Decreased excretion of water and sodium 2. Stasis of blood in circulation, venous congestion, and decreased renal blood flow lead to decreased renal excretion of fluid and sodium 3. Rapid infusion or excessive infusion of isotonic fluid exceeds heart and kidneys' ability to compensate 4. Sodium and water are retained 5. Sodium and water are retained
Hypotonic	1. Repeated administration of plain water enemas, NG irrigation, or bladder irrigation 2. Excess use or rapid infusion of hypotonic IV fluids, such as D_5W, 0.0225% saline, and 0.045% saline 3. Excessive intake of free water without electrolyte replacement 4. Inappropriately prepared infant formula and/or excess water; frequent use of a water bottle as a pacifier 5. SIADH: Syndrome of Inappropriate Antidiuretic Hormone; excessive release of ADH can be precipitated by stress, surgery, anesthesia, opioid analgesics, pain, and lung and brain tumors 6. Psychogenic polydipsia, a compulsive drinking of excess water associated with psychiatric disorders	1. The free water can be drawn into cells and expelled water takes electrolytes with it 2. Excess free water is taken into cells too quickly; when D_5W is infused, the dextrose is quickly metabolized, leaving free water 3. If isotonic fluids and/or electrolytes are lost, they need to be replaced with water and electrolytes, especially sodium 4. Parents may dilute infant formula or give excessive free water in effort to stretch formula; both result in excess ingestion of free water 5. Excessive ADH causes kidneys to retain large amounts of water without sodium; in turn, the excessive hypotonic extracellular fluid is drawn into cells by osmosis 6. Excessive intake of free water leads to water intoxication
Interstitial	1. Increased blood hydrostatic pressure 2. Decreased blood colloid osmotic pressure secondary to low plasma proteins; associated with liver failure, malnutrition, nephritic syndrome 3. Increased capillary permeability, caused by damage to capillaries; associated with trauma, burns, and crushing injuries 4. Impaired lymphatic drainage associated with lymphedema and tumors *Note:* Some causes are the same as those associated with hypotonic excess	1. Extracellular fluid excess increases fluid volume in vascular space leading to increased pressure against capillary walls with movement of fluid into interstitial spaces 2. Plasma proteins hold fluid in the capillary spaces; when low, the pulling force is lost and fluid seeps into interstitial spaces 3. The capillaries become permeable to protein, which leaks into interstitial spaces, carrying fluid with it 4. Lymph vessels normally return small proteins and excess fluid to the vascular compartment; when blocked, the fluid remains in the interstitial space

      a. Increased pushing pressure within the capillary (blood pressure) forces more fluid out of arterial end of capillary and draws less fluid back into venous end, resulting in excess fluid accumulation (edema) in tissues

      b. Hypertension and vascular fluid volume overload (hypervolemia) are causes of edema

   2. Decreased capillary oncotic pressure also disrupts normal movement of fluid into and out of capillaries

      a. Weaker pulling pressure within the capillary (because of decreased albumin, plasma proteins) allows more fluid to be pushed out of arterial end of capillary and draws less fluid back into venous end, resulting in excess fluid accumulation (edema) in tissues

      b. Causes of low capillary oncotic pressure

1) Injury or inflammation (e.g., trauma, burns, sepsis, bacterial infections, allergic reactions, cancer, intestinal obstruction), which increases capillary permeability, allowing fluid and proteins to leak from vessels

2) Malnutrition or liver dysfunction (e.g., starvation, cirrhosis, chronic alcoholism) reduces liver production of albumin, decreasing capillary oncotic pressure (which normally helps keep adequate fluid inside vessels)

3) Lymphatic obstruction or surgical removal of lymph nodes impairs lymph drainage and normal flow of lymph fluid from body tissues to venous system, creating local edema distal to obstruction or node removal

4) Sodium excess (e.g., due to renal failure, decreased renal perfusion, or excess aldosterone or corticosteroids) causes water retention that elevates BP, increasing hydrostatic pressure within capillaries; this forces more fluid into tissues, resulting in edema

C. Assessment

1. Clinical manifestations of FVE (see Table 1-5)

2. A weight gain of 1.4 kg (3lb) or more can occur over 2–5 days in adults; see Table 1-3 again for correlation of weight gain to degree of fluid volume excess; note that infants and children are more susceptible to complications of fluid gains and may exhibit more severe symptoms with a mild fluid excess

3. Diagnostic and laboratory findings

   a. Hct and BUN are decreased due to **hemodilution** (plasma has more water than normal); the percentage of RBCs and urea particles per liter of plasma is lower than normal in dilute plasma even though actual number of cells and particles has not dropped; once extra fluid is removed, Hct and BUN return to normal

   b. In hypotonic fluid volume excess (water intoxication):

      1) Serum osmolality (concentration) is low (<275 mOsm/kg)

      2) Serum sodium is very low (<125 mEq/L)

   c. Chest x-ray may show pleural effusions

   d. Arterial blood gases

      1) Low pO_2 indicates hypoxemia, which usually occurs before pCO_2 is affected (carbon dioxide diffuses more easily than oxygen)

      2) Low pCO_2 (hyperventilation) is often present in early phases of compensation but will be low (hypoventilation) in later phases when compensation is failing

      3) As pulmonary edema progresses to hypoventilation and respiratory failure, respiratory acidosis causes the pH to drop

4. Identification of risk factors predisposing to fluid volume excess

   a. Age

      1) Because of decreased heart and kidney function, older adult clients are not able to compensate as easily for fluid volume excess

      2) Infants (up to age 2 years) have immature kidneys and cannot dilute urine well to eliminate excess fluid as efficiently as adults

      3) Children 2–12 years of age have less stable regulatory responses to fluid imbalances

   b. Acute illness

      1) Surgery stimulates stress response, with release of cortisol, ADH, and aldosterone, which promotes water and sodium retention

      2) Clients with medical problems (acute or preexisting) receiving IV fluids are prone to develop fluid imbalances, leading to FVE

   c. Chronic illness

      1) Cardiovascular disease reduces pumping strength of heart and results in diminished blood flow to kidneys, which causes sodium and water retention, leading to fluid volume excess

Practice to Pass

A young mother who comes to the clinic with her two-month-old infant for a well-baby visit tells the nurse that she has been mixing the formula half-strength because it is so expensive. What fluid imbalance does this predispose the infant to develop? Why? How should the nurse respond to the mother?

Table 1-5	Clinical Manifestations Consistent with Fluid Volume Excess
Assessment Parameter	**Signs Consistent with Fluid Volume Excess (Fluid Overload)**
Urine	Increasing urine output (polyuria); if cause of fluid retention is impaired cardiac or renal function, urine output may be decreased
Edema	Edema tends to follow gravity, so is often seen in legs, ankles, feet, and hands of ambulatory clients and on sacrum and back of clients confined to bed Edema from local obstruction of veins, such as when legs and feet swell after prolonged sitting, usually resolves with walking and/or leg elevation Edema that is present in legs and feet even after a period of elevation (e.g., upon awakening in morning) and in face (including periorbital edema and puffy eyelids) is more indicative of generalized edema (**anasarca**) related to fluid overload associated with a heart or kidney problem Edematous skin is often tight and shiny due to decreased circulation in swollen tissue Edema severity can be estimated on a scale from 1+ (minimal) to 4+ (severe) Pitting edema occurs when a finger pressed into edematous area leaves an imprint that does not resolve immediately when finger is removed In infants, edema is often generalized; edema in children occurs in dependent parts and may be evident in sacral areas if child is supine in bed; scrotum or labia may also be edematous
Fontanelles	Tense or bulging fontanels in children <18 months old; not applicable after fontanelles close
Vital signs	*Heart rate:* normal to increased (because of increased cardiac output) depending on severity of state *Heart sounds:* gallop rhythm in adults (S_3 heart sound) is evident when ventricles become overdistended due to venous congestion *Respirations:* usual and regular rate, progressing to signs of pulmonary edema (see section later in table) *Blood pressure:* normal to increased because of increased circulating volume to pump
Peripheral vascular	Full or bounding peripheral pulses, warm extremities, capillary refill less than 3 seconds Distended neck veins when head of bed is elevated to 45 degrees or higher; infants often do not display distended neck veins Delayed or absent hand vein emptying when hand is raised above heart (normally 3–5 seconds); engorged veins are evident
Pulmonary edema	Tachypnea and dyspnea, irritated cough (often early sign of fluid in alveoli) Hacking cough that eventually becomes moist and productive (clear to white sputum); a late sign of fluid in alveoli and larger airways Labored breathing (seen as intercostal and substernal retractions, nasal flaring, and expiratory grunting in infants) Wet lung sounds (moist crackles) on auscultation (first appear in bases bilaterally when client is in upright or semi-Fowler position and progresses upward as lung water increases) Decreased O_2 saturation due to inadequate or mismatched ventilation and perfusion as a result of FVE Cyanosis (a late sign of hypoxemia) *Note:* Acute pulmonary edema is a life-threatening medical emergency caused by large amounts of fluid pooling in alveoli from fluid retention; respiratory signs are severe and immediate action is required to prevent death
Miscellaneous	Hepatomegaly and splenomegaly (signs of venous congestion) Third-space fluid accumulations may be present as fluid is forced from vessels into spaces that normally do not contain much fluid (ascites, pleural effusion, pericardial effusion)

     2) Renal disease can lead to abnormal retention of water, sodium, potassium, and other electrolytes

    d. Medications: long-term glucocorticoid therapy predisposes to sodium and fluid retention

    e. See Table 1-6 for specific examples of age-related concerns with fluid volume excess

Table 1-6	Lifespan Considerations for Health Maintenance	
Lifespan Considerations	**Common Risk Factors for Imbalances**	**Nursing Implications**
Infants	**FVE** Dilution of infant formula Use of free water in bottles	Instruct parents to follow directions for formula dilution closely Explain dangers of "stretching the formula" by adding excessive water Discourage the excessive use of free water in bottles as pacifiers
Children	**FVE** Excessive use of free water when treating flu and diarrhea Nephrotic syndrome	Instruct parents to replace electrolytes using an electrolyte solution such as Pedialyte Impaired kidney function leads to fluid retention Monitor child closely for signs of FVE Instruct parents on sodium restriction
Adults	**FVE** Psychogenic polydipsia SIADH Excessive use of hypotonic solutions Excessive intake of water without electrolyte replacement Heart failure	Supervise clients with psychiatric disorders closely for excessive intake of fluids Monitor clients at risk for SIADH for decreased urine output and fluid retention Monitor clients receiving hypotonic solutions for signs of FVE Educate clients of the need to replace electrolytes along with water when engaging in activities that produce excessive sweating and diuresis Monitor clients with a history of HF for signs of FVE

Source: London, Marcia L.; Ladewig, Patricia W.; Ball, Jane W.; Bindler, Ruth C.; Cowen, Kay J., *Maternal & Child Nursing Care*, 3rd Ed © 2011. Reprinted and Electronically reproduced by permission of Pearson Education, Inc., Upper Saddle River, New Jersey.

D. Priority nursing concerns
   1. Fluid volume excess because of excessive fluid or sodium intake and/or retention
   2. Risk for development of pulmonary edema because of hypervolemia
   3. Reduced client comfort associated with manifestations of fluid excess
   4. Possible interruption of skin integrity because of edema
   5. Inadequate client knowledge of risk factors and therapeutic interventions
E. Therapeutic management
   1. Restrict fluid intake
      a. Fluid intake by all routes may be limited, sometimes as low as 1000–1500 mL per 24-hour period; plan for greater fluid intake over daytime hours (including breakfast and lunch), with less for evening (including supper), and approximately 100 mL (or enough for medications) during night
         1) Sodium-restricted diets help decrease water retention
         2) Level of sodium restriction commonly varies from mild (4–5 grams sodium per day) to moderate (2 grams per day)
         3) Stricter (0.5-gram sodium per day) restrictions are reserved for very severe conditions but are difficult to adhere to
      b. IV access is often maintained with a "saline lock" device to avoid administering any excess IV fluids
   2. Promote excretion
      a. Diuretics promote excretion of water through urine
         1) Loop diuretics are commonly used (e.g., furosemide)
         2) Potassium-sparing diuretics may also be used (e.g., spironolactone)
         3) Thiazide diuretics may also be used (e.g., hydrochlorothiazide)
      b. Human B-type natriuretic peptide (hBNP) such as nesiritide may be administered in acute heart failure to facilitate smooth muscle relaxation, renal perfusion, and thus urinary elimination

    c. Medications such as digoxin, low-dose beta blockers, and angiotensin-converting enzyme (ACE) inhibitors used in clients with heart failure may promote urinary excretion by improving cardiac efficiency

    d. Protein intake may be increased in clients who are malnourished and have low serum proteins to increase capillary oncotic pressure, thus pulling fluid out of tissues into vessels where it can be eliminated by kidneys

3. Monitor during therapy

    a. Monitor respiratory status, assessing for signs of worsening gas exchange, such as increased respiratory effort, lung crackles, falling O_2 and saturation (SaO_2)

    b. *Note:* Pulse oximetry values below 95% are considered low in people with healthy lungs; trend ABG results, assessing for decreasing PaO_2 and increasing $PaCO_2$

    c. Assess for improving or worsening venous engorgement

    d. Assess fluid I&O carefully, looking for improved UO in response to therapy

    e. Monitor daily weights (same time, same clothing, same scale), looking for acute weight gain

    f. Assess for peripheral edema, especially in morning before client arises or after client has reclined with feet elevated for some time (to differentiate dependent, or stasis, edema from more generalized edema related to heart, kidney, or liver problems)

    g. Observe for signs of developing or worsening water intoxication (hypotonic fluid volume excess), often associated with neurological changes

    h. Evaluate for overcorrection, in which signs of fluid volume deficit begin to appear

    i. Monitor lab values for normalizing BUN, Hct, serum sodium, and arterial blood gases; watch for electrolyte imbalances (low sodium, low or high potassium) due to drug therapy

F. Client-centered nursing care

1. Monitor assessment parameters, observe response to therapy, note any sign of improvement, and watch for signs of hypovolemia due to overcorrection

2. Restrict fluids as prescribed

    a. Teach clients to measure items that are liquid at room temperature and include them in fluid intake totals

    b. Involve client in dividing fluid allowances over 24-hour period; plan for more fluids during times for meals and taking oral medications

    c. Use an infusion pump to help prevent inadvertent administration of excess fluid

    d. Provide mouth care and use measures to moisten mouth regularly to decrease thirst; ice chips can be soothing, but count as fluid intake (1 cup ice chips = ½ cup water), so calculate them into the allowed fluid intake

    e. Encourage cool fluids, which tend to decrease thirst better than warm ones; avoid or limit sweet or salty foods to minimize thirst

3. Measure fluid losses/gains

    a. Measure I&O, noting color and concentration of urine

    b. Weigh daily and monitor patterns of weight loss/gain (remember, a change of 2.2 lbs [1 kg] is equivalent to a 1 L water loss or gain)

4. Institute measures to prevent fluid volume excess

    a. Irrigate NG tube and bladder with normal saline rather than plain water

    b. Avoid repeated plain tap water enemas

    c. Mix infant formula according to package directions; do not use a water bottle as a pacifier for infants

    d. Monitor infusion rates closely; use a volume control device and pump and use only small bags (250–500 mL) for infants and young children

5. Remain alert for acute pulmonary edema, an emergency requiring prompt action

    a. Anxious client with labored breathing

    b. Moist crackles on auscultation, bilaterally from bases into upper lung fields

Practice to Pass

A 2-month-old infant is being treated for gastroenteritis and dehydration. The infant has received normal saline boluses and has just been switched to D5¼NS at 40 mL/hour. What monitoring and nursing measures should be implemented at this time? Why?

    c. Productive cough with frothy, clear sputum

    d. SaO_2 below 95%; blood gases likely reveal low pO_2 (hypoxia); if impending respiratory failure, high pCO_2 (hypercarbia and respiratory acidosis)

    e. Prompt action: stop or limit any ongoing fluid intake; assess client (e.g., vital signs, lung sounds, pulse oximetry, mental status); implement actions to increase gas exchange (e.g., high-Fowler position, supplemental oxygen); and notify healthcare provider as soon as possible

  6. Skin care

    a. If edema is present, provide skin care and protection to prevent tissue trauma and skin breakdown

G. Medication therapy

  1. Diuretic therapy

    a. Loop diuretics and thiazide diuretics cause potassium and sodium loss while potassium-sparing diuretics can cause hyperkalemia

    b. Monitor electrolytes during diuretic therapy

    c. Give diuretics in the morning to avoid sleep disruption; if prescribed twice per day, administer second dose by midafternoon

  2. Treat underlying disease processes that place client at risk for developing FVE, such as congestive heart failure, or treatment with low-dose beta-blocking agents and/or ACE inhibitors

  3. Evaluate client for potential fluid and electrolyte imbalances that may result from overcorrection

H. Client education

  1. Teach clients risk factors for development of FVE

  2. Teach adults to weigh themselves daily and report a gain of more than 0.9 kg (2 lb) per week

  3. Teach clients with peripheral edema to elevate extremities and change position frequently

  4. Dietary education

    a. Teach clients about possible sodium-restricted diet, including rationale, limitations, and dietary choices (see Chapter 2 for listing of foods high and low in sodium)

      1) Suggest use of alternative seasonings, such as natural sodium-free herbs and spices

      2) Clients taking potassium-sparing diuretics and/or ACE inhibitors (which cause potassium retention) should not use salt substitutes because most contain potassium

    b. Teach clients to avoid adding salt while cooking or at the table

    c. Teach clients to assess sodium content by reading food/OTC drug labels

    d. Consult dietitian for more detailed dietary information regarding sodium and fluid restrictions

I. Evaluation

  1. Client regains fluid volume balance

    a. Peripheral edema is resolved; in a young pediatric client fontanels are soft and nonbulging

    b. Unlabored breathing; lungs clear to auscultation; chest x-ray shows no infiltrates or effusion

    c. Vital signs, level of consciousness, and orientation return to baseline

    d. Hct, BUN, serum osmolality, and serum electrolytes return to client's baseline

    e. Weight returns to baseline

  2. Underlying cause of fluid volume excess is resolved

  3. Client/family verbalize understanding of risk factors, prevention, and follow-up care for fluid volume excess

NWTC Library
2740 W. Mason St.
Green Bay, WI 54307

Case Study

A 9-month-old infant is brought to the emergency department by the infant's mother. During the intake assessment, the mother reports the infant has had a fever, vomiting, and diarrhea for the past 2 days. You are the nurse assigned to the care of the infant.

1. What questions will you ask the mother about the child initially?

2. What assessment findings will alert you to a serious fluid imbalance?

3. If intravenous fluids are prescribed, what are the priorities of care and monitoring during the intravenous infusion?

4. What rehydration instructions should be given to the mother in preparation for discharge?

5. When the mother asks about the BRAT diet her friends have told her to follow until the diarrhea is gone, how would you respond?

For suggested responses, see page 190.

POSTTEST

1 A 78-year-old client is admitted with dehydration and urinary tract infection. After IV infusion of 750 mL normal saline, the client begins to cough and asks for the head of the bed to be raised to ease breathing. The nurse assesses jugular vein distention (JVD) and increased respiratory rate. How should the nurse interpret this data?

1. The fluid volume deficit is worsening.
2. Hypervolemia is developing.
3. Hypotonic water intoxication is beginning.
4. Ascites is causing respiratory compromise.

2 The nurse is helping a client who was recently placed on a low-sodium diet to reduce fluid retention to choose foods for lunch. The nurse recommends which lunch menu that would be most beneficial for this client?

1. Grilled chicken sandwich on white bread, apple, salad, and iced tea
2. Tuna salad sandwich on wheat bread, canned fruit cocktail, salad, and a soda
3. Ham and bean soup, fresh fruit salad, low-sodium crackers, and a diet soda
4. Cheeseburger, grapes, fresh pineapple, and tomato juice

3 A 28-year-old client is admitted with severe bleeding from a fractured femur. Which intravenous (IV) fluid does the nurse anticipate as the most appropriate for use to replace potential fluid losses?

1. 0.9% sodium chloride (0.9% NaCl)
2. 3% sodium chloride (3%NaCl)
3. 5% dextrose in water (D_5W)
4. 5% dextrose in 0.225% sodium chloride ($D_5\frac{1}{4}NS$)

4 The nurse is preparing to administer 25 mg furosemide intravenously to a client with peripheral edema and lung crackles. The 2-mL vial is labeled 20 mg/mL. How many mL of solution should the nurse draw up? Record your answer rounding to two decimal places.

Fill in your answer below:
_____ mL of solution

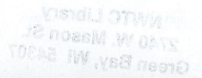

5 The nurse caring for the following group of clients considers which client to be at highest risk for developing fluid volume deficit?

1. A thin, 52-year-old female receiving corticosteroid therapy for bronchitis
2. A 60-year-old male who had a left inguinal herniorrhaphy 12 hours ago
3. A 76-year-old male who has diarrhea caused by gastroenteritis for 3 days
4. A 68-year-old female who is NPO for a flexible sigmoidoscopy procedure

6 A 17-year-old client who sustained a head injury in a motorcycle crash 2 days ago is responsive only to pain. Which intravenous (IV) fluid prescription would the nurse question because it could increase the risk of complications from increased intracranial pressure?

1. Ringer's solution
2. 5% dextrose in water (D_5W)
3. 0.9% sodium chloride (0.9% NaCl)
4. Lactated Ringer's solution

7 The nurse is caring for a client admitted with heart failure (HF). When assessing the client's risk for fluid imbalance, the nurse should check which laboratory values? Select all that apply.

1. Hemoglobin (Hgb)
2. Hematocrit (Hct)
3. Atrial natriuretic peptide (ANP)
4. Blood glucose
5. Liver enzymes

8 A client who was admitted to the hospital with fluid overload has been treated with diuretics and fluid restriction. Which set of findings is most indicative that fluid balance is not yet fully restored?

1. Client's S_3 heart sounds and moist lung crackles are resolving.
2. Client exhibits return to coherent conversation and appropriate behavior.
3. Oral mucous membranes are no longer sticky and cracked, and skin is warm and dry.
4. Skin tenting decreases and conjunctiva of eyes are moist.

9 A client is receiving an intravenous (IV) infusion of 0.0225% sodium chloride at 50 mL/hour. It is most important for the nurse to monitor which assessment parameter to detect complications of therapy?

1. Urine output and concentration
2. Legs and arms for edema
3. Tongue and mouth for dryness
4. Mental status and orientation

10 A father telephones the clinic nurse asking what he should do for his 3-year-old son who developed fever, vomiting, and diarrhea today. What would be an appropriate recommendation by the nurse?

1. "Have him drink as much water as you can get him to swallow."
2. "Give small sips of commercial oral rehydration fluids frequently."
3. "Provide frequent sips of fruit juice and commercial sports drinks."
4. "Have him eat only bananas, rice, applesauce, and toast (BRAT diet)."

➤ *See pages 29–31 for Answers and Rationales.*

POSTTEST

ANSWERS & RATIONALES

Pretest

1 **Answer: 1 Rationale:** Infants and older adults cannot compensate as well for fluid losses. Clients with NG suction (loss of fluids and electrolytes in fairly proportional amounts) are at greater risk for fluid volume deficit. The older adult with NG suction has both risk factors, while the child's age is the only risk factor. The client taking glucocorticoids is predisposed to sodium and fluid retention rather than fluid loss. The 30-year-old jogger is a healthy adult in a moderate climate, which lowers the risk from exertion alone. **Cognitive Level:** Analyzing **Client Need:** Physiological Adaptation **Integrated Process:** Nursing Process: Diagnosis **Content Area:** Adult Health **Strategy:** Recall concepts of fluid balance and factors contributing to losses. Eliminate one option because fluid is retained with steroids and eliminate two others because they have fewer risk factors than the correct option. **Reference:** LeMone, P., Burke, K., Bauldoff, G., & Gubrud, P. (2015). *Medical surgical nursing: Clinical reasoning in patient care* (6th ed.). New York, NY: Pearson, pp. 183–185.

2 **Answer: 3 Rationale:** Items that are liquid at body temperature are also considered part of the fluid intake, so ice pops, gelatin, and ice cream can be considered as part of overall fluid intake. The color of urine is only one indicator of hydration and some older adults take a diuretic, which would produce more dilute urine, falsely reassuring the client. The client should drink a variety of fluids, not just water. With aging, the thirst mechanism becomes less effective. Significant fluid can be lost before thirst is triggered, so older adults should not rely solely on thirst to indicate a need to drink fluids. **Cognitive Level:** Applying **Client Need:** Health Promotion and Maintenance **Integrated Process:** Communication and Documentation **Content Area:** Adult Health **Strategy:** Note the critical words *older adult* and *remain hydrated* Recall knowledge of risk factors for dehydration in older adults and of fluid intake to make a final selection. **Reference:** LeMone, P. T., Burke, K. M., Bauldoff, G., & Gubrud, P. (2015). *Medical surgical nursing: Clinical reasoning in patient care* (6th ed.). New York, NY: Pearson, pp. 187–189.

3 **Answer: 2, 4 Rationale:** The client has symptoms of fluid volume deficit (FVD) and hypovolemia. An increase in heart rate would accompany hypovolemia. The presence of postural hypotension (a drop in BP when rising from a lying position to a standing position) indicates the presence of significant hypovolemia. Skin temperature is a general assessment that can be affected by many variables, especially environmental temperature. Dyspnea is not a sign of fluid volume deficit, although

it may be present with fluid overload. Oxygen saturation reflects the adequacy of oxygen circulation to peripheral tissues, which can be adversely influenced by nutrition and disorders of red blood cells. **Cognitive Level:** Analyzing **Client Need:** Physiological Adaptation **Integrated Process:** Nursing Process: Assessment **Content Area:** Adult Health **Strategy:** Recognize that the client has signs and symptoms of an intravascular FVD and recall clinical manifestations of such. Eliminate options that are general assessments that do not reflect intravascular fluid losses. **Reference:** LeMone, P. T., Burke, K. M., Bauldoff, G., & Gubrud, P. (2015). *Medical surgical nursing: Clinical reasoning in patient care* (6th ed.). New York, NY: Pearson, pp. 184–185.

4 **Answer: 1, 4, 5 Rationale:** Neck veins are normally flat when the bed is elevated; distended neck veins reflect FVE in the vascular system. An accumulation of fluid in the alveoli and blood vessels will often cause shortness of breath with activity, reflecting FVE. Pitting edema reflects an accumulation of fluid in the interstitial tissues as seen with FVE. Hand veins would remain full or empty slowly if FVE is present. Rapid and weak peripheral pulses reflect a fluid volume deficit, not an excess. **Cognitive Level:** Analyzing **Client Need:** Physiological Adaptation **Integrated Process:** Nursing Process: Evaluation **Content Area:** Adult Health **Strategy:** Note the critical words *hydration status* and *fluid volume excess*. Choose those options that reflect a full vascular bed, which in this case are peripheral edema, venous engorgement, and excessive pulmonary fluid. **Reference:** LeMone, P. T., Burke, K. M., Bauldoff, G., & Gubrud, P. (2015). *Medical surgical nursing: Clinical reasoning in patient care* (6th ed.). New York, NY: Pearson, pp. 189–190.

5 **Answer: 3 Rationale:** 0.9% sodium chloride is an isotonic solution that does not produce fluid shifts and would be the best choice of solutions. 10% dextrose is a hypertonic solution and would pull water from the GI tract into the vascular space, possibly leading to a fluid volume excess. 5% dextrose is metabolized to a hypotonic solution and could contribute to fluid shifts into the GI tissue. 0.45% sodium chloride is a hypotonic solution and could contribute to fluid shifts into the GI tissue. **Cognitive Level:** Applying **Client Need:** Physiological Adaptation **Integrated Process:** Nursing Process: Planning **Content Area:** Adult Health **Strategy:** Recall principles of osmosis and diffusion and differences among hypotonic, isotonic, and hypertonic fluids. Eliminate incorrect options since fluid shifts will occur with hypotonic and hypertonic solutions. **Reference:** Berman, A., Snyder, S., & Frandsen, G. (2016). *Kozier & Erb's fundamentals of nursing: Concepts, process, and practice* (10th ed.). New York, NY: Pearson, p. 1336.

6 **Answer: 4 Rationale:** A moist cough, dyspnea, and a falling pulse oximetry reading in a client with a history of heart disease are signs of developing pulmonary edema secondary to fluid volume excess (FVE). The first action should be to reduce IV fluid intake to prevent more fluid from accumulating in the lungs, then further assessment can be done, emergency actions taken, and the healthcare provider contacted. **Cognitive Level:** Analyzing **Client Need:** Reduction of Risk Potential **Integrated Process:** Nursing Process: Implementation **Content Area:** Adult Health **Strategy:** Note the critical word *first*, indicating one option has a priority action. Use knowledge of cardiovascular disease and EFV to choose correctly. **Reference:** LeMone, P. T., Burke, K. M., Bauldoff, G., & Gubrud, P. (2015). *Medical-surgical nursing: Clinical reasoning in patient care* (6th ed.). New York, NY: Pearson, pp. 207–213.

7 **Answer: 2 Rationale:** Explaining the functioning of the kidneys provides the client with information as to why the fluid restriction is necessary. The client already knows the healthcare provider prescribed the restriction. There is no evidence that the client drank excessive fluids before becoming ill; this explanation is not accurate. Although explaining effects of excess fluid is accurate information, it is presented in an alarming fashion. **Cognitive Level:** Applying **Client Need:** Physiological Adaptation **Integrated Process:** Communication and Documentation **Content Area:** Adult Health **Strategy:** Note the critical words *best* and *response*. Use knowledge of communication skills and regulation of fluid imbalances to choose the correct option. **Reference:** LeMone, P. T., Burke, K. M., Bauldoff, G., & Gubrud, P. (2015). *Medical surgical nursing: Clinical reasoning in patient care* (6th ed.). New York, NY: Pearson, pp. 189–190.

8 **Answer: 1 Rationale:** An excess response to diuretic therapy results in an excess loss of water and electrolytes in the urine, leaving the blood hemoconcentrated and causing a high BUN (normal 8–22 mg/dL) and Hct (normal approximately 38–45%). The water loss results in an acute weight loss. Weight gain indicates ineffective response to diuretic therapy. **Cognitive Level:** Analyzing **Client Need:** Physiological Adaptation **Integrated Process:** Nursing Process: Evaluation **Content Area:** Adult Health **Strategy:** Note the critical words *excessive response*, indicating a greater than desired action is achieved. Use knowledge of diuretic action and recall normal values for BUN and Hct to eliminate incorrect options. **Reference:** LeMone, P. T., Burke, K. M., Bauldoff, G., & Gubrud, P. (2015). *Medical surgical nursing: Clinical reasoning in patient care* (6th ed.). New York, NY: Pearson, pp. 189–190.

9 **Answer: 1 Rationale:** DI is associated with insufficient ADH production, which would lead to excessive fluid losses. DI would lead to excessive fluid losses, not fluid volume excesses. Diabetes mellitus, not DI, is associated with poor insulin production. Hypoglycemia can be a complication of diabetes mellitus, not DI. **Cognitive Level:** Analyzing **Client Need:** Physiological Adaptation **Integrated Process:** Nursing Process: Diagnosis **Content Area:** Adult Health **Strategy:** The critical words are *diabetes insipidus* and *at risk for*. Eliminate two options because they relate to diabetes mellitus. Discriminate appropriately between DI and SIADH to choose correctly between the remaining two. **Reference:** LeMone, P. T., Burke, K. M., Bauldoff, G., & Gubrud, P. (2015). *Medical surgical nursing: Clinical reasoning in patient care* (6th ed.). New York, NY: Pearson, p. 184.

10 **Answer: 1, 4, 5 Rationale:** Priority should be placed on assessment of the neurological system since the 3% NaCl infusion can lead to cellular dehydration and could lead to mental status changes and possibly seizures. 3% NaCl is very hypertonic and, if infused too rapidly, will increase serum sodium and osmolality, causing high volumes of water to be pulled into vessels from cells. This results in cellular dehydration and vascular volume overload. The serum sodium level should be monitored to ensure adequate therapy without too rapid an increase. Urine specific gravity would not provide the most important information regarding onset of complications as it would be affected later. Serum glucose levels are an indicator of pancreatic function. **Cognitive Level:** Analyzing **Client Need:** Physiological Adaptation **Integrated Process:** Nursing Process: Evaluation **Content Area:** Adult Health **Strategy:** Note critical words *priority* and *detect*. Recall physiology of fluids shifts from hypertonic solutions to choose correctly. Note the wording of the question indicates that more than one option is correct. **Reference:** LeMone, P. T., Burke, K. M., Bauldoff, G., & Gubrud, P. (2015). *Medical surgical nursing: Clinical reasoning in patient care* (6th ed.). New York, NY: Pearson, pp. 187–189.

Posttest

1 **Answer: 2 Rationale:** Dyspnea and increased respirations are most likely caused by fluid accumulation in the lungs, both signs of fluid volume excess. The jugular vein distention is also a sign of fluid accumulation related to hypervolemia. The client is exhibiting signs of fluid volume excess, not fluid volume deficit. The client is receiving an isotonic solution, not a hypotonic solution. The client does not display fluid accumulation in the abdomen related to ascites, but rather in the lungs and jugular veins. **Cognitive Level:** Analyzing **Client Need:** Physiological Adaptation **Integrated Process:** Nursing Process: Diagnosis **Content Area:** Adult Health **Strategy:** Note the client is an older adult and has received too much fluid, indicating high risk for fluid overload. Recall knowledge of fluid volume excess to eliminate options that are incorrect or irrelevant to the client. **Reference:** LeMone, P. T., Burke, K. M., Bauldoff, G., & Gubrud, P. (2015). *Medical surgical nursing: Clinical*

ANSWERS & RATIONALES

reasoning in patient care (6th ed.). New York, NY: Pearson, pp. 189–193.

2 Answer: 1 Rationale: Processed and/or canned foods, such as tuna, soup, tomato juice, and sodas, are more likely to be high in sodium. Fresh foods, such as grilled chicken, fruit, and vegetables, are lower in sodium. **Cognitive Level:** Applying **Client Need:** Health Promotion and Maintenance **Integrated Process:** Nursing Process: Implementation **Content Area:** Adult Health **Strategy:** Note the critical word *best* is used, indicating one of the choices is better than the others. Recall knowledge of the sodium content of various foods to eliminate the incorrect options. **Reference:** LeMone, P. T., Burke, K. M., Bauldoff, G., & Gubrud, P. (2015). *Medical surgical nursing: Clinical reasoning in patient care* (6th ed.). New York, NY: Pearson, p. 191.

3 Answer: 1 Rationale: Acute bleeding results in isotonic fluid loss and can quickly lead to shock and vascular collapse. The priority is to expand vascular volume and restore circulation using isotonic IV fluid. Hypertonic solutions such as 3% saline are not indicated because isotonic solutions are appropriate. Hypotonic (D_5W, $D_5\frac{1}{4}NS$) solutions are not indicated because isotonic solutions would be appropriate. **Cognitive Level:** Applying **Client Need:** Pharmacological and Parenteral Therapies **Integrated Process:** Nursing Process: Planning **Content Area:** Adult Health **Strategy:** The critical words are *most appropriate* and *fluid losses*. Recognize the client needs replacement of isotonic fluids to eliminate incorrect options, since these are either hypertonic or hypotonic. **Reference:** LeMone, P. T., Burke, K. M., Bauldoff, G., & Gubrud, P. (2015). *Medical surgical nursing: Clinical reasoning in patient care* (6th ed.). New York, NY: Pearson, pp. 187–188.

4 Answer: 1.25 Rationale:

$$\frac{\text{Desired dose}}{\text{Dose on hand}} \times \text{Quantity}$$

$$\frac{25\ mg}{20\ mg} \times 1\ mL$$

25 divided by 20 $\times$ 1 = x

$x = 1.25$

Cognitive Level: Applying **Client Need:** Pharmacological and Parenteral Therapies **Integrated Process:** Nursing Process: Planning **Content Area:** Adult Health **Strategy:** Specific knowledge of formulas for calculating medication dosage is needed to answer this question. Recall the formula and check calculations carefully. **Reference:** Kee, J., & Marshall, S. (2013). *Clinical calculations with applications to general and specialty areas* (7th ed.). St. Louis, MO: Elsevier, p. 76.

5 Answer: 3 Rationale: The 76-year-old client is most at risk for a fluid volume deficit secondary to increasing age and 3 days of fluid losses caused by diarrhea. Clients receiving corticosteroids often retain sodium and fluid, placing them at risk for a fluid volume excess, not deficit. An inguinal herniorrhaphy is not considered major surgery and the client is not at risk for large volumes of fluid loss. Although the 68-year-old client has been NPO for the procedure, fluid replacement will be resumed and the risk for deficit is low. **Cognitive Level:** Analyzing **Client Need:** Physiological Adaptation **Integrated Process:** Nursing Process: Assessment **Content Area:** Adult Health **Strategy:** Critical words are *at highest risk* and *fluid volume deficit*. Recall knowledge of risk factors contributing to fluid deficits and determine one option has the greater number of them. **Reference:** LeMone, P. T., Burke, K. M., Bauldoff, G., & Gubrud, P. (2015). *Medical surgical nursing: Clinical reasoning in patient care* (6th ed.). New York, NY: Pearson, pp. 184–186.

6 Answer: 2 Rationale: 5% dextrose in water (D_5W) has a hypotonic effect when infused, providing free water to cells, which would worsen this client's cerebral edema. The other fluids listed (Ringer's solution, 0.9% sodium chloride, and Lactated Ringer's solution) are isotonic and would primarily remain in the extracellular spaces. **Cognitive Level:** Analyzing **Client Need:** Pharmacological and Parenteral Therapies **Integrated Process:** Nursing Process: Implementation **Content Area:** Adult Health **Strategy:** Note the client has a head injury and recognize the danger of hypotonic fluids that could contribute to cerebral edema. Also note the question requires the nurse to question a prescription, indicating that one option will be incorrect and three are correct. Consider tonicity of IV fluids to make a selection. **Reference:** LeMone, P. T., Burke, K. M., Bauldoff, G., & Gubrud, P. (2015). *Medical surgical nursing: Clinical reasoning in patient care* (6th ed.). New York, NY: Pearson, pp. 185–187.

7 Answer: 1, 2, 3 Rationale: Hemoglobin and hematocrit can decrease or increase secondary to hemoconcentration or hemodilution. ANP is a cardiac hormone released when atria are stretched by increased blood volume, which would occur in HF. Glucose and liver enzymes would not be affected by fluid volume. **Cognitive Level:** Applying **Client Need:** Physiological Adaptation **Integrated Process:** Nursing Process: Assessment **Content Area:** Adult Health **Strategy:** Note that the client has HF. Recall knowledge of fluid imbalances and correlate lab studies associated with them. Eliminate two options since they are not affected by fluid volume. **Reference:** LeMone, P. T., Burke, K. M., Bauldoff, G., & Gubrud, P. (2015). *Medical surgical nursing: Clinical reasoning in patient care* (6th ed.). New York, NY: Pearson, pp. 189–190.

8 Answer: 1 Rationale: S_3 heart sounds are associated with increased workload on the heart and lung crackles are associated with fluid accumulation in the lungs. Since these sounds are resolving, it would support that fluid volume is decreasing, but not yet fully achieved. Although a client with a fluid overload may become confused and incoherent, this would not be the best choice to support resolution of a fluid volume excess. The client may have been inappropriate for reasons unrelated to the fluid excess. Cracked and sticky mucous membranes are associated with a fluid volume deficit, not an excess. A decrease in skin tenting indicates an improvement from a fluid volume deficit, not excess. **Cognitive Level:** Analyzing **Client Need:** Physiological Adaptation **Integrated Process:** Nursing Process: Evaluation **Content Area:** Adult Health **Strategy:** Note the critical phrases *fluid overload* and *has not yet been achieved*. Recall signs and symptoms of fluid excess and eliminate one option because it indicates full resolution of these signs. Eliminate two other options because they indicate resolution of deficient fluid volume, which is not the focus of the question. **Reference:** LeMone, P. T., Burke, K. M., Bauldoff, G., & Gubrud, P. (2015). *Medical surgical nursing: Clinical reasoning in patient care* (6th ed.). New York, NY: Pearson, pp. 190–191.

9 **Answer: 4 Rationale:** A solution of 0.225% sodium chloride ¼NS is a hypotonic solution that provides free water to the cells. Cerebral cells are especially sensitive to fluid gains from hypotonic fluids. If infused too rapidly, the cerebral cells will be the first to gain fluid too quickly, resulting in neurologic changes. Monitoring the client for urine output, edema, and oral cavity dryness are important, but this reflects a response to IV therapy rather than detection of

a complication. **Cognitive Level:** Analyzing **Client Need:** Physiological Adaptation **Integrated Process:** Nursing Process: Assessment **Content Area:** Adult Health **Strategy:** Note critical words *complications of therapy* and *most important*, indicating one of the options is of higher priority. Recall knowledge of fluid shifts with hypotonic fluids to choose correctly. **Reference:** Berman, A., Snyder, S., & Frandsen, G. (2016). *Kozier & Erb's fundamentals of nursing: Concepts, process, and practice* (10th ed.). New York, NY: Pearson, pp. 1318–1320.

10 **Answer: 2 Rationale:** Oral rehydration fluids contain electrolytes that will help to replace what is lost with vomiting and diarrhea. Replacing fluid losses with plain water could lead to electrolyte imbalances since electrolytes are lost with perspiration, vomiting, and diarrhea. Fruit juices and commercial sports drinks are often high in sugar and could worsen the vomiting. Solid foods should not be encouraged when the child is vomiting. **Cognitive Level:** Applying **Client Need:** Physiological Adaptation **Integrated Process:** Nursing Process: Implementation **Content Area:** Child Health **Strategy:** Recall knowledge of age-appropriate fluids. Determine symptoms reflect risk for fluid volume deficit to choose correctly. **Reference:** LeMone, P. M., Burke, K. T., Bauldoff, G., & Gubrud, P. (2015). *Medical surgical nursing: Clinical reasoning in patient care* (6th ed.). New York, NY: Pearson, pp. 188, 626–627.

References

Ball, J., Bindler, R., & Cowen, K. (2014). *Child health nursing: Partnering with children and families* (3rd ed.). Upper Saddle River, NJ: Pearson.

Berman, A., Snyder, S., & Frandsen, G. (2016). *Kozier & Erb's fundamentals of nursing: Concepts, process, and practice* (10th ed.). New York, NY: Pearson.

Ignatavicius, D. D., & Workman, M. L. (2016). *Medical-surgical nursing: Patient-centered collaborative care* (8th ed.). Philadelphia, PA: Elsevier Saunders.

Kee, J. L. (2017). *Pearson's handbook of laboratory and diagnostic tests* (8th ed.). New York, NY: Pearson.

Kee, J., & Marshall, S. (2013). *Clinical calculations with applications to general and specialty areas* (7th ed.). St. Louis, MO: Elsevier.

LeMone, P. T., Burke, K. M., Bauldoff, G., & Gubrud, P. (2015). *Medical surgical nursing: Clinical reasoning in patient care* (6th ed.). New York, NY: Pearson.

London, M., Ladewig, P., Ball, J., Bindler, R., & Cowen, K. (2016). *Maternal and child nursing care* (5th ed.). New York, NY: Pearson Education.

Sole, M. L., Klein, O. G., & Moseley, M. J. (2016). *Introduction to critical care nursing* (7th ed.). St. Louis, MO: Elsevier Saunders.

ANSWERS & RATIONALES

2 Sodium and Chloride Balance and Imbalances

Chapter Outline

Overview of Sodium Regulation
Hyponatremia
Hypernatremia

Overview of Chloride
  Regulation
Hypochloremia

Hyperchloremia

NCLEX-RN® Test Prep

Access the NEW Web-based app that provides students with additional practice questions in preparation for the NCLEX experience.

Objectives

➤ Identify the basic functions of sodium and chloride in the body.
➤ Explain the pathophysiology and etiology of sodium and chloride imbalances.
➤ Identify specific assessment findings in sodium and chloride imbalances.
➤ Identify priority nursing concerns for a client experiencing a sodium imbalance.
➤ Describe the therapeutic management of sodium and chloride imbalances.
➤ Describe the management of nursing care for clients experiencing sodium or chloride imbalance.

Review at a Glance

anion an ion with a negative charge

cation an ion with a positive charge

cerebral demyelination an adverse outcome of hyponatremia that causes demyelination of the pons in the brain and leads to dysphagia, delirium, coma, and even death

chloride anion found in the ECF that is linked to sodium, bicarbonate, and water in the body and participates in osmotic pressure regulation and acid–base balance

diabetes insipidus (DI) an endocrine disturbance whereby ADH is either not secreted (central DI) or there is kidney failure (nephrogenic DI) that leads to an increased dilute urine, hypernatremia, and thirst

dilutional hyponatremia a term used to describe hyponatremia where the serum sodium level is diluted by excess fluid

euvolemia normal fluid volume in the body

halogen a nonionized form of a halide that combines with alkali metals in the body to form salts such as sodium chloride or potassium chloride

hyperchloremia a serum chloride level greater than 108 mEq/L

hypernatremia a serum sodium level above 145 mEq/L

hyperosmolar osmotic pressure greater than normal plasma pressure

hypochloremia a serum chloride level less than 95 mEq/L

hyponatremia a serum sodium level below 135 mEq/L; also called dilutional hyponatremia or water intoxication

syndrome of inappropriate antidiuretic hormone secretion (SIADH) excessive release of ADH hormone that causes fluid and electrolyte imbalances resulting in fluid retention, increased ECF volume, hyponatremia, and concentrated urine

water intoxication another term to describe hyponatremia where the serum sodium level is diluted by excess fluid

PRETEST

1 Which serum electrolyte imbalances would the nurse assess for in a child admitted with a high fever and severe dehydration? Select all that apply.

1. Hypercalcemia
2. Hypokalemia
3. Hypernatremia
4. Hyperchloremia
5. Hypophosphatemia

2 Which client would the nurse identify as being most at risk of developing a sodium imbalance?

1. An adult client taking corticosteroid therapy
2. An older adult client who drinks eight glasses (8 ounces each) of water each day
3. A school-age client with diabetes mellitus who is under glycemic control
4. A teenager who is drinking Gatorade during exercise workouts

3 When caring for a 79-year-old client who has a sodium level of 149 mEq/L, the nurse identifies that which factor increases the client's risk of developing dehydration?

1. A diminished thirst drive
2. An increased level of aldosterone
3. A decrease in muscle mass
4. ADH (antidiuretic hormone) is no longer produced

4 Which intervention should the nurse complete when caring for a client admitted with a sodium level of 152 mEq/L?

1. Provide extra blankets for warmth.
2. Observe client for nausea and malaise.
3. Observe and prepare for possible seizures.
4. Restrict fluids to 1200 mL per day.

5 The nurse is teaching a client who is on a low-sodium diet how to read food labels and check for hidden sodium content. The nurse informs the client that sodium is contained in higher amounts in which products? Select all that apply.

1. Baking goods containing baking powder
2. Seasonings using monosodium glutamate (MSG)
3. Over-the-counter cold and cough preparations
4. Canned vegetables
5. Salad oil

6 The nurse is caring for a client who is experiencing a steady decline in sodium level. The nurse places highest priority on which aspect of care?

1. Close monitoring of neurologic status
2. Preventing weakness and fatigue
3. Spacing activities to conserve energy
4. Providing oral hygiene and skin care

7 A client is being discharged with a prescription for prednisone. Which statement would indicate the client understands the side effects of prednisone that could affect the client's serum sodium and chloride levels?

1. "I should limit my salt intake."
2. "I will not need to take my diuretic now."
3. "It will be important to eat more vegetables."
4. "I should increase my intake of spinach and celery, which I enjoy."

8 Lab chemistry results reveal a client's serum sodium is within normal range. Based on this finding, the nurse estimates the client's serum (plasma) osmolality to be no higher than _____ mOsm/kg.

Fill in your answer below:
_____ mOsm/kg

9 A client with abnormal sodium loss is receiving a regular diet. To encourage foods high in sodium, the nurse would recommend which menu selections for lunch? Select all that apply.

1. A ham and cheese sandwich
2. Chicken salad in a lettuce wrap
3. Tossed salad with vinegar dressing
4. White fish and plain baked potato
5. Hot dog and baked beans

10 Which intervention should the nurse anticipate implementing in a client who is experiencing dilutional hyponatremia?

1. Administration of hypotonic intravenous solutions
2. Restriction of additional oral fluids
3. Increasing sodium intake in the diet
4. Encouraging intake of tap water

➤ *See pages 56–57 for Answers and Rationales.*

I. OVERVIEW OF SODIUM REGULATION

A. **Sodium balance and function**: major extracellular fluid (ECF) **cation** (positively charged ion), making up about 99% of body's sodium level; the remaining 1% is in intracellular fluid (ICF) and is responsible for water balance and determination of plasma osmolality; movement of **chloride** (major **anion**—negatively charged ion—in the ECF) is also closely associated with movement of sodium

1. Serum levels
   a. Normal ECF range is 135–145 mEq/L; normal intracellular level is 10 mEq/L
   b. Sodium works with chloride in body to affect electrolyte changes; they may occur at same time or independently
   c. Serum sodium level has a profound effect on cellular fluid dynamics
   d. Serum sodium level is used to monitor electrolyte, water, and acid–base balance in body

2. Determinant of plasma osmolality
   a. Sodium is the major determinant of plasma osmolality
   b. Osmolality determines movement of water between ECF and ICF; water moves from a lower concentration of solute (hypotonic) to a higher concentration of solute (hypertonic)
   c. Osmolality of ECF and ICF are roughly equal (isotonic) at 270–290 mOsm/kg water
   d. Osmotic force helps to move water across cell membrane to equalize osmotic pressure; water follows sodium, so a sodium imbalance is usually accompanied by an associated imbalance in water
   e. Plasma osmolality can be roughly estimated by doubling the plasma sodium value
   f. Formula used to determine serum osmolality:

$$2 \times \text{serum Na} + \frac{\text{BUN}}{3} + \frac{\text{glucose}}{18} = \text{serum osmolality}$$

   g. Free water (pure water) is available to all body compartments and helps to maintain osmotic balance

3. Functions of sodium in body
   a. Determines plasma osmolality and regulates water balance and distribution
   b. Helps maintain electrolyte balance by exchanging for potassium and attracting chloride
   c. Assists with acid–base balance by combining with bicarbonate and chloride to alter pH

Practice to Pass

What methods can the nurse use to get an estimate of a client's plasma osmolality?

        d. Promotes neuromuscular response and stimulates conduction of nerve impulses and muscle fiber impulse transmission through the sodium–potassium pump

    4. System interactions

        a. Sodium concentration is primarily regulated by renal tubules in kidneys

        b. In addition, posterior pituitary and adrenal glands of endocrine system help to regulate sodium levels by hormonal control

           1) Aldosterone (a mineralocorticoid) and cortisone increase serum sodium by increasing tubular reabsorption

           2) Antidiuretic hormone (ADH) increases sodium and water renal tubular reabsorption

        c. Sodium movement and regulation is also affected by sodium–potassium pump, which is located in the cell membrane; ATP helps to actively move sodium from cell into ECF; the process of diffusion offsets the continual movement

        d. Cerebral cells are very sensitive to changes in serum sodium levels and exhibit adaptive changes to sodium imbalances

           1) In acute situations where there is a dramatic change in sodium levels, brain tries to adapt with a corresponding change in water to maintain fluid balance

           2) It is important to recognize both the rapid onset and acuity of a severe sodium disturbance

        e. Since brain readily responds to sodium imbalances to maintain homeostasis, restoration of a normal sodium level must be done carefully; too rapid a correction can cause further fluid and cellular shifting, which can further compromise the client's condition; for example, too rapid a correction of hypernatremia leads to fewer particles in serum than in brain, causing fluid to shift into brain with resultant brain swelling

        f. Sodium imbalances can exist in different volume states: **euvolemia** (normal volume), hypovolemia, and hypervolemia

B. Sources of sodium

    1. Cellular level

        a. A greater amount of sodium is found in bones than in ECF, but it is not involved in electrolyte exchange

        b. Sodium is found in all body fluids, including blood, bile, gastric and intestinal secretions, pancreatic fluid, and saliva

        c. Sodium is found normally in body perspiration

    2. Dietary level

        a. Most people in the United States eat more sodium (average of 4–6 grams on a daily basis) than is needed; safe minimum levels have been established for infants and children, adults, and pregnant and lactating women; 500 mg is the minimally safe recommended sodium intake for an adult client (refer to current findings of the National Research Council–National Academy of Sciences for further information)

        b. Table salt (NaCl) is the primary dietary source of sodium; it contains approximately 40% sodium

        c. Sodium is found in a variety of foods in Western diet such as cheese, eggs, fish, milk, poultry, shellfish, canned foods, and processed foods

        d. Hidden sources of dietary sodium are found in processed foods, preservatives, seasonings, and flavorings; in addition, hidden sodium may also be found in medications; although this may not be considered a dietary form, it still contributes to overall dietary intake (see Box 2-1 for hidden sources of sodium)

Practice to Pass

Where does the chief regulation of sodium occur?

Box 2-1	The following items should be evaluated for their hidden sodium content:
Hidden Sources of Sodium	• Processed foods: contain increased amounts of sodium used in the processing and preserving process • Medications: such as OTC cold products, cough syrups, antacids, and Alka-Seltzer • Canned food items: often contain increased amounts of sodium, especially soups • Seasonings: such as MSG (monosodium glutamate), seasoned salts, and soy sauce • Baking products: such as baking powder and baking soda

II. *HYPONATREMIA*

A. Definition, etiology, and pathophysiology

1. Sodium level below 135 mEq/L (135 mmol/L)
2. Cellular-level transport
   a. Sodium deficit is usually associated with hypervolemia (increased volume) states and can also be referred to as **dilutional hyponatremia** or **water intoxication** (excess fluid that dilutes serum sodium)
   b. Sodium deficit can also occur in euvolemia and hypovolemia states (see Table 2-1 for a summary of this disorder)
   c. Water will shift from ECF (area of lower volume of solutes) to ICF (area of higher volume of solutes) in an attempt to restore equilibrium, resulting in decreased circulating plasma volume and an increased intracellular fluid volume
   d. Body responds to low sodium level using these compensatory mechanisms:
      1) Decreased circulating plasma volume leads to activation of pressure receptors (baroreceptors) in cardiac atria and thoracic veins in an attempt to increase plasma volume; ADH hormone responds to changes in extracellular volume (ECV) and plasma osmolality
      2) Renal sodium excretion is decreased in order to prevent further sodium depletion
      3) Hormonal response of aldosterone helps to promote sodium retention and potassium excretion

> **Practice to Pass**
>
> What happens to the fluid balance of the body when the sodium level is decreased?

Table 2-1	**Hyponatremia in Various Fluid Volume States**		
	Description	**Clinical Presentation**	**Treatment**
Euvolemia	Decrease in fluids in both intravascular and interstitial space Use of sodium-free solutions that dilute the ECF Serum osmolality remains normal	Medications, hypothyroidism, psychiatric disorders, cerebral salt-wasting syndrome	Water restriction, correction of underlying cause; treat SIADH with demeclocycline (unlabeled use) and increase dietary salt intake
Hypervolemia	High glucose states that pull water from cells, leading to cellular dehydration as seen in diabetic ketoacidosis (DKA) Fluid loss from ECF greater than solute loss leading to increased serum osmolality	Congestive heart failure (CHF), cirrhosis, syndrome of inappropriate ADH (SIADH), nephrotic syndrome, and renal failure	Water restriction, treat existing disease states, loop diuretics, and restrict dietary salt intake
Hypovolemia	Glucose in isotonic solutions is oxidized, leading to cellular swelling Loss of solute from ECF is greater than excess of water, resulting in a decreased serum osmolality	GI fluid loss, diuretic therapy, osmotic diuresis, adrenal insufficiency, burns, sweating, and hypotonic dehydration	NS to correct ECF deficits, increase dietary salt intake; hypertonic saline to raise sodium level

Figure 2-1

Cellular dynamics in response to sodium levels. **A.** Hyponatremia (cells edematous). **B.** Hypernatremia (cells shrink).

Cell swells as water is pulled in from ECF

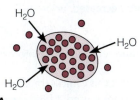

Cell shrinks as water is pulled out into ECF

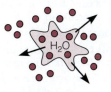

A Hyponatremia:
Na less than 135 mEq/L

B Hypernatremia:
Na greater than 145 mEq/L

    e. Cellular response results in cellular swelling/edema (see Figure 2-1A)

    f. Cerebral cell response

        1) Osmotic force that causes water to be drawn into brain cells leads to development of cerebral edema in hyponatremic disorders

        2) If hyponatremia is severe (acuity and severity of onset), **cerebral demyelination** can occur; this is a serious complication whereby the pons is severely affected, leading to mutism, dysphagia, delirium, coma, and possibly death

3. Predisposing clinical conditions

    a. Conditions that cause loss of body fluids and sodium

        1) Renal losses through excretion, diuretic administration, and renal disease (salt-wasting nephropathy)

        2) Gastrointestinal (GI) losses through vomiting, diarrhea, suctioning, tap water enemas (TWE), GI surgery, and bulimia

        3) Skin losses through perspiration, environmental conditions, burns, and tissue destruction

        4) Wound drainage; wound suctioning

    b. Conditions that increase extracellular water

        1) Hormone regulation response of ADH and aldosterone, leading to fluid shifting and water gain

        2) Disease states that add to increased volume such as congestive heart failure (CHF), cirrhosis, and nephrotic syndrome

        3) Disease states such as psychiatric disorders that involve compulsive water drinking

        4) Disease states such as tumors, **syndrome of inappropriate antidiuretic hormone secretion** or **SIADH**, and adrenal insufficiency affect hormonal response, leading to increased secretion (refer to Box 2-2 for additional information on SIADH)

        5) Hyperglycemic states such as diabetic ketoacidosis (DKA) that cause cellular dehydration

        6) Medications can promote development of hyponatremia (refer to Table 2-2 for sample medications that affect serum sodium levels)

        7) Prolonged or excessive administration of hypotonic fluids can lead to hyponatremia

    c. Conditions that lead to inadequate dietary intake of sodium

        1) Prolonged intake of fluids without sodium replacement

        2) Anorexia and other eating disorders can lead to inadequate intake of dietary sodium

4. See Table 2-3 for age-related risk factors for hyponatremia

Box 2-2	
Syndrome of Inappropriate Antidiuretic Hormone Secretion (SIADH)	• Increased ADH secretion occurs due to malignancies, CNS disorders, pulmonary disorders, medications, and in postoperative states. • Plasma osmolality and sodium are decreased, urine sodium is high, and urine osmolality is increased. • Hyponatremia is present. • Clients present with significant fluid retention, GI symptoms, and neurologic symptoms related to fluid retention. • Free water restriction is used to treat this clinical condition. • Demeclocycline (blocks ADH secretion) is used if fluid restriction alone does not correct the disturbance. Lithium also blocks ADH secretion, but it is not commonly used as it can reach toxic levels in the body and cause additional complications. • Clients can be placed on a high-salt, high-protein diet to restore normal sodium level and allow the kidneys to excrete more urine (increased solute load). • It is important to identify and correct the underlying cause of the problem. • It is important when restoring normal sodium balance that the correction is done per protocol so as not to cause further complications.

Table 2-2   Medications That Can Affect Sodium Levels

Increase Sodium Levels	Decrease Sodium Levels
Corticosteroids (cortisone, prednisone)	Diuretics
Hypertonic saline solutions	Lithium
Sodium bicarbonate, sodium phosphate, and sodium salicylate	Antineoplastic agents* (cisplatin, vincristine)
Antibiotics* (such as penicillin Na)	ACE inhibitors* (captopril, lisinopril)
Amphotericin B	Psychotropic medications* (amitriptyline, thioridazine)
Demeclocycline	Antidiabetic agents* (chlorpropramide, tolbutamide)
Lactulose	CNS depressants* (morphine, barbiturates)
Some cough syrups and cold preparations	Oxytocin

* For these medications, please refer to a drug textbook for specific names as there are many different types of drugs in each category.

Table 2-3   Lifespan Considerations for Health Maintenance: Hyponatremia

Lifespan Considerations	Fluids	Electrolytes	Acid–Base Balance
Infants	Mature breast milk is present by 2 weeks postpartum; establish an "on-demand" feeding schedule	Sodium (Na^+) is essential for fluid balance, nerve, and muscle function	Acid–base imbalance in infants is primarily due to respiratory disorders related to respiratory insufficiency
Children	Give isotonic fluids and avoid hypotonic fluids such as D_5W; possible fluid restriction	Monitor for decreased level of consciousness, anorexia, nausea and vomiting, confusion, headache, respiratory distress, muscle weakness, agitation, and lethargy	Acidosis can occur through the loss of fluid in clients with cystic fibrosis
Adults	Due to a loss of sodium or a gain of water; monitor fluid losses and gains; check urine specific gravity	Hyponatremia leads to swelling of the cells, with resulting confusion, hypotension, edema, muscle cramps, weakness, and dry skin	If the imbalance is due to a loss of sodium, replace the sodium with appropriate fluids; if the imbalance is due to a gain of water (edema), expect to administer diuretics

B. Assessment
1. Clinical manifestations
   a. Common signs are related to shift of water into cells from vascular space and to sodium's role in nerve impulse transmission and muscle contraction
   b. Cardiovascular: tachycardia, hypotension (with decreased ECV), hypertension with bounding pulse (with increased ECV)
   c. Integument: pale, dry skin and dry mucous membranes (with decreased ECV), edema, "doughy" skin, and weight gain (with increased ECV)
   d. Renal: thirst (decreased ECV), renal failure (increased ECV)
   e. Neuromuscular: lethargy and weakness, headache, confusion, agitation, dizziness, seizures
   f. Gastrointestinal: vomiting, diarrhea, abdominal cramps
2. Diagnostic and laboratory findings
   a. Plasma levels and urinary levels
      1) Plasma level less than 135 mEq/L
      2) Change in urine sodium level reflects the deficit's cause; see Box 2-3 for procedure for collecting 24-hour urine sodium specimen
      3) Urine sodium levels >20 mEq/L correlate to renal etiology or SIADH
      4) Urine sodium levels <10 mEq/L correlate with edema etiology (CHF, cirrhosis, and nephrotic syndrome)
   b. Associated electrolyte and other levels
      1) Serum osmolality <270 mOsm/kg
      2) Serum chloride may be decreased
      3) Urine specific gravity (SG)<1.010 (except in SIADH)
      4) Decreased blood urea nitrogen (BUN), unless CHF is the cause, and hematocrit (Hct)
      5) An increase of 100 mg/dL in blood glucose will decrease serum sodium by 1.7–2.4 mEq/L
   c. Trending of results
      1) Identify primary cause of mechanism for sodium deficit
      2) Confirm compensatory response to sodium loss
      3) Determine client fluid balance status and response to treatment measures
3. Identification of risk factors
   a. Aging and gender variables
      1) Very young and older adult clients are more prone to sodium deficit
      2) There is an increased risk for development of acute hyponatremia in female clients and those with human immunodeficiency virus (HIV)
   b. Medications
      1) Obtain pertinent client history of medications that can alter sodium levels (refer again to Table 2-2 for sample medications that cause sodium deficit)
      2) Treatment measures that include hypotonic intravenous solutions (such as D_5W), hypotonic fluids, irrigations, and tap water enema (TWE) as part of therapeutic plan of care can lead to hyponatremia

Practice to Pass

The pathophysiological effects of hyponatremia are most evident in which areas of the body?

Box 2-3	• Obtain large urine collection container labeled with start and stop times.
	• Explain procedure to client and family to ensure all urine is placed in container.
Measurement of Urine Sodium (24-hour Specimen)	• Place container in refrigerator or on ice.
	• Instruct not to mix/contaminate specimen with bathroom tissue or feces.
	• Discard specimen voided at start time but save specimen voided at end time.

3) Clients undergoing operative procedures involving irrigations (such as endometrial ablation and transurethral resection of the prostate [TURP])may develop hyponatremia

c. Dietary

1) Prolonged NPO status

2) Overcorrection with nonelectrolyte solutions, causing free water accumulation

d. Medical disorders such as heart failure, cancer, or GI disorders

C. **Priority nursing concerns:** possible fluid volume excess, possible alterations in mental status and/or injury, possible interruption in skin integrity

D. **Therapeutic management:** treatment focuses on restoring normal levels, preventing complications, and treating underlying problems

1. Replacement therapies

a. Encourage inclusion of high-sodium foods in diet

b. Referral to a dietitian for assistance in meal planning to include adequate sources of dietary sodium (refer to Table 2-4 for sodium food sources)

c. If a client has hyponatremia with normal fluid volume (euvolemic), use water restriction and treat underlying cause to correct deficit

d. If a client has hyponatremia with hypovolemic volume, treat with normal saline (NS) or Lactated Ringer's (LR) solution to correct ECF deficit

e. If a client has hyponatremia with hypertonic dehydration, treat with fluid restriction and treat underlying cause to correct deficit

f. If a client requires irrigation (such as via nasogastric tube) as a part of therapy, use of appropriate solutions (isotonic saline) should prevent further fluid shifting and sodium deficit

g. A client with acute hyponatremia can be treated with 3% hypertonic saline (refer to healthcare provider prescription, pharmacy, and hospital protocols for rate of infusion) and loop diuretics to promote water excretion if indicated by clinical picture

h. Loop diuretics, sodium and fluid restrictions, and possibly dialysis may be used to treat fluid excess if clinical picture dictates

2. Continued monitoring of client

a. Monitor laboratory results

b. Keep accurate intake and output (I&O) records

c. Obtain daily weights

d. Perform neurologic assessment; monitor for central nervous system (CNS) changes, such as confusion, lethargy, and seizures, and maintain safe environment

e. Monitor and document routes of fluid loss

Practice to Pass

You are providing care to a client who is NPO and has intermittent nasogastric suctioning. What will you monitor for and why?

Table 2-4   Dietary Sources of Sodium

High-Sodium Foods	Low-Sodium Foods
Canned, processed, and pickled foods are *higher* in sodium content	Fresh foods are *lower* in sodium content
• Foods prepared in brine (e.g., pickles, olives, sauerkraut)	• Fresh meat and fish
• Salty or smoked meats (e.g., bologna, hot dogs, ham, lunch meats, bacon, sausage)	• "No added salt" snack items
• Salty or smoked fish (e.g., anchovies, herring, sardines, smoked salmon)	• Sodium-free spices and flavorings
• Salty snacks (e.g., potato chips, popcorn, nuts, crackers, pretzels)	• Soups made with fresh items
• Salty seasonings (e.g., seasoned salts, soy sauce, Worcestershire sauce, barbecue sauces)	• Fresh fruits and vegetables
• Processed cheeses	• Low-sodium canned products
• Canned and instant soups	
• Canned vegetables and fruits	

3. Restoration of balance
   a. Depending on acuity and severity of deficit, client may be either asymptomatic or symptomatic; correlate laboratory values with client's overall physical condition in order to maintain sodium and fluid balance
   b. If client's sodium deficit is acute and symptomatic, prompt management should be initiated
      1) Follow healthcare provider prescription, pharmacy, and hospital protocol for rate of infusion and length of therapy
      2) It is critical to raise sodium levels per established protocols as cerebral cell adaptation can cause further complications
      3) A target goal of 120–125 mEq/L should be aimed for, and sodium levels should be raised no more than 25 mEq/L in first 48 hours with a rate not to exceed 1–2 mEq/L/hr
   c. It is important to identify and treat underlying cause in order to prevent reoccurrence of deficit and restore sodium and fluid balance

E. **Client-centered nursing care**
   1. Monitor pertinent client assessment data for potential effects related to hyponatremia and for response to treatment
      a. Assess for confusion, changes in the level of consciousness, and seizures
      b. As clinical condition progresses, signs and symptoms may become more acute, ranging from anorexia, nausea, and lethargy in early phase to disorientation, agitation, focal neurologic deficits, coma, and seizures in advanced phase
   2. Protect client from injury and maintain a safe environment if client experiences neurologic changes due to hyponatremia
   3. Employ dietary interventions to promote normal sodium levels
      a. Encourage use of high-sodium foods in diet
      b. Give appropriate amounts of fluids in diet to prevent dehydration
      c. Avoid caffeinated beverages (such as coffee, tea, sodas)
   4. Provide replacement therapy as prescribed by healthcare provider, paying attention to baseline laboratory results, client's response, and therapeutic benefits
      a. Keep accurate fluid I&O records, looking at shift and 24-hour totals to determine fluid balance
      b. Depending on acuity and severity, hourly monitoring may be indicated
      c. Weigh client daily, at same time using same scale and in similar clothing
      d. A weight loss of >0.5 pounds in 24 hours is considered to be due to fluid loss

F. **Medication therapy**
   1. Oral replacement therapy
      a. Salt tablets can be used to correct sodium deficits
      b. Numerous medications contain sodium (refer again to Table 2-2 for medications that can affect sodium levels)
      c. Depending on the nature of volume status, diuretic therapy may either be restricted (such as no thiazide diuretics because they promote ADH activity) or used (loop diuretics) to promote fluid loss and regain sodium balance
   2. Parenteral replacement therapy
      a. LR or 0.9% sodium chloride (NS) can be used to treat hyponatremia with isotonic dehydration
      b. 3% or 5% hypertonic saline can be used to treat clients with a more severe deficit
   3. Dietary therapy
      a. Encourage foods high in sodium (see Table 2-4) and possibly table salt
      b. Judiciously use processed foods and foods containing preservatives as one way to add sodium to diet

G. Client education

1. Awareness of predisposing factors
   a. Older adult and very young clients are at risk for hyponatremia due to potential fluid volume disturbances
   b. Fluid restriction, if applicable
   c. Recognition of environmental conditions (heat and humidity) that may increase sodium and fluid loss, and use of appropriate oral replacement therapies to prevent further electrolyte depletion
   d. Daily weight
2. Dietary education: provide a list of high-sodium foods (see again Table 2-4) and collaborate with dietitian as indicated
3. Report early signs and symptoms of hyponatremia such as abdominal cramps, muscle weakness, and nausea
4. Teach clients and family members to report changes in mental status, especially if client already has contributory medical conditions such as cardiac, renal, and endocrine problems that might exacerbate hyponatremia

H. Evaluation

1. Serum sodium level returns to a normal range (135–145 mEq/L or mmol/L)
2. Client is free of injury and alert and oriented to time, place, and person
3. Client is free of any signs or symptoms of hyponatremia
4. Client is euvolemic
5. Vital signs are within normal limits

III. *HYPERNATREMIA*

A. Definition, etiology, and pathophysiology

1. Serum sodium level higher than 145 mEq/L
2. Cellular-level transport
   a. Sodium excess always exists in a **hyperosmolar** (osmotic pressure greater than normal plasma pressure) state
   b. Sodium excess can exist in hypovolemic, euvolemic, and hypervolemic states (see Table 2-5 for summary of this disorder)
   c. To restore equilibrium between ECF and ICF, water will shift from ICF to ECF, which results in cellular shrinkage/dehydration (refer back to Figure 2-1B)
    d. Cerebral cells shrink in response to high-sodium levels as osmotic pressure drives fluid out of cells, leading to a decreased brain volume
   e. High serum sodium levels lead to an increase in neurologic activity
   f. In response to high-sodium levels, thirst mechanism is stimulated
3. Predisposing clinical conditions
   a. Disturbances in water regulation such as decreased intake, increased insensible loss, or watery diarrhea
   b. Water loss due to fever, hyperventilation, diuretic therapy, hypertonic tube feedings, and burns
   c. Increased sodium intake (through dietary intake or infusion of sodium-containing fluids)
   d. Renal losses or disease/hormonal states such as Cushing syndrome (increased cortisol production) or **diabetes insipidus** or **DI** (a defect in ADH secretion causing sodium retention and increased secretion of a dilute urine) are prone to develop hypernatremia (refer to Box 2-4 for more information on DI)
   e. Near drowning in salt water (infrequent cause)

Table 2-5 | **Hypernatremia in Various Fluid Volume States**

	Description	Clinical Presentation	Treatment
Euvolemia	Decrease in water that leads to elevation of serum sodium levels Does not present with contracted volume unless there is a severe water loss	Increased fluid loss via skin or lungs (hyperventilation)	Free water replacement either orally or by fluid-hydrating solutions
Hypervolemia	Greater gain of sodium in relation to fluids that leads to elevation of serum sodium levels	Seen with administration of hypertonic saline solutions or $NaHCO_3$, in primary hyperaldosteronism or hypertonic dehydration	Remove sodium source, administer diuretics, and replace water
Hypovolemia	Greater loss of water than sodium, leading to elevation of serum sodium levels	Renal losses with osmotic diuresis, diabetes insipidus (DI), insensible loss with sweating and/or fever, GI losses with diarrhea More prone to develop in young and older adult clients	Normal saline to correct intra-vascular volume deficit, then hypotonic fluids can be used to restore sodium level

Note: All hypernatremic states are hyperosmolar.

B. **Assessment**
1. Clinical manifestations
   a. Common signs are related to water shift from cells (cellular dehydration) into vascular space and sodium's role in nerve impulse transmission and muscle contraction
   b. Cardiovascular: tachycardia, hypertension, decreased cardiac contractility

---

Box 2-4

Diabetes Insipidus (DI)

- DI is characterized by decreased secretion of ADH or failure to respond to ADH secretion due to malignancies, excessive water intake, medications (demeclocycline and lithium), and genetic defects.
- DI can be further classified as central (insufficient production) or nephrogenic (related to decreased renal sensitivity).
- Plasma osmolality is increased, urine osmolality and specific gravity are decreased; water deprivation test reveals inability to concentrate urine.
- Hypernatremia is present.
- Clients present with polyuria (increased dilute urine) and polydipsia (increased thirst).
- Treatment for central DI consists of desmopressin acetate nasal spray administration or, if critically ill, vasopressin IV.
- Treatment for nephrogenic DI consists of a low-salt diet and thiazide diuretics to increase sodium excretion, as well as fluid replacement.
- Assessing I&O is critical to clients with this disorder.
- Complications of treatment: therapy can lead to water intoxication so client must be closely monitored by looking at labs/diagnostics and performing frequent physical assessment.
- Continued monitoring of fluid status upon discharge is necessary for clients who experience this type of disorder to prevent further recurrences.
- Correction of underlying disorder and recognition of clients at risk in clinical setting will lead to better client outcomes.

    c. Integument: dry and sticky mucous membranes, rough dry tongue, flushed skin that has poor turgor and tenting

    d. Renal: thirst, increased urine output

    e. Neuromuscular: twitching, tremor and hyperreflexia, agitation, hallucinations, CNS irritability, seizures, coma; worsening hypernatremia can result in hyporeflexia, paralysis, and coma

    f. Gastrointestinal: watery diarrhea, nausea, thirst

    g. Clients whose levels rise slowly may be asymptomatic for some time

2. Diagnostic and laboratory findings

    a. Plasma levels and urinary levels

      1) Plasma levels greater than 145 mEq/L

      2) May see increased urine output

    b. Associated electrolyte and other levels

      1) Chloride may be elevated

      2) Serum osmolality greater than 290 mOsm/kg

      3) Urine SG greater than 1.015 unless diabetes insipidus is present, which leads to dilute urine with SG of less than 1.005

      4) Increased BUN and Hct

    c. Trending of results

      1) Identify primary cause of sodium excess

      2) Confirm compensatory response to sodium excess

      3) Determine client fluid balance status and response to treatment measures

3. Identification of risk factors

    a. Age-related risk factors (see also Table 2-6)

      1) Very young clients can be at risk for fluid deprivation due to poor nutritional care or having an activity level that overlooks hydration (so busy playing that they don't eat or drink enough)

      2) Older adult clients are at risk due to decreased thirst mechanism and renal functioning

      3) Infant clients can be placed at risk due to improper reconstitution, usage, and storage of prepared formula

Table 2-6   **Lifespan Considerations for Health Maintenance: Hypernatremia**

Lifespan Considerations	Fluids	Electrolytes	Acid–Base Balance
Infants	Breastfeeding (colostrum); formula; whole milk	Sodium (Na^+) is essential for fluid balance, nerve and muscle function	Acid–base imbalance in infants is primarily due to respiratory disorders related to respiratory insufficiency
Children	Increase water intake; do not give undiluted formula concentrate or evaporated milk due to high-sodium content; popsicles, both hypotonic and isotonic fluids	Monitor for diarrhea, vomiting, and excessive sweating without fluid replacement	Isotonic fluids may be prescribed first to replenish the volume, followed by hypotonic fluid to correct the osmolality
Adults	Hypotonic and isotonic fluids; increase water intake	Sodium is the most abundant electrolyte in the ECF; increased risk: heart failure, tuberculosis, cirrhosis, head injury, surgical clients	Central nervous system is especially affected, resulting in signs of neurologic impairment (e.g., restlessness, weakness, disorientation, delusion, and hallucinations)

    b. Medications

        1) Obtain complete medication history because some medications have hidden sodium that client may not be aware of (refer again to Table 2-2 for sample medications that can affect sodium levels); high-sodium OTC medications such as Alka-Seltzer and cough and cold products may contribute to increased sodium levels

        2) Treatment measures that include use of sodium, such as sodium bicarbonate administration during a code, use of hypertonic saline solutions, and saline-induced abortions, can contribute to increased sodium levels

        3) Cortisone therapy and loop diuretics can contribute to increased sodium levels

    c. Dietary: high levels of sodium-containing foods or salt as a flavoring agent

C. Priority nursing concerns: possible fluid volume deficit, possible injury, possible altered oral mucous membranes

D. Therapeutic management: treatment focuses on restoring normal levels, preventing complications, and treating underlying problems

  1. Decrease sodium intake

    a. Restrict dietary sodium; restriction varies depending on severity of clinical condition and may be set at 2 grams, 1 gram, or 500 mg/day

    b. Refer client to a dietitian to evaluate dietary intake for hidden sodium sources

  2. Promote sodium excretion

    a. If client has hypernatremia with normal fluid volume (euvolemic), use water replacement and treat underlying cause to promote sodium loss

    b. If client has hypernatremia with hypovolemia, treat with NS initially to correct intravascular deficit

    c. If client has hypernatremia with hypervolemia, remove source of sodium excess, administer diuretics, and replace water as needed

  3. Continued monitoring of client

    a. Monitor laboratory results

    b. Keep accurate I&O records, assessing for trends

    c. Obtain daily weights at the same time using same equipment and similar clothing in order to accurately trend results

    d. Assess CNS for neurologic changes such as agitation, hallucinations, and seizures, and maintain a safe environment

  4. Restoration of balance

    a. With hypernatremia, it is important to gradually reduce serum sodium levels to normal because cerebral cells are both adaptive and sensitive to changes in sodium levels

    b. Typical protocol with chronic hypernatremia is to correct 50% of calculated water deficit in first 12–24 hours with remainder corrected in 1–2 days; follow healthcare provider prescription and pharmacy and hospital protocols when correcting hypernatremia in clinical setting

    c. Continue to monitor volume status of client before and during attempts to restore sodium balance in order to prevent further complications

    d. If client has hypernatremia because of solute excess, then use of diuretics with water replacement may be warranted

    e. It is important to identify and treat underlying cause in order to restore sodium and fluid balance and prevent recurrence of excess

E. Client-centered nursing care

  1. Monitor pertinent client assessment data for potential effects related to hypernatremia and for response to treatment

    a. Serum sodium levels and plasma osmolality

    b. Urine sodium levels and urine osmolality

! c. Monitor neurologic status closely as client is likely to have CNS irritability, possibly leading to seizures

! 2. Maintain safe environment as a result of CNS irritability and risk of seizure activity; initiate seizure precautions

3. Dietary interventions to decrease sodium levels
   a. Place client on a salt-restricted diet (refer again to Table 2-4 for high- and low-sodium foods and to Box 2-5 for tips to aid client adherence)
   b. Refer client to a dietitian as needed to assist with dietary measures

4. Provide therapy as prescribed by healthcare provider, paying attention to baseline labs, client's response, and therapeutic benefits

5. Assess I&O
   a. Keep accurate fluid I&O records looking at shift and 24-hour totals to determine fluid balance
   b. Depending on acuity and severity, hourly monitoring may be indicated
   c. Weigh client on daily basis using the same equipment and similar clothing
   d. Weight gain can be a consequence of fluid retention from hypernatremia, which could lead to further clinical compromise

F. Medication therapy
1. Diuretic therapy
   a. Loop diuretics can be used to treat sodium excess
   b. Thiazide diuretics can be used in the treatment of diabetes insipidus
2. Parenteral administration of fluids
   a. NS to correct intravascular volume deficit
   b. D_5W solution can be used once volume deficit has been restored

G. Client education
1. Awareness of predisposing factors
   a. Older adult clients are also at risk for hypernatremia due to limited mobility, multiple medication profile, and possible restricted access to fluids
   b. Teach clients potential signs and symptoms of hypernatremia and have them report problems to their healthcare provider
2. Dietary education (refer again to Box 2-5)
   a. Teach clients about daily dietary sodium requirement along with proper fluid management; daily intake for a majority of individuals exceeds needed RDA
   b. Teach clients about sodium content of foods and sources of hidden sodium as previously described

Practice to Pass

In caring for a client with hypernatremia, what should the nurse do to help ensure client safety?

Box 2-5	The following client actions should be taken when following a sodium-restricted diet:
Client Tips for Adhering to Sodium-Restricted Diet	• Note sodium restriction prescribed by healthcare provider.
	• Do not routinely add salt to foods prior to tasting.
	• Limit or avoid use of bottled or canned sauce products, as they are usually higher in sodium than homemade preparations.
	• Use lemon, pure herbs, seasonings, and wine in cooking preparation, as many "seasoned" products and cooking wine contain sodium.
	• When eating outside the home at restaurants, have food items prepared without salt.
	• Eat freshly prepared bakery products; commercially prepared and frozen products contain more sodium due to processing and use of preservative agents.
	• Be aware that artificial sweeteners used in soft drinks and other products can contain additional sodium. Limit your intake of such products.
	• There is a wide range of "low-sodium" and "sodium-free" products available. Learn to read and interpret nutrition labels to make wise food selections.

   c. Teach client to read all labels for sodium content prior to ingestion
   d. Explain that salt substitutes are useful but should be avoided by clients with impaired renal function because they contain potassium
H. Evaluation
   1. Serum sodium level returns to normal range (135–145 mEq/L or mmol/L)
   2. Client is free of any signs or symptoms of hypernatremia
   3. Client is alert and oriented to time, place, and person and free of injury
   4. Client is euvolemic
   5. Vital signs are within normal limits

IV. OVERVIEW OF CHLORIDE REGULATION

   A. Chloride balance and function: major extracellular anion (average level 104 mEq/L) that also exists in a lesser concentration in cells (average 4 mEq/L); it is closely associated with serum sodium levels and affects acid–base balance
   1. Normal chloride levels
   a. See Table 2-7 for normal serum chloride levels
   b. Normal urinary chloride ranges from 110 to 254 mEq/24 hours in adults and varies in children depending on age
   c. Chloride sweat levels: 10–70 mEq/L in adults and 5–45 mEq/L in children
   2. Functions in body
   a. Chloride is a **halogen** (nonionized form of a halide) that combines with alkali metals to form salts in body, such as sodium chloride or potassium chloride
   b. Chloride circulates primarily with sodium and water and aids cellular integrity by maintaining a balance between intracellular and extracellular fluids; it also helps to control osmotic pressure
   c. Chloride is a passive transport companion for sodium and potassium in body, although active transport mechanisms may also be involved
   d. Chloride is essential for maintaining acid–base and electrolyte balance and is an enzyme activator; it serves as a buffer in oxygen and carbon dioxide exchange in red blood cells
   e. When joined with hydrogen (a cation), chloride anions play an important role in digestion by forming hydrochloric acid (HCl) in stomach; chloride regulates pH of stomach acid and aids protein digestion
   f. In conjunction with calcium and magnesium, chloride helps to maintain nerve transmission and normal muscle contraction and relaxation
   g. Kidneys eliminate or retain chloride mainly as sodium chloride to regulate acid–base levels
   h. Chloride may also assist liver in clearing waste products
   i. Chloride is also found in significant amounts in sweat
   3. System interactions
   a. There is a correlation between chloride levels and serum osmolality and sodium levels

Table 2-7 **Normal Serum Chloride Levels**	
Age	**Normal Range**
Adult	95–108 mEq/L
Child	98–105 mEq/L
Newborn	96–106 mEq/L

1) When serum osmolality is increased to >295 mOsm/kg, there are a greater number of sodium and chloride ions in proportion to body water, leading to elevated serum chloride levels
2) When serum osmolality is decreased to <280 mOsm/kg, there are relatively fewer sodium and chloride ions in proportion to body water, leading to decreased serum chloride levels
3) Chloride is frequently retained when sodium is retained; sodium retention leads to water retention

    b. Kidneys excrete chloride anions and bicarbonate, and sodium reabsorbs either chloride or bicarbonate to maintain acid–base balance

4. See Table 2-8 for lifespan factors affecting chloride balance

B. Sources of chloride

    1. Cellular level

        a. Chloride passively diffuses from renal glomeruli into renal tubules along with other electrolytes; reabsorption of chloride into renal capillaries is usually proportional to active reabsorption of sodium

        b. Chloride regulation in kidney affects acid–base balance in body

        c. Chloride is absorbed from small intestine and is primarily found in extracellular fluid

        d. It is secreted in gastric juice as hydrochloric acid

    2. Dietary level

        a. Chloride is obtained primarily from salt, such as standard table salt or sea salt

        b. Foods with high chloride levels include canned vegetables, dates, bananas, cheese, spinach, milk, eggs, celery, crabs, fish, olives, and rye (refer to Table 2-9 for a list of foods high in chloride)

Table 2-8	Lifespan Considerations for Health Maintenance: Chloride Balance	
Lifespan Considerations	**Common Risk Factors for Imbalances**	**Nursing Implications**
Infants	*Hypochloremia* Severe diarrhea, tube-feedings, failure to thrive, burns	Prolonged diarrhea/vomiting can quickly lead to dehydration and arrhythmias Electrolyte solution replacements are needed
	Hyperchloremia Renal tubular acidosis, ileal loops, dehydration	Administer hypotonic IV solutions as prescribed
Children	*Hypochloremia* Diarrhea, poor dietary intake, cystic fibrosis, excessive sweating/fever, gastroenteritis, congenital chloride-losing diarrhea, burns	Close assessment for manifestations of electrolyte imbalance Electrolyte solution replacements are needed
	Hyperchloremia Renal failure, loss of pancreatic secretions, renal compromise, prolonged diarrhea	Administer hypotonic IV solutions or diuretics as prescribed; dialysis is needed for renal failure
Adults	*Hypochloremia* Increased use of diuretics, heart failure, poor dietary intake, laxative abuse, renal tubular acidosis, Addison disease, SIADH, thiazide diuretics	Educate client on manifestations of low chloride and sources of chloride as well as sodium supplements
	Hyperchloremia Hyperparathyroidism, metabolic acidosis, hypernatremia, ureteral colonic anastomosis, bromide intoxication, acetazolamide, boric acid, ammonium chloride	Monitor for manifestations of hyperchloremia Provide hypotonic IV solutions as prescribed Educate client on proper use of medications

Table 2-9	Foods High in Chloride
Food Group	**Examples**
Fruits	Dates and bananas only
Dairy products	Cheese, milk
Vegetables	Canned vegetables and soup, spinach, celery, olives, and rye
Meat, fish, and poultry	Eggs, crabs, fish, turkey

     c. Processed foods are high in chloride content

     d. Chloride is a constituent part of sodium chloride as well as other dietary salts

     e. There is no RDA for chloride, but there is an adult estimated minimum requirement of 750 mg/day

V. *HYPOCHLOREMIA*

  A. Definition, etiology, and pathophysiology

    1. A serum chloride level below 95 mEq/L

    2. Cellular level

      a. Decreases in chloride usually accompany decreases in sodium and potassium

      b. A reduction in hydrochloric acid decreases chloride

      c. Chloride is excreted with cations during massive diuresis and when bicarbonate level is elevated

      d. When serum level falls, urinary chloride excretion is decreased to promote retention

    3. Predisposing clinical conditions (see Table 2-10)

      a. Fluid and electrolyte imbalances

        1) Hyponatremia

        2) Metabolic alkalosis (from ingestion of alkaline substances such as antacids or from elevated bicarbonate concentration in certain disease processes—can be chloride responsive or chloride resistant depending on urinary chloride levels)

        3) Hypokalemia

        4) Prolonged administration of D_5W IV therapy

Table 2-10	Chloride Imbalances with Abnormal Values and Etiologies	
Etiology	**Hypochloremia (serum level <95 mEq/L adults)**	**Hyperchloremia (serum level >108 mEq/L adults)**
Metabolic imbalance	Metabolic alkalosis	Metabolic acidosis
Gastrointestinal disorders and dietary changes	GI suctioning, vomiting, diarrhea, GI surgery, hypokalemia, excessive ingestion of alkaline substances	Increased retention or intake, hyperkalemia, hypernatremia, severe vomiting, salicylate intoxication, stomach cancer, dehydration
Renal disorders	Advanced renal disorders, diuretics	Reduced glomerular filtration, renal failure
Hormonal influences	SIADH, Addison disease, diabetic ketoacidosis	Excess adrenocortical hormone production (Cushing syndrome), IV or oral cortisone therapy
Altered cellular function	Hypervolemic CHF and cirrhosis	
Skin/environmental changes	Burns, fever, large skin wounds, profuse perspiration	
Head injury		Head trauma

Table 2-11	Pharmacological Agents Affecting Chloride Balance

Decrease Serum Chloride Levels	Increase Serum Chloride Levels
Aldosterone	Acetazolamide
Amiloride	Ammonium chloride
Bumetanide	Boric acid
Corticotropin	Chlorothiazide
Dextrose infusion (prolonged)	Cyclosporine
Furosemide	Glucocorticoids
Mercurial diuretics	Phenylbutazone
Prednisolone	Sodium bromide
Sodium bicarbonate	0.9% Sodium chloride solution
Thiazide diuretics	3% Sodium chloride solution
	Triamterene

   b. Chronic respiratory acidosis (clients with chronic lung disease have high pCO_2 levels with chronic elevation of bicarbonate levels, which results in a decreased serum chloride)
   c. Diabetic acidosis because of increased anion gap
   d. Acute infections, although the mechanism by which they lower serum chloride level is unclear
   e. Vomiting (loss of HCl), GI suctioning, perspiration, diarrhea, and presence of fistulas, bulimia, and tap water enemas
   f. Metabolic stress conditions, such as severe burns, fever, and heat and exhaustion states
   g. Disease states such as Addison disease, anorexia, salt-wasting renal nephropathy, syndrome of inappropriate antidiuretic hormone (SIADH), and hypervolemic states such as congestive heart failure (CHF) and cirrhosis
   h. Various medications that promote electrolyte loss, have diuretic activity, or promote alkalosis (see Table 2-11 for medications that contribute to hypochloremia)
   i. Low sodium diet, anorexia nervosa
B. **Assessment**
   1. Clinical manifestations (refer to Table 2-12)
      a. Hyperexcitability of nerves and muscles leads to tremors and twitching
      b. Respiratory abnormalities include slow and shallow breathing
      c. Cardiac abnormalities include hypotension when there are severe chloride and ECF losses

Table 2-12	Clinical Manifestations of Chloride Imbalances	

System Alteration	Hypochloremia	Hyperchloremia
Respiratory	Slow and shallow respirations (signs of metabolic alkalosis due to bicarbonate retention)	Deep rapid respirations (signs of metabolic acidosis due to loss of bicarbonate)
Cardiac	Hypotension with severe chloride and extracellular fluid loss	
Neurologic	Muscle tremors and twitching	Weakness, lethargy, stupor, unconsciousness
Serum laboratory value	<95 mEq/L	>108 mEq/L

> **d.** Alterations in serum chloride levels are seldom a primary problem; there are usually associated electrolyte imbalances (such as hyponatremia or hypokalemia) and acid–base disturbances such as metabolic alkalosis and hypokalemic alkalosis
>
> **e.** Decreased levels are associated with diarrhea, emphysema, gastric suction, fluid volume excess states (such as CHF, hyponatremia, and SIADH), pyloric obstruction, malabsorption syndrome, diabetes with ketoacidosis, excess of mineralocorticoids, and salt-wasting renal disease
>
> **f.** Decreased chloride sweat levels are seen in hypoaldosteronism, sodium depletion, and the administration of mineralocorticoids

2. Diagnostic and laboratory findings
   a. Serum chloride level is <95 mEq/L
   b. Panic (critical) value for serum chloride level is <80 mEq/L
   c. Urinary chloride concentration varies with salt intake and urine volume and is helpful when discriminating between chloride-responsive (<10 mEq/L) and chloride-resistant (>10 mEq/L) metabolic alkalosis disturbances
   d. ABG results and serum sodium and potassium levels may provide information needed to manage clients with chloride deficit
   e. Trending of results
      1) Helpful in differentiating between types of metabolic alkalosis
      2) Hypochloremia should be considered in relation to presenting clinical manifestations or other electrolyte imbalances, such as hyponatremia or hypokalemia
3. Identification of risk factors: dietary insufficiency or previously identified coexisting medical conditions that lead to or exacerbate hypochloremia

C. Priority nursing concerns
   1. Insufficient nutritional intake if there is decreased chloride intake or increased loss
   2. Possible related fluid overload (hemodilution)
   3. Sensory-perceptual (neurologic) changes
   4. Risk for client injury if concurrent muscle weakness, general weakness, or lethargy

D. Therapeutic management
   1. Replacement therapies
      a. If chloride levels are slightly low and client can tolerate oral intake, then administer oral salt tablets or increase chloride dietary sources
      b. Provide IV infusion containing chloride if levels are critical or if client is unable to tolerate oral administration
   2. Continued monitoring of client
      a. Serum and urinary chloride levels
      b. I&O, because excess water administration can cause dilutional hypochloremia and hyponatremia
      c. Blood pressure, which can decrease if hypochloremia is due to ECF volume loss
      d. ABG results if client's clinical presentation or underlying medical history suggests accompanying acid–base imbalance
   3. Restoration of balance
      a. Promote dietary changes to increase chloride intake
      b. Administer chloride supplements or parenteral replacement as prescribed
      c. Continue to assess those clients at risk
      d. Monitor the client with underlying or contributory disease processes and/or medication therapy that would lead to chloride deficiencies

E. Client-centered nursing care
   1. Identify risk factors specific to development of chloride loss, such as dietary factors, GI losses, renal losses, altered hormone secretion, altered cellular states, and metabolic alkalosis

Practice to Pass

A client is being treated for metabolic alkalosis and is at risk for altered serum chloride level, which can occur concurrently with this condition. Would you expect the serum chloride level to be increased or decreased? Why?

2. Monitor client during therapy, looking at pertinent lab values and clinical manifestations
3. Monitor vital signs (VS) and I&O parameters
4. Maintain safety precautions by keeping bedrails up and assisting client with ambulation if client presents with muscle tremors and/or decreased blood pressure

F. Medication therapy

1. Oral replacement therapy: use salt tablets or potassium chloride salts to raise serum chloride level because chloride is found in these products or in others as an additive/buffer
2. Parenteral replacement therapy
   a. Chloride can be given parenterally as a constituent part of a medication such as potassium chloride or sodium chloride
   b. Monitoring of IV solutions containing chloride follows same principles as monitoring IV therapy in general
3. Dietary therapy: include foods that are high in chloride, such as salt, processed foods, canned vegetables, dates, bananas, cheese, spinach, milk, eggs, celery, crabs, fish, olives, and rye (refer back to Table 2-9)

G. Client education

1. Teach awareness of predisposing factors, including contributory conditions
   a. Endocrine states that result in adrenocortical insufficiency or primary aldosteronism
   b. Acid–base imbalances that result in metabolic acidosis (high anion gap), such as diabetic ketoacidosis, Addison disease, and nephritis
   c. Acid–base imbalances that result in metabolic alkalosis, such as pyloric obstruction, or as compensation for chronic respiratory acidosis
   d. Use of medications that would likely increase chloride loss (refer back to Table 2-11)
2. Dietary education
   a. Review foods that are high in chloride
   b. Advise client that electrolyte replacement as well as fluid replacement is important during exercise leading to prolonged perspiration
   c. Collaborate with dietitian as needed

H. Evaluation

1. Chloride serum levels and other pertinent electrolyte levels return to normal baseline
2. Acid–base balance returns to normal baseline
3. Clinical manifestations resolve

VI. HYPERCHLOREMIA

A. Definition, etiology, and pathophysiology

1. A serum chloride level above 108 mEq/L
2. Cellular level
   a. Cellular chloride shifts are seen in response to acid–base changes and volume disturbances
   b. Increases in serum chloride are seen in conjunction with other electrolyte imbalances and are usually assessed with sodium, potassium, water, and CO_2 levels
3. Predisposing clinical conditions (refer again to Table 2-10)
   a. Fluid and electrolyte imbalances
      1) Hypernatremia
      2) Metabolic acidosis (loss of sodium bicarbonate because of prolonged diarrhea), hyperchloremic metabolic acidosis (renal disease that causes decreased excretion of hydrogen ions and prevents reabsorption of bicarbonate), or respiratory alkalosis (hyperventilation)
   b. Ingestion or administration of drugs that promote chloride retention, such as IV saline, certain diuretics, salicylate intoxication, and corticosteroids (refer back to Table 2-11)

Practice to Pass

A client is diagnosed with hypochloremia. How would you explain the disorder? What strategies can be used to correct the problem?

    c. Fluid volume losses that result in dehydration (hemoconcentration)

    d. Endocrine disturbances that result in diabetes insipidus (DI) and certain cases of hyperparathyroidism (seen in association with hypercalcemia)

    e. Renal changes that manifest as renal tubular acidosis or acute kidney injury

B. Assessment

  1. Clinical manifestations (refer again to Table 2-12)

    a. Neuromuscular symptoms include weakness and lethargy and can progress to significant CNS damage

    b. Respiratory abnormalities include deep, rapid breathing that can lead to unconsciousness (compensation for acidotic state due to loss of bicarbonate)

    c. Cardiac abnormalities include risk of dysrhythmias due to retained chloride and accompanying acid–base disturbances

    d. Fluid volume disturbances can lead to increased chloride levels, including dehydration, retention of salt and water due to drug administration, and a greater sodium loss than chloride loss, leading to imbalance

    e. Presence of disease states such as DI, certain types of hyperparathyroidism, and renal tubular diseases result in hydrogen ion retention and decreased reabsorption of bicarbonate

    f. Increased chloride sweat levels are seen in DI, hypothyroidism, malnutrition, acute kidney injury, and certain genetic disorders such as cystic fibrosis and glucose-6-phosphate-dehydrogenase (G6PD) deficiency

  2. Diagnostic and laboratory findings

    a. Serum chloride level above 108 mEq/L; panic value is >115 mEq/L

    b. Urine chloride level >250 mEq/L in 24 hours is significant and is associated with sodium and fluid imbalances

    c. In dehydration states, serum chloride levels are increased due to hemoconcentration

    d. Increased chloride sweat levels are seen in many disease states and can be used as a diagnostic tool in the workup for cystic fibrosis

    e. Associated electrolyte imbalances that usually occur with elevated chloride levels are elevated potassium and sodium levels and decreased bicarbonate levels

    f. Trending of results

      1) Monitor acid–base values and trend results by examining anion gap

      2) Hyperchloremic acidosis is associated with a normal anion gap

      3) Because there can be artifact disturbances in acid–base imbalances resulting in falsely elevated chloride levels, trend results and evaluate the client using complete assessment parameters

C. Priority nursing concerns

  1. Changes in respiratory pattern such as tachypnea

  2. Possible risk for skin breakdown in presence of dehydration

  3. Possible risk for client injury in presence of weakness and lethargy

D. Therapeutic management

  1. Decrease chloride intake; withdraw all chloride-containing agents used as treatment measures

  2. Promote chloride excretion by administering diuretics

  3. Continue monitoring client, including acid–base, respiratory, and cardiac status

  4. Restoration of balance

    a. Administer appropriate IV therapy to restore fluid and electrolyte balance

    b. Correct dehydration states with oral and parenteral fluids as needed

    c. Promote dietary changes to decrease chloride intake

    d. Increase water intake

    e. Continue to assess clients at risk because of underlying or contributory disease and implement appropriate therapies to decrease serum chloride levels

Practice to Pass

A client is taking both furosemide for treatment of hypertension and a steroid methylprednisolone dose pack for an allergic reaction. Which of these medications would intensify hyperchloremia?

Practice to Pass

A client with hyperchloremia should be monitored for respiratory abnormalities. Which symptoms should the nurse assess for?

   E. **Client-centered nursing care**
      1. Identify risk factors for chloride excess, such as dietary factors, specific disease states, medical therapies, and acidotic states
      2. Monitor client during therapy, trending pertinent laboratory test results and response to treatment
      3. Monitor VS and I&O parameters
      4. Promote client safety, especially fall prevention measures, because of possible lethargy and weakness
   F. **Medication therapy**
      1. Parenteral administration
         a. Hypotonic solutions such as 0.45% NaCl or D_5W to restore balance
         b. IV diuretics may be prescribed to restore acid–base disturbances
      2. Additional drug therapies may be indicated based on underlying clinical conditions and presence of contributory disease
   G. **Client education**
      1. Awareness of predisposing factors
         a. Educate client to avoid medications and supplements containing chloride
         b. If client is experiencing other electrolyte imbalances (high sodium, high potassium), have a high index of suspicion for possible development of hyperchloremia
      2. Dietary education
         a. Avoid foods that are high in chloride and restrict use of processed foods (high in both sodium and chloride content)
         b. Maintain adequate hydration
         c. Collaborate with dietitian as needed
   H. **Evaluation**
      1. Serum chloride level and other pertinent electrolyte levels return to normal baseline
      2. Client can identify restricted foods, medications, and therapies that would elevate serum chloride
      3. Underlying disease states and contributory clinical conditions are corrected (assist in returning chloride levels to normal)
      4. Resolution of symptoms associated with hyperchloremia

Case Study

A 45-year-old construction company owner was brought from work to the emergency department reporting dizziness, nausea, weakness, abdominal cramps, and headache. During the admission assessment, the following information was obtained:

- *Onset of symptoms occurred 3 days ago but were mild until today when client stated that he "almost fell off a building at work."*
- *Previously diagnosed with hypertension (HTN) 6 weeks ago.*
- *Has been following a low-sodium diet and has been taking hydrochlorothiazide as directed since being diagnosed 6 weeks ago.*

1. What does the initial data provided by the client suggest?
2. What questions will you ask of the client prior to performing your physical examination?
3. What data do you expect your physical assessment to reveal?
4. What do you expect the laboratory tests to reveal?
5. What discharge teaching would be important to perform?

For suggested responses, see pages 190–191.

POSTTEST

1 When assessing a client with diabetes insipidus (DI), the nurse expects to find which clinical manifestations?

1. Nausea and vomiting
2. Polyuria and polydipsia
3. Dysuria and urgency
4. Confusion and disorientation

2 A client is receiving treatment for hypernatremia. The nurse should assess this client for signs and symptoms of which complication of therapy?

1. Cellular dehydration
2. Cerebral edema
3. Red blood cell (RBC) destruction
4. Renal shutdown

3 A client is semiconscious and restless and exhibits tremors and muscle weakness. Physical examination reveals a dry, swollen tongue and a body temperature of 37.7°C (99.8°F). The nurse anticipates that the client is most likely to have which serum sodium value?

1. 120 mEq/L
2. 132 mEq/L
3. 142 mEq/L
4. 155 mEq/L

4 When a client is admitted with a chloride level of 80 mEq/L, the nurse anticipates administration of which intravenous solution?

1. 5% dextrose and water
2. 0.9% sodium chloride
3. 0.45% sodium chloride with 20 mEq of potassium
4. 3% sodium chloride with 10 mEq of potassium

5 When caring for an adult client diagnosed with hyponatremia, the nurse plans to restrict which item during client intake?

1. Water
2. Sodium
3. Potassium
4. Chloride

6 Which manifestations should the nurse assess for when developing a plan of care for a client with hypernatremia? Select all that apply.

1. Restlessness
2. Dry mucous membranes
3. Subnormal temperature
4. Report of thirst
5. Weight gain

7 The nurse is providing care to a client with syndrome of inappropriate antidiuretic hormone (SIADH). What should the nurse explain to the unlicensed assistant about water intake?

1. It should be encouraged.
2. It should be restricted.
3. It is given according to the client's preference.
4. It is given via intravenous fluids only.

8 A client with a diagnosis of bipolar disorder has been drinking copious amounts of water and voiding frequently. The client is experiencing a bounding pulse and confusion and is reporting a headache. The nurse checks laboratory test results for which anticipated alteration?

1. Decreased platelet count
2. Decreased sodium level
3. Increased serum osmolality
4. Increased urine specific gravity

9 A client with a feeding tube has been experiencing severe watery diarrhea. The client is lethargic with decreased skin turgor, a pulse rate of 110, and hyperactive reflexes. The nurse would include which interventions on the client's plan of care? Select all that apply.

1. Monitor and record intake, output, and daily weights.
2. Administer salt tablets.
3. Withhold tube feedings until diarrhea subsides.
4. Avoid adding additional water before and after tube feedings.
5. Initiate seizure precautions.

10 The nurse assigned to a client with hyponatremia would conclude that which client factors may have contributed to this electrolyte imbalance? Select all that apply.

1. Osmotic diuretic therapy
2. Fever
3. Fluid retention
4. Excessive hypertonic intravenous infusion
5. Heart failure

➤ *See pages 58–59 for Answers and Rationales.*

ANSWERS & RATIONALES

Pretest

1 **Answer: 3, 4 Rationale:** The combination of high fever and severe dehydration leads to insensible water loss (a loss of pure water that does not contain electrolytes). Excessive insensible water loss results in a hypertonic dehydration that leads to a state of hypernatremia and hyperchloremia. Calcium levels usually decrease in the presence of dehydration and fever. Phosphate levels usually increase in the presence of dehydration and fever. Potassium levels can usually remain normal in the serum and are increased in the urine. **Cognitive Level:** Applying **Client Need:** Physiological Adaptation **Integrated Process:** Nursing Process: Assessment **Content Area:** Child Health **Strategy:** The critical words in this question are *imbalance*, *high fever*, and *severe dehydration*. Systematically eliminate options containing an imbalance not associated with water losses and dehydration. **Reference:** LeMone, P., Burke, K., Bauldoff, G., & Gubrud, P. (2015). *Medical surgical nursing: Clinical reasoning in patient care* (6th ed.). New York, NY: Pearson, pp. 195–196.

2 **Answer: 1 Rationale:** The use of corticosteroids can lead to the development of hypernatremia because they cause sodium to be retained and potassium to be excreted. The older adult client who drinks eight glasses of water each day is within a normal range of fluid intake and is not at risk for developing sodium imbalances. The diabetic client whose blood glucose is within normal range is not at risk for developing sodium imbalances. The teenager who is using Gatorade as an oral replacement therapy to compensate for fluid and electrolyte loss during exercise is not at risk for developing sodium imbalances. **Cognitive Level:** Analyzing **Client Need:** Physiological Adaptation **Integrated Process:** Nursing Process: Assessment **Content Area:** Adult Health **Strategy:** The critical word

most indicates all or some of the options are correct, but one will have a greater influence on creating the imbalance. Eliminate one option because it is not an abnormal amount of water to consume. Eliminate another as it is not associated with sodium, and a third because the client is young and better able to accommodate an imbalance. **Reference:** LeMone, P., Burke, K., Bauldoff, G., & Gubrud, P. (2015). *Medical surgical nursing: Clinical reasoning in patient care* (6th ed.). New York, NY: Pearson, pp. 195–196.

3 **Answer: 1 Rationale:** The thirst mechanism is decreased in older adults and would normally serve as a compensatory mechanism to provide water intake. Aldosterone production would be decreased in the presence of hypernatremia. Muscle mass may be reduced in older adults but the decreased thirst poses a greater risk. ADH is still produced. **Cognitive Level:** Analyzing **Client Need:** Reduction of Risk Potential **Integrated Process:** Nursing Process: Assessment **Content Area:** Adult Health **Strategy:** Critical items to note include an older adult client, hypernatremia, and risk for dehydration. Knowledge of compensatory mechanisms of fluid balance is required to answer this question. **Reference:** LeMone, P., Burke, K., Bauldoff, G., & Gubrud, P. (2015). *Medical surgical nursing: Clinical reasoning in patient care* (6th ed.). New York, NY: Pearson, pp. 195–196.

4 **Answer: 3 Rationale:** Clients with hypernatremia (normal 135–145 mEq/L or mmol/L) should be assessed for potential development of neurological complications such as seizures. Blankets are not needed because temperature is often elevated with hypernatremia. Malaise and nausea are symptoms of hyponatremia. Clients with hypernatremia have an increased need for fluids, not a decreased need. **Cognitive Level:** Analyzing **Client Need:** Reduction of Risk Potential **Integrated Process:** Nursing Process: Implementation **Content Area:** Adult Health

Strategy: The core concept of the question is knowledge of interventions that are necessary when a client has hypernatremia. Recall high sodium levels cause temperature elevations to eliminate one option, and eliminate another because fluids need to be encouraged. Remember that seizures are a risk with high sodium levels in order to choose correctly between the remaining two options. **Reference:** LeMone, P., Burke, K., Bauldoff, G., & Gubrud, P. (2015). *Medical surgical nursing: Clinical reasoning in patient care* (6th ed.). New York, NY: Pearson, pp. 195–196.

5 **Answer: 1, 2, 3, 4 Rationale:** Processed foods and some baking products contain sodium. Clients need to be taught to look for products containing sodium as part of the ingredient. Monosodium glutamate has the word *sodium* as part of its name. Many over-the-counter cough, cold, and flu remedies contain sodium. Canned goods often contain sodium and these food labels should be read carefully. Salad oil is typically low in sodium and is a good diet option. **Cognitive Level:** Applying **Client Need:** Health Promotion and Maintenance **Integrated Process:** Teaching and Learning **Content Area:** Adult Health **Strategy:** Recall knowledge of foods or products containing sodium. The wording of the question indicates that more than one option is correct. **Reference:** LeMone, P., Burke, K., Bauldoff, G., & Gubrud, P. (2015). *Medical surgical nursing: Clinical reasoning in patient care* (6th ed.). New York, NY: Pearson, pp. 195–196.

6 **Answer: 1 Rationale:** As sodium levels decrease, fluid shifts in the brain can lead to cerebral edema and seizures. Clients should be assessed for headaches, lethargy, decreased responsiveness, and seizure activity. Hyponatremia will also cause weakness and fatigue, and the client needs to conserve energy, but neurologic status is of highest priority. Energy conservation is important with fatigue, but is not the greatest concern at this time. Oral and skin care are routine aspects of care. **Cognitive Level:** Analyzing **Client Need:** Physiological Adaptation **Integrated Process:** Nursing Process: Planning **Content Area:** Adult Health **Strategy:** Critical words are *highest priority*, indicating all options will be appropriate, but one is more important. Note similarity in two options to eliminate them. Choose correctly, recalling neurologic status is higher priority than skin care. **Reference:** LeMone, P., Burke, K., Bauldoff, G., & Gubrud, P. (2015). *Medical surgical nursing: Clinical reasoning in patient care* (6th ed.). New York, NY: Pearson, pp. 193–195.

7 **Answer: 1 Rationale:** Glucocorticoids cause retention of chloride and sodium, leading to fluid retention. It is still important for the client to take a prescribed diuretic. The client needs to maintain vegetable intake, but this does not assist with managing side effects of prednisone. Eating increased amounts of high-chloride foods such as spinach and celery may increase the serum chloride level. **Cognitive Level:** Application **Client Need:** Pharmacological and Parenteral Therapies **Integrated Process:** Teaching and Learning **Content Area:** Adult Health **Strategy:** The

critical words are *prednisone* and *side effects*. Recall that this drug is a corticosteroid, and that this type of drug causes retention of sodium and chloride to direct you to the correct option. **Reference:** Holland, L., Adams, M., & Brice, J. (2018). *Core concepts in pharmacology* (5th ed.). New York, NY: Pearson, pp. 400–401.

8 **Answer: 290 Rationale:** An estimate of serum osmolality is obtained by multiplying the sodium level by two. The normal range of sodium is 135–145. If the highest normal sodium value is 145, then the highest normal serum osmolality should be no higher than 290. **Cognitive Level:** Applying **Client Need:** Reduction of Risk Potential **Integrated Process:** Nursing Process: Assessment **Content Area:** Adult Health **Strategy:** Recall normal serum sodium level and multiply by two. **Reference:** LeMone, P., Burke, K., Bauldoff, G., & Gubrud, P. (2015). *Medical surgical nursing: Clinical reasoning in patient care* (6th ed.). New York, NY: Pearson, p. 194.

9 **Answer: 1 Rationale:** Cheese can be high in sodium and ham is high in sodium because it is cured as a preservative process. Ingestion of hot dogs and baked beans will supply extra sodium in the diet. Chicken salad on lettuce is lower in sodium content. Tossed salad with vinegar dressing is not high in sodium. White fish and plain baked potato do not provide excessive sodium. **Cognitive Level:** Applying **Client Need:** Health Promotion and Maintenance **Integrated Process:** Nursing Process: Implementation **Content Area:** Adult Health **Strategy:** The question requires knowledge of sodium content of foods. Note foods high in sodium is the correct answer. Choose the first option because processed and preserved foods contain a lot of sodium. **Reference:** LeMone, P., Burke, K., Bauldoff, G., & Gubrud, P. (2015). *Medical surgical nursing: Clinical reasoning in patient care* (6th ed.). New York, NY: Pearson, p. 192.

10 **Answer: 2 Rationale:** Hyponatremia is caused by an excess of water, which dilutes the amount of sodium present in the plasma, leading to a fluid volume excess (FVE). It is important to restrict additional fluids as they can further increase the sodium deficit. In addition, the client already is in an FVE state, which can lead to development of further disturbances of fluid balance. Hypotonic fluids would further complicate the hyponatremia. Sodium usually does not need to be replaced in dilutional states. When the excess fluid is removed, the sodium is often within normal range. Tap water is a hypotonic fluid and hypotonic fluids would further complicate the hyponatremia. **Cognitive Level:** Applying **Client Need:** Physiological Adaptation **Integrated Process:** Nursing Process: Planning **Content Area:** Adult Health **Strategy:** The critical word is *dilutional*. Eliminate two options because additional water is not needed. Eliminate a third option because additional sodium is not needed. **Reference:** LeMone, P., Burke, K., Bauldoff, G., & Gubrud, P. (2015). *Medical surgical nursing: Clinical reasoning in patient care* (6th ed.). New York, NY: Pearson, pp. 193–195.

Posttest

1 **Answer: 2 Rationale:** DI is characterized by a decrease in ADH secretion, resulting in loss of fluids through polyuria. Polyuria in turn leads to increased thirst. Nausea and vomiting are not characteristic of DI. Dysuria would occur with a disorder or infection of the bladder. Confusion has many causes, but DI is not among them. **Cognitive Level:** Applying **Client Need:** Physiological Adaptation **Integrated Process:** Nursing Process: Assessment **Content Area:** Adult Health **Strategy:** Recall physiology of DI. If you have trouble recalling information, a clue might be the common word *diabetes*—although diabetes mellitus is different from diabetes insipidus, they share the common symptoms of polyuria and polydipsia. **Reference:** LeMone, P., Burke, K., Bauldoff, G., & Gubrud, P. (2015). *Medical surgical nursing: Clinical reasoning in patient care* (6th ed.). New York, NY: Pearson, pp. 193–195.

2 **Answer: 2 Rationale:** Too rapid a correction of hypernatremia can lead to changes in vascular tone, which can affect blood vessels and cause increased fluid entry into the brain, thereby causing cerebral edema. Cellular dehydration is caused by hypernatremia. RBC destruction is not viewed as a risk when treating hypernatremia. Renal shutdown could be of concern because of the original state of hypernatremia but not because of treatment. **Cognitive Level:** Analyzing **Client Need:** Physiological Adaptation **Integrated Process:** Nursing Process: Assessment **Content Area:** Adult Health **Strategy:** Critical words are *hypernatremia* and *complications*. Note the question addresses the complications of treatment. Recall treatment involves fluid replacement and increasing risks of fluid shifts so choose the option correctly. **Reference:** LeMone, P., Burke, K., Bauldoff, G., & Gubrud, P. (2015). *Medical surgical nursing: Clinical reasoning in patient care* (6th ed.). New York, NY: Pearson, pp. 195–196.

3 **Answer: 4 Rationale:** This client has signs and symptoms of hypernatremia, and the serum sodium level of 155 mEq/L matches the expected value, which would be greater than 145 mEq/L. A value of 120 mEq/L indicates a significant state of hyponatremia, which does not match the client's symptoms. A value of 132 mEq/L reflects a mild decrease and is not consistent with the client's symptoms. A value of 142 mEq/L reflects a normal serum sodium level. **Cognitive Level:** Applying **Client Need:** Reduction of Risk Potential **Integrated Process:** Nursing Process: Assessment **Content Area:** Adult Health **Strategy:** Recognize that symptoms in the question reflect hypernatremia. Systematically eliminate options less than 145 mEq/L. **Reference:** LeMone, P., Burke, K., Bauldoff, G., & Gubrud, P. (2015). *Medical surgical nursing: Clinical reasoning in patient care* (6th ed.). New York, NY: Pearson, pp. 195–196.

4 **Answer: 3 Rationale:** The client presents with hypochloremia and most likely is experiencing other electrolyte deficiencies as well, most notably sodium and potassium. A solution with 0.45% saline with added potassium would correct expected fluid and electrolyte imbalances. Dextrose 5% and water is a hypotonic solution once dextrose is metabolized and can further dilute the plasma and the serum chloride level. A solution of 0.9% sodium chloride would not be the most appropriate solution because it does not address the issue of additional electrolyte deficiencies, which are most likely occurring in addition to the chloride deficiency. Hypertonic saline is usually administered in cases of severe hyponatremia. **Cognitive Level:** Analyzing **Client Need:** Pharmacological and Parenteral Therapies **Integrated Process:** Nursing Process: Planning **Content Area:** Adult Health **Strategy:** First recognize the level is dangerously low and recall sodium and potassium occur with low chloride and will need to be replaced. Only one option provides both of these electrolytes. **Reference:** LeMone, P., Burke, K., Bauldoff, G., & Gubrud, P. (2015). *Medical surgical nursing: Clinical reasoning in patient care* (6th ed.). New York, NY: Pearson, pp. 193–195.

5 **Answer: 1 Rationale:** In hyponatremia, water is already present in an excessive amount compared to the amount of sodium present. This can result in water intoxication or dilutional hyponatremia; therefore, water restriction is a primary cornerstone of therapy. Sodium should not be restricted but rather should be included in the treatment plan to prevent further electrolyte imbalances from occurring. Potassium should not be restricted but rather should be included in the treatment plan so as to prevent further electrolyte imbalances from occurring. Chloride intake usually accompanies sodium intake. **Cognitive Level:** Applying **Client Need:** Physiological Adaptation **Integrated Process:** Nursing Process: Planning **Content Area:** Adult Health **Strategy:** The critical word is *restrict*. Recall dangers related to further dilution of sodium to choose correctly. **Reference:** LeMone, P., Burke, K., Bauldoff, G., & Gubrud, P. (2015). *Medical surgical nursing: Clinical reasoning in patient care* (6th ed.). New York, NY: Pearson, pp. 193–195.

6 **Answer: 1, 2, 4 Rationale:** Restlessness is a common neurologic alteration when a client has hypernatremia. Dry mucous membranes indicate decreased fluid volume, which can accompany hypernatremia if the cause of the increased sodium level is hemoconcentration. The client's temperature would not be low with hypernatremia. Thirst is a primary indicator of sodium excess (hypernatremia) and should be assessed for in a plan of care for a client with hypernatremia. Weight gain would be expected with excess fluid volume, which would more likely be accompanied by hyponatremia from hemodilution. **Cognitive Level:** Applying **Client Need:** Physiological Adaptation **Integrated Process:** Nursing Process: Assessment **Content Area:** Adult Health **Strategy:** Critical words are *manifestations* and *hypernatremia*. Recall the primary compensatory mechanism for fluid balance to choose correctly. **Reference:** LeMone, P., Burke, K.,

ANSWERS & RATIONALES

Bauldoff, G., & Gubrud, P. (2015). *Medical surgical nursing: Clinical reasoning in patient care* (6th ed.). New York, NY: Pearson, pp. 195–196.

7 **Answer: 2 Rationale:** In SIADH, the antidiuretic hormone is present in excess amounts. This causes excessive water reabsorption. Water must be restricted to avoid water intoxication. Giving additional fluids would only further serve to increase fluid levels and increase sodium deficit. While it is important to consider a client's preference in fluid selection, fluid restriction is the major priority. While fluid therapy can be given via IV, it is important to allow the client to take PO fluids even if they are on a restricted basis. **Cognitive Level:** Applying **Client Need:** Management of Care **Integrated Process:** Nursing Process: Implementation **Content Area:** Adult Health **Strategy:** The question addresses the relationship between water and SIADH. Note the incorrect options are similar in that all provide fluids in some form; therefore, these should be eliminated. **Reference:** LeMone, P., Burke, K., Bauldoff, G., & Gubrud, P. (2015). *Medical surgical nursing: Clinical reasoning in patient care* (6th ed.). New York, NY: Pearson, pp. 498–499.

8 **Answer: 2 Rationale:** The client has consumed excessive amounts of water, which is hypotonic and contributes to fluid intoxication, and is actually exhibiting signs of hyponatremia. The nurse would check the electrolyte levels, expecting to find a low sodium level. Monitoring the CBC for a platelet level is not indicated, as there is no correlation between sodium levels and platelet activity. The client's serum osmolality would be low due to water intoxication. The client's urine specific gravity is expected to be low because of water intoxication. **Cognitive Level:** Applying **Client Need:** Physiological Adaptation **Integrated Process:** Nursing Process: Assessment **Content Area:** Adult Health **Strategy:** Recognize that symptoms are reflective of a fluid volume excess and hyponatremia to choose correctly. **Reference:** LeMone, P., Burke, K., Bauldoff, G., & Gubrud, P. (2015). *Medical surgical nursing: Clinical reasoning in patient care* (6th ed.). New York, NY: Pearson, pp. 193–195.

9 **Answer: 1, 5 Rationale:** The client is exhibiting signs of hypernatremia and dehydration. Appropriate nursing interventions are to measure and record I&O (intake and output) and daily weight. The client is at risk to develop seizures secondary to an elevated sodium level. Administering salt tablets would further contribute to the client's hypernatremic state. Restricting fluid intake and holding feedings could worsen the hypernatremia and fluid volume deficit (hypertonic dehydration) as the client already has extensive fluid loss due to diarrhea, elevated pulse rate, and decreased skin turgor. Avoiding adding additional water would worsen the hypertonic dehydration. **Cognitive Level:** Analyzing **Client Need:** Reduction of Risk Potential **Integrated Process:** Nursing Process: Implementation **Content Area:** Adult Health **Strategy:** Recognize that symptoms reflect dehydration and hypernatremia. Eliminate two options because fluids need to be replaced. Eliminate a third option because additional salt is not needed. **Reference:** LeMone, P., Burke, K., Bauldoff, G., & Gubrud, P. (2015). *Medical surgical nursing: Clinical reasoning in patient care* (6th ed.). New York, NY: Pearson, pp. 195–196.

10 **Answer: 3, 5 Rationale:** Fluid retention can result in hyponatremia through a dilutional effect. Fluid is retained in heart failure leading to dilutional hyponatremia. Osmotic diuretic therapy could lead to hypernatremia. Fever could result in hypernatremia secondary to increased metabolism and loss of free water. Excessive hypertonic intravenous infusion would lead to hypernatremia. **Cognitive Level:** Applying **Client Need:** Physiological Adaptation **Integrated Process:** Nursing Process: Assessment **Content Area:** Adult Health **Strategy:** Analyze options to identify potential for sodium losses or dilution. Eliminate two options since more water than sodium is lost. Eliminate a third option since sodium would be gained. **Reference:** LeMone, P., Burke, K., Bauldoff, G., & Gubrud, P. (2015). *Medical surgical nursing: Clinical reasoning in patient care* (6th ed.). New York, NY: Pearson, pp. 193–195.

References

Ball, J., Bindler, R., & Cowen, K. (2014). *Child health nursing: Partnering with children and families* (3rd ed.). Upper Saddle River, NJ: Pearson.

Berman, A., Snyder, S., & Frandsen, G. (2016). *Fundamentals of nursing: Concepts, process, and practice* (10th ed.).New York, NY: Pearson.

Ignatavicius, D., & Workman, M. (2015). *Medical-surgical nursing: Patient-centered collaborative care* (8th ed.). Philadelphia, PA: Elsevier Saunders.

Kee, J. L. (2017). *Pearson's handbook of laboratory and diagnostic tests* (8th ed.). New York, NY: Pearson Education.

LeMone, P., Burke, K., Bauldoff, G., & Gubrud, P. (2015). *Medical surgical nursing: Clinical reasoning in patient care* (6th ed.). New York, NY: Pearson.

London, M., Ladewig, P., Davidson, M., Ball, J., Bindler, R., & Cowen, K. (2017). *Maternal and child nursing care* (5th ed.). New York, NY: Pearson.

Sole, M., Klein, O., & Moseley, M. (2016). *Introduction to critical care nursing* (7th ed.). St. Louis, MO: Elsevier Saunders.

ANSWERS & RATIONALES

3 Potassium Balance and Imbalances

Chapter Outline

Overview of Potassium Regulation

Hypokalemia

Hyperkalemia

 NCLEX-RN® Test Prep

Access the NEW Web-based app that provides students with additional practice questions in preparation for the NCLEX experience.

Objectives

➤ Identify the basic functions of potassium in the body.
➤ Explain the pathophysiology and etiology of potassium imbalances.
➤ Identify specific assessment findings in potassium imbalances.
➤ Identify priority nursing concerns for a client experiencing a potassium imbalance.
➤ Describe the therapeutic management of potassium imbalances.
➤ Describe the management of nursing care for a client who is experiencing a potassium imbalance.

Review at a Glance

hyperkalemia serum potassium level above the laboratory normal value (usually 5.1 mEq/L)

hypokalemia serum level of potassium falls below 3.5 mEq/L

relative hyperkalemia movement of potassium from the intracellular fluid to the extracellular fluid, leading to elevated serum potassium levels without a true

body increase of potassium, such as occurs with acidosis

relative hypokalemia movement of potassium from the extracellular fluid to the intracellular fluid, leading to lowered serum potassium levels without a true decrease of potassium in the body, such as occurs with insulin therapy

sodium-potassium pump controls the concentration of potassium by removing three sodium ions from the cell for every two potassium ions that return to the cell; fueled by the breakdown of ATP and responsible for causing muscle cells to generate action potentials and transmit impulses

PRETEST

1 Which potassium levels would be of concern to the nurse if noted in the laboratory results for a client who is taking furosemide?

1. 5.4 mEq/L
2. 4.3 mEq/L
3. 3.7 mEq/L
4. 3.1 mEq/L
5. 2.8 mEq/L

- -

2 Which statement should the nurse include when teaching a client about oral potassium supplementation?

1. "When you take your potassium pill, if you cannot swallow it, you can crush it up and put it in orange juice."
2. "Potassium should only be taken in the morning on an empty stomach."
3. "Take your potassium tablet after you have eaten breakfast."
4. "You can continue to use a salt substitute while you are taking your potassium supplement."

- -

3 The nurse anticipates the client with which condition would be most at risk to develop hyperkalemia?

1. Chronic renal failure
2. Newly diagnosed cirrhosis
3. Partial bowel obstruction requiring nasogastric suctioning
4. Diarrhea for the last 4 days

- -

4 The nurse should place highest priority on which nursing intervention for a client with renal failure who has a potassium level of 6.8 mEq/L?

1. Obtain an electrocardiogram (ECG).
2. Evaluate level of consciousness.
3. Measure urinary output.
4. Draw arterial blood gases.

- -

5 The nurse should include dietary teaching regarding addition of potassium-rich foods if the client is receiving which diuretic? Select all that apply.

1. Hydrochlorothiazide
2. Spironolactone
3. Triamterene with hydrochlorothiazide
4. Amiloride
5. Furosemide

- -

6 A client has a potassium level of 6.2 mEq/L. The nurse identifies which ECG tracing to correlate with this electrolyte level?

1.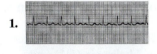
2.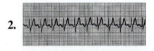
3.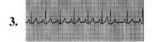
4.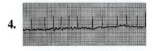

Source: LeMone, Priscilla; Burke, Karen M.; Bauldoff, Gerene, *Medical Surgical Nursing: Critical Thinking in Patient Care*, 5th Ed, © 2011. Reprinted and Electronically reproduced by permission of Pearson Education, Inc., Upper Saddle River, New Jersey..

7 When caring for a client who has a potassium level of 2.8 mEq/L, the nurse should assess for which possible resulting health problem?

1. Perforated bowel
2. Paralytic ileus
3. Renal failure
4. Diabetes mellitus

- -

8 The nurse should determine that an intravenous (IV) administration of calcium gluconate to a client with hyperkalemia has been effective after noting which assessment finding?

1. Urine output has increased.
2. Bowel movements are loose.
3. Cardiac dysrhythmia is corrected.
4. Muscles are relaxed and weak.

9 Which statement by a client indicates a need for further instruction regarding treatment for hypokalemia?

1. "I will eat more bananas and cantaloupes for breakfast."
2. "I will eat more bran flakes to increase my potassium level."
3. "I will take my potassium in the morning after breakfast so it does not upset my stomach."
4. "I will tell my primary care provider if I start having muscle cramps or weakness."

10 What is the best response by the nurse to the 22-year-old daughter of a 56-year-old client admitted with hypokalemia and who reports being dizzy upon standing?

1. "Your mother has been lying in bed too long and when she stands up she will get dizzy."
2. "Once we correct your mother's potassium level, the dizziness should improve."
3. "Your mother is probably dizzy because her heart is not pumping as effectively, making her blood pressure low."
4. "Your mother is dizzy because her nervous system is not functioning correctly; once her potassium level goes up, she will improve."

➤ *See pages 76–78 for Answers and Rationales.*

I. OVERVIEW OF POTASSIUM REGULATION

A. **Potassium (K^+) balance and function:** major cation of intracellular fluid (ICF); 98% of body's K^+ store is located in ICF; the remaining 2% is in the extracellular fluid (ECF) (i.e., intravascular and interstitial spaces outside cells; responsible for neuromuscular function)

1. Serum levels
   a. Normal serum concentration ranges:
      1) Newborn: 3.7–5.9 mEq/L
      2) Infant: 4.1–5.3 mEq/L
      3) Child: 3.4–4.7 mEq/L
      4) Adult: 3.5–5.1 mEq/L
   b. Even small changes in K^+ level have a profound effect on body and are poorly tolerated

2. Role in acid–base balance
   a. Hydrogen (H^+) and K^+ ions shift back and forth between ICF and ECF to maintain pH
   b. H^+ ions move out of cells in alkalotic states to help correct a high pH, and K^+ ions move in to maintain an electrically stable state; the reverse happens in acidosis

3. Functions in body

Practice to Pass

A client asks the nurse why potassium levels are so important in the body. How will the nurse respond?

   a. ECF K^+ is responsible for maintaining action potentials in excitable cells of muscles, neurons, and other tissues
   b. ECF K^+ assists in controlling cardiac rate and rhythm, nerve impulse conduction, skeletal muscle contraction, and function of smooth muscles and endocrine tissues
   c. Intracellular K^+ has a role in cellular metabolism and functions in regulation of protein and glycogen synthesis
   d. Because K^+ is the primary intracellular cation, it has some control over intracellular osmolarity and volume via sodium–potassium ion exchange mechanism

Table 3-1	Lifespan Considerations for Health Maintenance: Potassium Balance
Lifespan Considerations	**Risk Factors for Imbalances**
Infants	Diarrhea, vomiting, pyloric stenosis
Children	Diarrhea, poor dietary intake
Adults	Increased use of diuretics Heart failure Poor nutrition

    4. System interactions
        a. Primary control of ECF K^+ concentration is **sodium-potassium pump** in cell membrane of all body cells
        b. Sodium-potassium pump controls K^+ concentration by removing three sodium (Na^+) ions from cell for every two potassium ions that return to cell
        c. Pump is fueled by breakdown of ATP and is responsible for causing muscle cells to generate action potentials and transmit impulses
    5. See Table 3-1 for lifespan factors affecting K^+ balance

B. Sources of potassium
    1. Cellular level: factors that affect movement in and out of cells contribute to level of K^+ in ICF and ECF
        a. Kidneys eliminate approximately 90% of K^+ lost
        b. Other 10% is excreted through stool and perspiration
        c. Cellular release can lead to additional K^+ circulating in body and may be due to disease processes and/or medications
    2. Dietary levels
        a. Adequate intake is approximately 40–60 mEq daily
        b. Western diets consist of adequate intake of K^+ daily in fruits, dried fruits, and vegetables
        c. Many salt substitutes contain K^+
        d. Intake can also occur when parenteral fluid with added K^+ is infused
        e. Excessive intake of black licorice can lead to decreased K^+ levels because of effect of glyceric acid (aldosterone effect)

II. *HYPOKALEMIA*

    A. Definition, etiology, and pathophysiology (see Table 3-2)
        1. Serum potassium level below 3.5 mEq/L
        2. Cellular-level transport
            a. Amount of K^+ in ECF is so small that small changes in K^+ level can lead to major alterations in membrane excitability in muscle and neural cells, making them less responsive to stimuli (such as in paralytic ileus) or can cause cardiac irritability (such as premature ventricular contractions [PVCs])
            b. Rapid changes in ECF K^+ cannot be compensated for quickly and can result in profound changes in body function
            c. If this decrease is not corrected very quickly, death can occur from cardiac and respiratory arrest
            d. **Relative hypokalemia** occurs when K^+ moves from ECF to ICF (total body level of K^+ remains unchanged), leading to abnormal distribution of K^+
                1) Alkalosis causes K^+ to migrate into cell as H^+ ions move out to correct high pH

Table 3-2	Overview of Hypokalemia	
Etiology	**Manifestations**	**Nursing Interventions**
Inadequate intake Use of potassium-wasting diuretics Excessive loss of GI fluid Heat-induced diaphoresis Starvation High glucose levels leading to diuresis Increased secretion of aldosterone as seen in adrenal adenomas, cirrhosis, nephrosis, heart failure, and hypertensive crisis Diabetes insipidus	Weak, thready pulse Pedal pulses difficult to palpate ECG changes—ST segment depression, flattened T wave, appearance of U wave, ventricular dysrhythmias (especially PVCs), heart block Enhanced effect of digoxin leading to toxicity at therapeutic levels Decreased breath sounds Shallow respiratory pattern Dyspnea Polyuria; difficulty in concentrating urine Decreased deep tendon reflexes Muscle weakness Anxiety Lethargy Depression Confusion Paresthesias Weakness Leg cramps Abdominal distention Hypoactive bowel sounds Vomiting Nausea Constipation Paralytic ileus	Monitor vital signs, especially blood pressure; orthostatic hypotension common Monitor serum potassium levels Assess heart rate and rhythm Assess ECG changes Assess respiratory rate, depth, and pattern Assess for signs of hypokalemia if client taking diuretics Protect from injury Monitor serum magnesium and calcium levels Monitor I&O (intake and output) Check for signs of metabolic alkalosis Give potassium supplements as prescribed with food to prevent gastric irritation Use an infusion pump when administering parenteral potassium and assess IV site frequently for infiltration, phlebitis, and tissue necrosis Assess mental status and cognition Client education about food sources of potassium (see Box 3-1, p. 68) and other measures (see Box 3-2, p. 69)

2) Increased secretion of insulin causes K^+ to move into skeletal muscles and hepatic cells when there is increased secretion of insulin

3) Tissue repair causes shifting of K^+ concentration

4) Water intoxication causes dilution of serum K^+

Practice to Pass

Why is an understanding of actual versus relative hypokalemia important to client safety?

3. Predisposing clinical conditions: actual hypokalemia is an actual loss of K^+ or lack of adequate intake of K^+

a. Increased secretion of aldosterone leads to excretion of K^+ from renal tubules and is seen in clients with these conditions:

1) Adrenal adenomas

2) Cirrhosis

3) Nephrosis

4) Heart failure and hypertensive crisis

5) Cushing syndrome

6) Diabetes insipidus

7) Hyperaldosteronism

b. Excessive loss of K^+ by use of certain medications, such as loop diuretics (e.g., furosemide), thiazide diuretics (e.g., hydrochlorothiazide), corticosteroids, cardiac glycosides (digoxin), penicillin derivatives (e.g., ampicillin, sodium penicillin, carbenicillin), amphotericin B, gentamicin, theophylline, cisplatin, and terbutaline (a tocolytic and respiratory agent); refer to Table 3-3 for a summary of medication classes that affect K^+ levels

Table 3-3	Common Medications That Affect Potassium Levels	
Increase Potassium Levels	**Decrease Potassium Levels**
Potassium chloride and salts	Laxatives, enemas, and sodium polystyrene sulfonate
Angiotensin converting enzyme (ACE) inhibitors*	Corticosteroids
Heparin	Antibiotics*
Barbiturates, sedatives, heroin, and amphetamines	Insulin and glucose
Nonsteroidal anti-inflammatory drugs (NSAIDs)*	Beta$_2$ agonists (terbutaline, estrogen, albuterol)
Beta blockers and alpha agonists*	Potassium-wasting diuretics*
Cyclophosphamide	Amphotericin
Potassium-sparing diuretics*	

For these medications, please refer to a drug textbook for specific names because there are many different types of drugs in each category.

    c. Gastrointestinal (GI) loss by vomiting, diarrhea, prolonged nasogastric (NG) suctioning, newly created ileostomy, villous adenoma on the intestinal tract, laxative abuse, or enema administration

    d. Heat-induced diaphoresis

    e. Renal disease affecting the reabsorption of K^+ seen in diuretic phase of acute kidney injury

    f. Hemodialysis and peritoneal dialysis

    g. Altered intake

        1) Potassium-restricted diets

        2) NPO status without sufficient IV replacement therapy

        3) Starvation, malnutrition, alcoholism, and anorexia

        4) High glucose levels, which increase osmotic pressure and lead to diuresis

        5) Large ingestion of black licorice (causes aldosterone effects)

    h. Intravenous insulin therapy to treat diabetic ketoacidosis, which drives K^+ into cells temporarily

B. Clinical manifestations

    1. Rarely develop before K^+ level falls below 3.0 mEq/L unless rate of fall is rapid

    2. See Table 3-4 for manifestations of hypokalemia in specific body systems

    3. See Figure 3-1 (p. 67) for electrocardiogram changes with hypokalemia

C. Assessment

    1. Monitoring expectations

        a. Serum K^+ levels

        b. ECG changes

        c. Electrolyte levels

        d. I&O

            1) Diuresis can lead to excessive loss of K^+

            2) One liter of urine contains about 40 mEq of K^+

    2. Identification of risk factors

        a. Assess for factors that increase risk of hypokalemia such as the following:

            1) Age: aging decreases kidneys' ability to concentrate urine, leading to diuresis; older adults are also more likely to be taking medications that can alter potassium levels

            2) Alcoholism

        b. Medications

            1) Obtain pertinent client history of medications that can alter potassium levels (refer back to Table 3-3)

Practice to Pass

How are you going to ensure client safety when that client has hypokalemia?

Table 3-4   **Clinical Manifestations of Hypokalemia**

Body System	Manifestations
Cardiovascular	Variable pulse rate Weak, thready pulse Decreased blood pressure Pedal pulses difficult to palpate *ECG changes:* ST segment depression, flattened T wave, appearance of U wave, ventricular dysrhythmias (especially premature ventricular contractions [PVCs]), and heart block Prolongs repolarization, leading to flattened, prolonged T waves and production of possible U waves (small, low-amplitude waveforms occurring after T wave) Digitalis toxicity is potentiated
Respiratory	Decreased breath sounds Shallow respiratory pattern Dyspnea
Renal	Polyuria and nocturia Decreased specific gravity
Neuromuscular	Deep tendon hyporeflexia Muscle weakness, paresthesias, leg cramps, and soft flabby muscles Fatigue and lethargy, proceeding to depression and coma with severe hypokalemia Coma Anxiety
Gastrointestinal	Hypermotility with hyperactive bowel sounds Abdominal cramping Nausea, vomiting, and diarrhea Weight loss

       2) Examine both prescription and over-the-counter client medications and supplements for possible interactions

    c. Dietary

       1) Obtain pertinent client history regarding food intake

       2) Determine whether client is taking nutritional supplements and check for potential interactions

D. Diagnostic and laboratory findings

  1. Plasma levels

    a. Hypokalemia is confirmed by a serum level less than 3.5 mEq/L (or the normal value indicated by a particular laboratory)

    b. Trending of serum K^+ levels is necessary in order to establish a baseline and monitor response to therapy

  2. Associated electrolyte levels

    a. Elevated pH and bicarbonate levels (alkalosis)

    b. Elevated serum glucose levels (increased insulin secretion and increased osmotic pressure)

    c. Decreased serum chloride levels

    d. Decreased magnesium levels (hypomagnesemia can potentiate hypokalemia)

    e. Decreased calcium levels can also be seen in conjunction with decreased potassium and magnesium levels

  3. Trending of results

    a. ECG tracings demonstrate characteristic changes with hypokalemia (described earlier in this chapter and as shown in Figure 3-1C on next page)

    b. Trending ECG changes can help to monitor a client's status and response to therapeutic treatment

Figure 3-1

Electrocardiogram (ECG) changes caused by altered potassium levels. **A.** Normal ECG. **B.** Changes resulting from hyperkalemia. **C.** Changes resulting from hypokalemia.

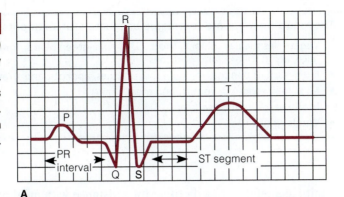

A

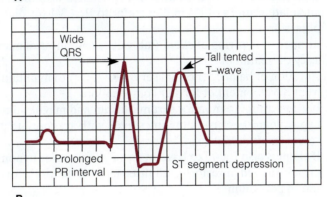

B

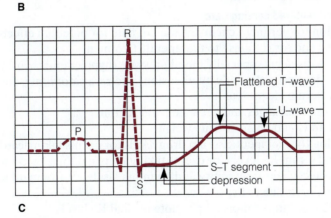

C

E. Priority nursing concerns
   1. Possible injury because of muscle weakness and hyporeflexia
   2. Possible adverse change in breathing pattern from neuromuscular impairment
   3. Possible reduced cardiac output if dysrhythmias occur
   4. Constipation as a response to smooth muscle atony
   5. Fatigue in response to neuromuscular weakness
   6. Possible reduction in mobility as a consequence of muscle weakness
F. Therapeutic management: treatment focuses on restoring normal levels, preventing complications, and treating underlying problems
   1. Replacement therapies
      a. For clients at risk, provide a diet containing adequate K$^+$, about 50–100 mEq daily
      b. If diet is insufficient to meet needs, administer K$^+$ supplements as prescribed

Box 3-1	The following foods are considered adequate sources of potassium:
Good Food Sources of Potassium	• Vegetables such as spinach, broccoli, carrots, green beans, tomatoes and tomato juice, acorn squash, and potatoes • Fruits such as bananas, cantaloupe, oranges, apricots, and strawberries • Milk, milk products, yogurt, and meat • Legumes, nuts, and seeds • Whole grains

    c. Initiate a referral to a dietitian for assistance with meal planning to ensure adequate sources of K^+ in diet (refer to Box 3-1 for dietary sources of potassium)

  2. Continued monitoring of client (lab values and physical manifestations) to assess efficacy of treatment

  3. Restoration of balance (normal serum K^+ level) to maintain homeostasis and prevent development of further complications

    a. It is important to monitor serum calcium and magnesium levels in clients who are hypokalemic because sometimes, even with appropriate potassium replacement, serum levels do not rise

    b. If client is also found to have hypocalcemia and/or hypomagnesemia, correction must be aimed at restoring all three electrolyte levels for successful correction of serum potassium

G. Client-centered nursing care

  1. Monitor pertinent client assessment data for potential effects related to hypokalemia and for response to therapeutic treatment

    a. Vital signs, especially blood pressure (hypokalemia can cause the client to develop orthostatic hypotension) and respiratory rate, depth, and pattern

    b. Serum electrolyte levels

    c. ECG changes and heart rate and rhythm

    d. I&O and possibly daily weight

  2. Monitor therapeutic serum drug levels for clients taking cardiac glycosides (digoxin) and serum K^+ levels for clients taking loop and thiazide diuretics

  3. Protect client from injury and maintain a safe environment as client may experience weakness due to hypokalemia

  4. Dietary interventions to promote normal K^+ levels

    a. Encourage use of high-fiber diets and increased fluid intake, if not on fluid restriction, to prevent constipation that can occur because of ileus secondary to hypokalemia

    b. Provide adequate dietary sources of K^+ in diet

    c. Maintain accurate I&O

  5. Check for signs of metabolic alkalosis (including irritability and paresthesias) because hypokalemia is present in alkalotic states

  6. Provide replacement therapy as prescribed by healthcare provider paying attention to baseline labs, client's response, and therapeutic benefit

  7. Always use an infusion pump when administering parenteral K^+

    a. Observe IV site frequently for signs of infiltration, phlebitis, and tissue necrosis as K^+-containing solutions are irritating to veins

    b. Verify additive K^+ in solution prior to hanging infusion

    c. Do not exceed maximum safe infusion rate (see section that follows)

  8. Observe client's mental status and cognition during course of therapy

H. **Medication therapy** (*Note:* potassium supplements should not be given unless the client has a urine output of at least 0.5 mL/kg/hour)
   1. Oral replacement therapy
      a. Clients should be started on oral supplements if they take K^+-wasting diuretics, have poor nutritional intake, and/or have disease processes that cause further K^+ losses
      b. Oral preparation is usually potassium chloride or KCl, which is available in many brands
      c. Daily prophylactic dose is 20 mEq
      d. Therapeutic treatment can be given at higher doses (up to 100 mEq in divided doses), depending on client's baseline
      e. Can be given in either liquid or pill form
      f. Refer to Box 3-2 for client teaching points regarding oral potassium therapy
   2. Parenteral replacement therapy
      a. Dilute K^+ in a solution that provides no more than 1 mEq/10 mL
      b. Most K^+ infusions are run at a rate not exceeding 5–10 mEq/hr unless there is moderate hypokalemia; peripheral IV K^+ should not be infused more quickly than 20 mEq/hr or in concentrations greater than 40 mEq/L unless severe hypokalemia exists; higher-concentration solutions should be administered through a central line, and client should have hemodynamic monitoring throughout course of K^+ replacement therapy
      c. Solution should be dextrose free, if possible, to prevent release of insulin
      d. If more than 20 mEq/hour is given, client should have continuous ECG monitoring, and serum K^+ levels should be checked every 4–6 hours until level normalizes
      e. Monitor IV site closely as KCl is irritating to blood vessels and can lead to infiltration, phlebitis, and tissue necrosis
      f. Use an infusion pump to control infusion, paying attention to rate, intake, and output
      g. Potassium should never be administered by IV push or intramuscular routes because this can lead to development of fatal dysrhythmias
   3. Diet therapy
      a. Foods high in K^+ include raisins, bananas, apricots, oranges, avocados, beans, beef, potatoes, tomatoes, cantaloupe, and spinach
      b. Avoid foods such as black licorice that, when eaten in large quantities, can cause hypokalemia

Practice to Pass

What nursing interventions should be used with clients receiving intravenous solutions containing KCl?

Box 3-2	Prior to discharge, teach client and family to do the following:
Client Education Regarding Hypokalemia	• Take potassium supplements with about 120 mL (at least 4 oz) of fluid or with food. • Never crush or break potassium tablets or capsules. • Dissolve powder form of potassium in about 120 mL (at least 4 oz) of water or juice (no carbonated beverages). • Take potassium after meals to prevent GI upset. • Do not use salt substitutes when taking potassium supplements. • Know the signs and symptoms of hyperkalemia and report any of these to the healthcare provider. • Get regular serum potassium levels drawn as per healthcare provider recommendations. • Teach client about side effects of potassium supplements and to report them to healthcare provider if they occur.

I. Client education

1. Teach awareness of predisposing factors

   a. Older adult clients are at risk for hypokalemia due to multiple medication profile

   b. Clients taking diuretics (loop and thiazide) and/or digoxin are at risk to develop K^+ depletion

2. Teach clients signs and symptoms of hypokalemia and have them report potential problems to healthcare provider

3. Teach clients about K^+ supplement medication

   a. Take with about 120 mL (at least 4 oz) of fluid or food to prevent GI upset

   b. Do not crush slow-release tablets, as this can trigger a quick release of potassium

4. Dietary education

   a. If client takes a potassium-sparing diuretic, do not encourage use of foods high in K^+

   b. Provide list of foods that are high in K^+ during client education (refer to Box 3-1 for a listing of adequate food sources of potassium)

   c. Collaborate with dietitian as needed

J. Evaluation

1. Client returns to and maintains a normal serum K^+ level
2. Client complies with drug and diet therapies as prescribed
3. Client states early signs and symptoms of hypokalemia
4. Client has normal bowel pattern
5. Client maintains adequate gas exchange
6. Client maintains regular cardiac rate and rhythm

Practice to Pass

What foods would you suggest to a client who is hypokalemic?

III. HYPERKALEMIA

A. Definition, etiology, and pathophysiology (see Table 3-5)

1. Serum K^+ level above 5.1 mEq/L
2. Cellular-level transport

Table 3-5	Overview of Hyperkalemia	
Etiology	**Manifestations**	**Nursing Interventions**
Excessive potassium intake from foods, medications, salt substitutes, IV infusions of KCl	Irregular, slow heart rate	Restrict potassium intake
Decreased excretion due to adrenal insufficiency, renal failure, potassium-sparing diuretics; decreased secretion of aldosterone	Decreased blood pressure	Monitor serum potassium levels
Massive tissue trauma	ECG changes—tall, peaked T waves, widened QRS, frequent ectopy, ventricular tachycardia or fibrillation, standstill	Assess for signs and symptoms
Metabolic acidosis	If levels are extremely high, can lead to muscle weakness, paralysis, and respiratory failure	Monitor cardiac status
Gastrointestinal bleeds	Muscle twitching, paralysis	Monitor for metabolic acidosis and implement treatment for same
Overdose	GI hypermotility	Monitor ECG changes
Insulin deficiency	Hyperactive bowel sounds	If blood transfusions necessary, give fresh packed red blood cells
Hyperuricemia	Abdominal cramping	Encourage compliance with therapeutic regimen
Burns	Diarrhea	Discontinue use of IV KCl
	Muscle cramps	Implement safety precautions
	Irritability	Administer diuretics or other medications that lower serum potassium levels
	Anxiety	
	Flaccid paralysis	
	Oliguria	

     a. K^+ moves from ECF to ICF and increases cell excitability, so that cells respond to stimuli of less intensity and may actually discharge independently without a stimulus

     b. Myocardium is most sensitive to increases in K^+ level

     c. Manifestations seen with hyperkalemia depend on how rapidly an increase occurs

        1) Sudden increases show profound functional changes at 6–7 mEq/L

        2) Slower increases may not lead to changes until levels of 8 mEq/L are reached

   3. Predisposing clinical conditions

     a. Actual hyperkalemia (K^+ level in ECF is elevated)

        1) Excessive K^+ intake due to overingestion of K^+-rich food or medications, use of salt substitutes, or rapid infusion of K^+-containing IV solutions

        2) Decreased excretion of K^+ from adrenal insufficiency (Addison disease), renal insufficiency or failure, K^+-sparing diuretics, or use of ACE inhibitors

     b. **Relative hyperkalemia** (movement of K^+ from ICF to ECF leading to elevated serum K^+ level without a true body increase of K^+)

        1) Conditions that affect cellular release

           a) Massive cell damage, crush injuries

           b) Burns

           c) Tumor lysis syndrome, in which K^+ is released from cells along with phosphates and uric acid

           d) Gastrointestinal bleeds

           e) Major surgeries and hypercatabolism

        2) Conditions that are considered to cause pseudohyperkalemia

           a) Hemolysis of blood sample due to prolonged tourniquet use

           b) Clenched fist during blood draws may cause RBC hemolysis

        3) Conditions that affect transcellular shifting

           a) Metabolic acidosis, which causes K^+ to move out of cell as H^+ ions move into cell to correct pH

           b) Insulin deficiency leads to a decrease in K^+ utilization

           c) Rapid increase in blood osmolality causes an increased blood concentration of K^+

        4) Conditions that result from medication therapy

           a) Overdose of replacement therapy

           b) Administration of stored blood, which causes hemolysis of RBCs in solution and increases serum K^+ level

           c) Use of K^+-sparing diuretics

        5) Addison disease due to decreased aldosterone that leads to Na^+ depletion and K^+ retention

     c. Hyperkalemia occurs rather rarely in clients who have normally functioning kidneys

B. Clinical manifestations (see Table 3-6)

C. Assessment

   1. Monitoring expectations

     a. Serum K^+ levels

     b. ECG changes (see Figure 3-1 again)

     c. I&O (adequate renal function is needed for K^+ excretion; measure I&O accurately and frequently)

   2. Identification of risk factors

     a. Assess for factors that increase risk for hyperkalemia, such as the following:

        1) Age: aging leads to a decrease in renal functioning

        2) Medications that can increase serum K^+ levels, such as K^+-sparing diuretics or K^+ supplements, blood products, ACE inhibitors, beta adrenergic

---

Practice to Pass

Why does a client who has massive tissue destruction get hyperkalemia?

Table 3-6	Clinical Manifestations of Hyperkalemia
Body System	**Manifestations**
Cardiovascular	Irregular, slow heart rate Decreased blood pressure *ECG changes* (refer again to Figure 3-1b): narrow, peaked T waves, widened QRS complexes, prolonged PR intervals, flattened P waves, frequent ectopy, ventricular fibrillation, and ventricular standstill
Respiratory	Unaffected until levels are very high, leading to muscle weakness and paralysis and causing respiratory failure
Renal	Oliguria (seen when renal failure is the cause of hyperkalemia)
Neuromuscular	Early: paresthesias, muscle twitching Muscle cramps Irritability Anxiety Difficulty with phonation Late: ascending flaccid paralysis involving arms and legs
Gastrointestinal	Hypermotility with hyperactive bowel sounds Abdominal cramping Nausea and vomiting and diarrhea Weight loss

  blockers, nonsteroidal anti-inflammatory drugs (NSAIDs), heparin, and sulfamethoxazole/trimethoprim

 b. Dietary

  1) High intake of K^+-rich foods

  2) Salt substitutes

  3) K^+ supplements

 c. Clients with disease states, both acute and chronic

  1) Diabetic ketoacidosis and renal failure can lead to hyperkalemia

  2) Acute disease such as massive trauma or burns can lead to hyperkalemia

 d. Clients undergoing therapeutic treatment: recent medical or surgical intervention, or blood transfusions

D. Diagnostic and laboratory findings

 1. Plasma levels: a value greater than 5.1 mEq/L confirms diagnosis of hyperkalemia

 2. Associated electrolyte levels

  a. If dehydration is causing hyperkalemia, then hematocrit, hemoglobin, Na^+, and chloride levels should be drawn

  b. If associated with renal failure, creatinine and BUN levels should also be drawn

  c. An arterial blood gas (ABG) is needed to monitor for metabolic acidosis

 3. Trending of results

  a. ECG monitoring to determine cardiac changes

  b. ABGs to determine acid–base balance

E. Priority nursing concerns

 1. Possible injury because of muscle weakness and hyporeflexia

 2. Possible decreased cardiac output as a consequence of dysrhythmias

 3. Diarrhea as a consequence of neuromuscular changes and irritability

F. Therapeutic interventions

 1. Decrease potassium intake

  a. Stress importance of adherence to prescribed K^+ restrictions

  b. Do not administer K^+ supplements either orally or in parenteral fluids

  c. Refer client to a dietitian to evaluate dietary intake for hidden K^+ sources

2. Promote K^+ excretion
   a. Increase urine output
   b. Ensure adequate renal function
3. Continued monitoring of client
   a. Serum K^+ levels; report abnormals
   b. Signs and symptoms of hyperkalemia
   c. Cardiac status
   d. Metabolic acidosis
4. Restoration of balance
   a. Because small elevations can lead to profound myocardial changes, a normal K^+ level should be restored as soon as possible to prevent lethal dysrhythmias
   b. Treatment is based on serum levels and client presentation; aggressive therapeutic management may be required to return serum levels to baseline in a timely manner
   c. Whenever possible, determine and treat underlying cause of hyperkalemia to restore balance
5. Dialysis may be performed for intractable conditions if hyperkalemia cannot be controlled in a timely manner to prevent development of potentially lethal problems or if client's clinical condition warrants immediate intervention

G. Client-centered nursing care

1. Monitor pertinent client assessment data for potential effects related to hyperkalemia and for response to therapeutic treatment
   a. Notify healthcare provider of levels exceeding 5.1 mEq/L as elevations can cause serious cardiac consequences
   b. Serum electrolyte levels
   c. ECG changes and heart rate and rhythm pattern
2. Monitor client for potential serum elevations due to concurrent drug therapy (as noted in Table 3-2)
3. Check for signs of metabolic acidosis because relative hyperkalemia frequently accompanies acidotic states (and often self-corrects when pH is corrected)
4. Do not provide any additional K^+ in form of medications (IV, supplements, and/or stored blood)
5. Dietary interventions to promote normal K^+ levels
   a. Decrease catabolism by encouraging client to consume prescribed amounts of dietary protein and carbohydrates
   b. Limit or stop additional K^+ sources in diet (such as salt substitutes)
   c. Refer client to a dietitian for individualized instruction as needed
6. Encourage adherence to therapeutic regimen, treat infections promptly, and decrease hypermetabolic responses

H. Medication therapy

1. Exchange resins
   a. Sodium polystyrene sulfonate can be given either as an enema or orally with an osmotic agent to decrease possible constipation
   a. Medication works to exchange Na^+ with potassium in GI tract and excrete resin formed with K^+ in the stool
   b. Sorbitol 70% can also be used as a cation exchange resin and is available in both oral and rectal forms
2. Intravenous medications
   a. Calcium gluconate
      1) Antagonizes effect of K^+ on myocardium and decreases myocardial irritability
      2) Calcium administration does not promote K^+ loss, thus it only temporarily manages symptoms
      3) Carefully monitor clients who are taking digoxin because calcium administration can promote digitalis toxicity

        b. Regular insulin and dextrose (usually 50%) solution

            1) Combination therapy is used to shift K^+ from ECF to ICF

            2) This is not a long-term treatment method but rather an emergency treatment to reduce K^+ level

        c. Sodium bicarbonate

            1) Makes cells more alkaline (elevating pH); should only be used with documented acidosis unresponsive to other treatment such as proper ventilation

            2) Shifts K^+ back into cells (transcellular shifting), and therefore is used to temporarily manage symptoms

    3. Diuretic therapy with K^+-wasting diuretics (loop, thiazide, and thiazide like diuretics) will promote K^+ excretion from renal tubules

    4. Aerosolized beta$_2$ agonist will drive K^+ into cells

    5. In presence of Addison disease, hydrocortisone succinate can be given via IV initially, then hydrocortisone by mouth plus fludrocortisone acetate

I. Client education

    1. Awareness of predisposing factors

        a. Older adult clients are at risk for hyperkalemia due to multiple medication profile as are clients with multiple disease profiles (such as diabetes and renal failure)

        b. Clients taking medications that promote K^+ retention should have periodic lab testing to determine serum levels

        c. Teach clients potential signs and symptoms of hyperkalemia and have them report problems to healthcare provider

    2. Dietary education

        a. Teach foods to avoid and permissible foods that contain very little K^+

        b. Teach clients to examine food labels and medication packages to determine K^+ content

        c. Teach clients to avoid salt substitutes

J. Evaluation

    1. Client returns to and maintains normal serum potassium level

    2. Client adheres to drug and diet therapies as prescribed

    3. Client states early signs and symptoms of hyperkalemia

    4. Client maintains adequate gas exchange

    5. Client maintains regular cardiac rate and rhythm

Case Study

A 68-year-old male client is admitted to the hospital after experiencing diarrhea for 3 days. The client reports being weak and feels like his heart is racing.

1. What questions will the nurse ask when assessing the client's medical history?

2. What other manifestations might be present?

3. What laboratory and diagnostic tests might be prescribed for this client?

4. What type of medical interventions would the nurse expect this client to receive?

5. What information will be provided to this client by the nurse before being discharged and what are the most effective teaching methods for this client?

For suggested responses, see page 191.

POSTTEST

1 Which serum potassium level would the nurse anticipate seeing in a child with a 3-day history of diarrhea?

1. 3.0 mEq/L
2. 3.6 mEq/L
3. 4.1 mEq/L
4. 5.8 mEq/L

---

2 The nurse is instructing a client diagnosed with hyperkalemia about foods to avoid. Which client statement indicates to the nurse a need for further instruction?

1. "I should avoid eating a lot of bananas."
2. "It will be nice to be able to eat lots of fresh tomatoes this summer."
3. "I will avoid using salt substitutes instead of real salt."
4. "It seems I will not be eating any more avocado salads."

---

3 A client is admitted to the hospital with a serum potassium level of 2.8 mEq/L. The nurse anticipates that client assessment will reveal which findings? Select all that apply.

1. Elastic skin turgor
2. Sinus rhythm at a rate of 76 beats/min
3. Two loose stools during the last 8 hours
4. Muscle weakness
5. Nausea and vomiting

---

4 The nurse instructs a client receiving hydrochloro-thiazide to report which symptoms to the healthcare provider? Select all that apply.

1. Leg cramps
2. Muscle weakness
3. Fatigue
4. Irritability
5. Anorexia

---

5 Which food should the nurse instruct the client with hyperkalemia from end stage renal disease (ESRD) to avoid?

1. Bread
2. Cantaloupe
3. Green beans
4. Apple juice

---

6 A client with a serum potassium level of 3.6 mEq/L is prescribed an IV with a potassium supplement (KCl) via a peripheral line. The nurse checks to determine that the amount of KCl prescribed does not exceed the standard hourly replacement rate of _____ mEq/hr. Record your answer rounding to the nearest whole number.

Fill in your answer below:
_____ mEq/hr

---

7 The nurse concludes that a client understands the side effects of furosemide and its relationship to potassium levels when the client makes which statement?

1. "I do not need to take my pulse anymore when I take my digoxin."
2. "I should call the doctor if I develop diarrhea."
3. "I should call my doctor if I feel myself becoming dizzy when I stand up."
4. "I do not need to eat bananas for breakfast anymore because I am taking this medication."

8 The nurse provides which instruction to a client going home with a prescription for spironolactone?

1. "Be sure to take this medication on an empty stomach."
2. "Take this pill just before you go to bed."
3. "Cut back on your intake of foods on your list that are high in potassium."
4. "You do not have to watch your intake of fluid while you are taking this medicine."

9 The nurse identifies which clients admitted to the hospital to be at risk for developing hypokalemia? Select all that apply.

1. A client whose arterial blood gases indicate metabolic acidosis
2. A client who had developed metabolic alkalosis
3. A client with acute renal failure
4. A client with adult respiratory distress syndrome (ARDS)
5. The client with a nasogastric tube to low intermittent suction

10 The nurse plans to administer which intravenous (IV) treatment to a client for treatment of hyperkalemia associated with severe acidosis?

1. Calcium gluconate to shift potassium from intracellular fluid (ICF) to extracellular fluid (ECF)
2. Insulin and dextrose to make client hypoglycemic
3. Sodium bicarbonate to make client alkalotic so potassium will shift into ICF
4. Normal saline (NS) to provide extra sodium so potassium will move out of ICF into ECF

➤ *See pages 78–79 for Answers and Rationales.*

ANSWERS & RATIONALES

Pretest

1 **Answer: 4, 5 Rationale:** Potassium is lost when taking a loop diuretic such as furosemide; a level of 3.1 mEq/L is below the normal range. A level of 2.8 mEq/L is well below the normal range. A level of 5.4 mEq/L is elevated, reflecting retention of potassium. A potassium level of 4.3 mEq/L is within the normal range. A potassium level of 3.7 mEq/L is within the normal range. **Cognitive Level:** Analyzing **Client Need:** Reduction of Risk Potential **Integrated Process:** Nursing Process: Assessment **Content Area:** Adult Health **Strategy:** The core issue of the question is recognition of low potassium levels in a client taking a potassium-losing diuretic. Evaluate each level as a true–false statement to choose the values that are below the normal range. **Reference:** LeMone, P., Burke, K., Bauldoff, G., & Gubrud, P. (2015). *Medical surgical nursing: Clinical reasoning in patient care* (6th ed.). New York, NY: Pearson, p. 196.

2 **Answer: 3 Rationale:** Potassium can irritate the stomach and should be taken just after eating. Many potassium supplements are time released and should not be crushed. To prevent gastric irritation, oral potassium supplements should be taken with 120 mL (at least 4 oz) of fluid or with food. Salt substitutes may contain potassium and, if taken with a potassium supplement, could cause hyperkalemia. **Cognitive Level:** Applying **Client Need:** Pharmacological and Parenteral Therapies **Integrated Process:** Teaching and Learning **Content Area:** Adult Health **Strategy:** Recall that potassium should not be crushed and is irritating to the stomach to eliminate two options. Recall that salt substitutes contain potassium to eliminate a third option. Note that two options are opposites, indicating that one could be true. **Reference:** LeMone, P., Burke, K., Bauldoff, G., & Gubrud, P. (2015). *Medical surgical nursing: Clinical reasoning in patient care* (6th ed.). New York, NY: Pearson, pp. 197–198.

3 **Answer: 1 Rationale:** Clients with renal failure have difficulty excreting potassium, leading to its accumulation in the bloodstream. Clients with cirrhosis tend to retain sodium and lose potassium, which would contribute to hypokalemia. Intestinal and nasogastric suctioning lead to the loss of potassium and hypokalemia. Potassium is lost with diarrhea, leading to hypokalemia. **Cognitive Level:** Analyzing **Client Need:** Physiological Adaptation **Integrated Process:** Nursing Process: Evaluation **Content Area:** Adult Health **Strategy:** The critical word is *hyperkalemia*. Review ways in which potassium is lost from the body to eliminate two options and choose the correct one. **Reference:** LeMone, P., Burke, K., Bauldoff, G., & Gubrud, P. (2015). *Medical surgical nursing: Clinical reasoning in patient care* (6th ed.). New York, NY: Pearson, p. 202.

4 **Answer: 1 Rationale:** A potassium level of 6.8 mEq/L is a critically high potassium level and could cause life-threatening cardiac arrhythmias; an ECG should be obtained. Although the client's level of consciousness may be affected by the hyperkalemia and decreased cardiac output, this is not of highest priority. The client with renal failure has a decreased urinary output that needs to be measured, but this is not the most critical nursing intervention with this critically high potassium level. Arterial blood gases may be indicated to determine state of acidosis and respiratory status, but is not a greater priority than obtaining an ECG. **Cognitive Level:** Analyzing **Client Need:** Reduction of Risk Potential **Integrated Process:** Nursing Process: Implementation **Content Area:** Adult Health **Strategy:** The critical words are *highest priority*. Eliminate one option since the client is in renal failure. Remember ABCs—airway, breathing, and circulation—to choose the correct option. **Reference:** LeMone, P., Burke, K., Bauldoff, G., & Gubrud, P. (2015). *Medical surgical nursing: Clinical reasoning in patient care* (6th ed.). New York, NY: Pearson, p. 202.

5 **Answer: 1, 5 Rationale:** Hydrochlorothiazide is a potassium-losing diuretic, so potassium supplementation may be indicated. Furosemide is a loop diuretic, which is potassium-wasting. Spironolactone is a potassium-sparing diuretic that does not require dietary supplementation of potassium. Triamterene with hydrochlorothiazide is a combination diuretic so dietary potassium supplementation would not be indicated. Amiloride is a potassium-sparing diuretic that does not require potassium supplementation in the diet. **Cognitive Level:** Analyzing **Client Need:** Pharmacological and Parenteral Therapies **Integrated Process:** Teaching and Learning **Content Area:** Pharmacology **Strategy:** The question is testing knowledge of potassium-wasting diuretics. Recall that thiazide and loop diuretics decrease potassium to choose correctly. **Reference:** LeMone, P., Burke, K., Bauldoff, G., & Gubrud, P. (2015). *Medical surgical nursing: Clinical*

reasoning in patient care (6th ed.). New York, NY: Pearson, p. 196.

6 **Answer: 2 Rationale:** A potassium level of 6.2 mEq/L reflects hyperkalemia. An ECG tracing associated with this electrolyte imbalance shows tall, tented T waves, which occur during repolarization of the cardiac conduction system. Normal sinus rhythm is a normal rhythm. Premature atrial contractions are not caused by hyperkalemia. Atrial fibrillation has a variety of causes, but hyperkalemia is not among them. **Cognitive Level:** Analyzing **Client Need:** Physiological Adaptation **Integrated Process:** Nursing Process: Diagnosis **Content Area:** Adult Health **Strategy:** First identify that a potassium level of 6.2mEq/L is elevated. Recall the ECG changes associated with hyperkalemia to choose the correct option. **Reference:** LeMone, P., Burke, K., Bauldoff, G., & Gubrud, P. (2015). *Medical surgical nursing: Clinical reasoning in patient care* (6th ed.). New York, NY: Pearson, pp. 200–201.

7 **Answer: 2 Rationale:** Hypokalemia can lead to alterations in smooth muscle functioning. Smooth muscle alterations in the gastrointestinal tract can lead to development of a paralytic ileus. Hyperkalemia, not hypokalemia, is associated with renal failure. Diabetes can lead to an increased potassium level if it causes diabetic nephropathy. A perforated bowel is more likely to lead to an increased potassium level. **Cognitive Level:** Analyzing **Client Need:** Physiological Adaptation **Integrated Process:** Nursing Process: Assessment **Content Area:** Adult Health **Strategy:** Recall action of potassium on body systems and its action on the neuromuscular system to choose the correct option. **Reference:** LeMone, P., Burke, K., Bauldoff, G., & Gubrud, P. (2015). *Medical surgical nursing: Clinical reasoning in patient care* (6th ed.). New York, NY: Pearson, pp. 196–197.

8 **Answer: 3 Rationale:** Calcium gluconate is given to antagonize the effects of potassium on the conduction system of the heart. Diuretics would increase urine output. Loose bowel movements are not caused or affected by calcium gluconate. Weak relaxed muscles do not indicate resolving hyperkalemia. **Cognitive Level:** Analyzing **Client Need:** Pharmacological and Parenteral Therapies **Integrated Process:** Nursing Process: Evaluation **Content Area:** Adult Health **Strategy:** The question requires recall of the use in calcium in treating hyperkalemia. Eliminate three options that are not relevant to the use of the drug in relation to hyperkalemia. **Reference:** LeMone, P., Burke, K., Bauldoff, G., & Gubrud, P. (2015). *Medical surgical nursing: Clinical reasoning in patient care* (6th ed.). New York, NY: Pearson, p. 201.

9 **Answer: 2 Rationale:** Bran flakes are not a source of potassium in the diet. It is important for the client to communicate to the healthcare provider if symptoms of hypokalemia, such as muscle cramps or weakness, develop during the course of therapy. Bananas and cantaloupe are excellent sources of dietary potassium. Taking potassium supplements on a full stomach will help to minimize gastric irritation, which is commonly associated with this medication. **Cognitive Level:** Analyzing **Client Need:** Reduction of Risk Potential **Integrated Process:** Teaching and Learning **Content Area:** Adult Health **Strategy:** The wording of the question has a negative stem, which indicates that the correct response is an incorrect statement. Recall that bran is not a good source of potassium, to choose bran as the correct response to the question. **Reference:** LeMone, P., Burke, K., Bauldoff, G., & Gubrud, P. (2015). *Medical surgical nursing: Clinical reasoning in patient care* (6th ed.). New York, NY: Pearson, pp. 198, 200.

10 **Answer: 3 Rationale:** Potassium works to maintain cardiac contractility and normal heart rate, which affects cardiac output and blood pressure; insufficient cardiac output can lead to orthostatic hypotension and dizziness. There is no information in the question to support that the client was on bedrest for a prolonged amount of time. Dizziness is not a symptom directly associated with the potassium level. The explanation about potassium level affecting the nervous system is vague and does not relate directly to the source of the client's dizziness. **Cognitive Level:** Analyzing **Client Need:** Physiological Adaptation **Integrated Process:** Communication and Documentation **Content Area:** Adult Health **Strategy:** The question asks for the best answer, indicating that all options may be completely or partially correct, but one is better. Eliminate one option since it does not relate to potassium. Eliminate two other options since they do not address the source or correct reason for the client's dizziness. **Reference:** LeMone, P., Burke, K., Bauldoff, G., & Gubrud, P. (2015). *Medical surgical nursing: Clinical reasoning in patient care* (6th ed.). New York, NY: Pearson, pp. 198–199.

Posttest

1 **Answer: 1 Rationale:** A client who has diarrhea will be more likely to develop hypokalemia. A serum potassium of 3.0 mEq/L indicates hypokalemia. A level of 3.6 mEq/L is just within the normal range but one would expect a greater K+ loss given the client's history of 3 days of diarrhea. A level of 4.1 mEq/L is within the normal range and does not reflect potassium loss. A level of 5.8 mEq/L reflects hyperkalemia. **Cognitive Level:** Applying **Client Need:** Reduction of Risk Potential **Integrated Process:** Nursing Process: Assessment **Content Area:** Child Health **Strategy:** Critical words are *3-day history of diarrhea*. Review normal potassium levels and recall that potassium is lost with diarrhea to choose the lowest level. **Reference:** LeMone, P., Burke, K., Bauldoff, G., &

Gubrud, P. (2015). *Medical surgical nursing: Clinical reasoning in patient care* (6th ed.). New York, NY: Pearson, pp. 200–203.

2 **Answer: 2 Rationale:** Tomatoes are high in potassium and should be limited in a client with hyperkalemia. The client statement about eating lots of tomatoes indicates a need for further teaching. The client should avoid eating many bananas, which are high in potassium. Salt substitutes tend to be high in potassium and should be avoided during hyperkalemia. Avocadoes are high in potassium and should be limited in a client with hyperkalemia. **Cognitive Level:** Applying **Client Need:** Reduction of Risk Potential **Integrated Process:** Teaching and Learning **Content Area:** Adult Health **Strategy:** Review foods high in potassium. Note the question asks for need for further instruction and look for the one incorrect response. **Reference:** LeMone, P., Burke, K., Bauldoff, G., & Gubrud, P. (2015). *Medical surgical nursing: Clinical reasoning in patient care* (6th ed.). New York, NY: Pearson, pp. 200–203.

3 **Answer: 4, 5 Rationale:** A serum level of 2.8 mEq/L reflects hypokalemia, which affects the resting potential of cell membranes, leading to skeletal muscle weakness. Nausea and vomiting can result from slowed peristalsis of the GI tract because of the effect of hypokalemia on smooth muscle cell membranes. Elastic skin turgor is a normal finding. Hypokalemia can cause cardiac dysrhythmias, while sinus rhythm at a rate of 76 beats/min is normal. The client would be more likely to have decreased bowel sounds and ileus because of hypokalemia, not loose stools. **Cognitive Level:** Analyzing **Client Need:** Reduction of Risk Potential **Integrated Process:** Nursing Process: Assessment **Content Area:** Adult Health **Strategy:** Recognize the value is indicative of severe hypokalemia. Eliminate one option since findings are normal and two other options since they are not as severe as those in the correct option. **Reference:** LeMone, P., Burke, K., Bauldoff, G., & Gubrud, P. (2015). *Medical surgical nursing: Clinical reasoning in patient care* (6th ed.). New York, NY: Pearson, pp. 196–200.

4 **Answer: 1, 2, 5 Rationale:** Hydrochlorothiazide is a potassium-wasting diuretic, and its use can lead to hypokalemia. Leg cramps can occur in a client with hypokalemia. Muscle weakness can be seen in a client with hypokalemia. Generalized fatigue is not a manifestation of hypokalemia. Irritability is not a sign of hypokalemia. Anorexia can occur in a client with hypokalemia because of its effect on smooth muscle cells of the GI tract. **Cognitive Level:** Analyzing **Client Need:** Pharmacological and Parenteral Therapies **Integrated Process:** Teaching and Learning **Content Area:** Pharmacology **Strategy:** Recall that hydrochlorothiazide is a potassium-wasting diuretic to direct you to options consistent with hypokalemia. **Reference:** LeMone, P.,

Burke, K., Bauldoff, G., & Gubrud, P. (2015). *Medical surgical nursing: Clinical reasoning in patient care* (6th ed.). New York, NY: Pearson, pp. 196–200.

5 **Answer: 2 Rationale:** Clients with ESRD are unable to excrete potassium and need to restrict intake of foods high in potassium. Cantaloupes are very high in potassium and should be avoided. Bread is not high in potassium and does not need to be restricted. Green beans are not a significant source of potassium. Apple juice is not a good source of potassium. **Cognitive Level:** Analyzing **Client Need:** Reduction of Risk Potential **Integrated Process:** Teaching and Learning **Content Area:** Adult Health **Strategy:** The core issue of the question is knowledge of foods that are high in potassium. Recall these foods to choose correctly. **Reference:** LeMone, P., Burke, K., Bauldoff, G., & Gubrud, P. (2015). *Medical surgical nursing: Clinical reasoning in patient care* (6th ed.). New York, NY: Pearson, pp. 200–203.

6 **Answer: 10 Rationale:** The maximum routine rate of infusion for KCl is 10 mEq/hour (may range from 5 to 10) via infusion pump. Clients who are moderately hypokalemic may have potassium administered at a rate between 10 and 20 mEq/hour, but this client is not moderately hypokalemic. Higher concentrations of potassium can be administered via a central line in critically ill clients who are hemodynamically monitored. **Cognitive Level:** Applying **Client Need:** Pharmacological and Parenteral Therapies **Integrated Process:** Nursing Process: Implementation **Content Area:** Adult Health **Strategy:** The critical words are *exceed* and *hourly replacement rate*. Note the question indicates a peripheral line to help you identify an amount that is not high. **Reference:** LeMone, P., Burke, K., Bauldoff, G., & Gubrud, P. (2015). *Medical surgical nursing: Clinical reasoning in patient care* (6th ed.). New York, NY: Pearson, p. 198.

7 **Answer: 3 Rationale:** Furosemide is a potassium-wasting diuretic that can cause the client to become hypokalemic. This can manifest as a weak, thready pulse and onset of orthostatic hypotension. Diarrhea is not usually seen as a side effect of this medication. Monitoring of one's pulse is not required for clients taking diuretic therapy but is necessary for clients taking digoxin or who have a pacemaker. Bananas are a good source of dietary potassium and may be warranted for this client in order to maintain normal serum potassium levels. **Cognitive Level:** Analyzing **Client Need:** Physiological Adaptation **Integrated Process:** Nursing Process: Evaluation **Content Area:** Adult Health **Strategy:** The core concept of the question is the relationship of low potassium to the diuretic. Eliminate two options as these are still important actions to take but do not necessarily indicate the client's understanding. Eliminate a third option that is not a usual effect of furosemide. **Reference:** LeMone, P., Burke, K., Bauldoff, G., &

Gubrud, P. (2015). *Medical surgical nursing: Clinical reasoning in patient care* (6th ed.). New York, NY: Pearson, pp. 197–200.

8 **Answer: 3 Rationale:** Spironolactone is a potassium-sparing diuretic and high intake of potassium-rich foods should be discouraged. Diuretics should be taken with food to decrease GI upset. Clients should not take diuretics before going to bed because this could lead to nocturia and interrupted sleep patterns. Clients taking diuretics should be aware of their fluid intake and monitor accordingly. **Cognitive Level:** Analyzing **Client Need:** Pharmacological and Parenteral Therapies **Integrated Process:** Teaching and Learning **Content Area:** Pharmacology **Strategy:** Recall knowledge of potassium-sparing diuretics to choose correctly. **Reference:** Adams, M. P., Holland, N., & Urban, C. (2017). *Pharmacology for nurses: A pathophysiologic approach* (5th ed.). New York, NY: Pearson, pp. 305–306.

9 **Answer: 2, 5 Rationale:** A client with metabolic alkalosis is at risk for developing hypokalemia because of the shift of potassium to ICF from ECF. Clients with NG tubes lose potassium from the stomach and the NPO status limits their intake. Clients with acute renal failure are usually hyperkalemic due to a decreased ability to excrete potassium. Clients with ARDS are usually hyperkalemic due to compromised ventilation, resulting in acidosis from hypoxia. Metabolic acidosis is associated with hyperkalemia because potassium shifts from ECF to ICF when there is increased hydrogen ion concentration. **Cognitive Level:** Analyzing **Client Need:** Physiological Adaptation **Integrated Process:** Nursing Process: Assessment **Content Area:** Adult Health **Strategy:** Recall knowledge of conditions in which potassium is lost or shifts into the cell to choose the correct options. **Reference:** LeMone, P., Burke, K., Bauldoff, G., & Gubrud, P. (2015). *Medical surgical nursing: Clinical reasoning in patient care* (6th ed.). New York, NY: Pearson, pp. 221–222.

10 **Answer: 3 Rationale:** Sodium bicarbonate will temporarily alkalinize the plasma, causing the potassium to move into the cells. NS is an isotonic solution and therefore will not cause fluid or electrolyte shifting. Calcium gluconate is given to blunt the effects on the myocardium; it does not decrease the serum K^+ level. Insulin and dextrose are given to decrease K^+ levels by increasing K^+ uptake at the cellular level. **Cognitive Level:** Applying **Client Need:** Reduction of Risk Potential **Integrated Process:** Nursing Process: Planning **Content Area:** Adult Health **Strategy:** A critical word is *acidosis*. Recall that potassium is increased in acidosis to direct you to the option in which alkalosis is the goal of treatment. **Reference:** LeMone, P., Burke, K., Bauldoff, G., & Gubrud, P. (2015). *Medical surgical nursing: Clinical reasoning in patient care* (6th ed.). New York, NY: Pearson, pp. 219–222.

ANSWERS & RATIONALES

References

Adams, M., Holland, N., & Urban, C. (2017). *Pharmacology for nurses: A pathophysiologic approach* (5th ed.). New York, NY: Pearson.

Ball, J., Bindler, R., & Cowen, K. (2014). *Child health nursing: Partnering with children and families* (3rd ed.). Upper Saddle River, NJ: Pearson.

Berman, A., Snyder, S., & Frandsen, G. (2016). *Kozier&Erb's fundamentals of nursing: Concepts, process, and practice* (10th ed.). New York, NY: Pearson.

Ignatavicius, D., & Workman, M. (2015). *Medical-surgical nursing: Patient-centered collaborative care* (8th ed.). Philadelphia, PA: Elsevier Saunders.

Kee, J. L. (2017). *Pearson handbook of laboratory and diagnostic tests* (8th ed.). New York, NY: Pearson.

LeMone, P., Burke, K., Bauldoff, G., & Gubrud, P. (2015). *Medical surgical nursing: Clinical reasoning in patient care* (6th ed.). New York, NY: Pearson.

London, M., Ladewig, P., Davidson, M., Ball, J., Bindler, R., & Cowen, K. (2017). *Maternal and child nursing care* (5th ed.). New York, NY: Pearson.

Calcium Balance and Imbalances

4

Chapter Outline

Overview of Calcium Regulation

Hypocalcemia

Hypercalcemia

Objectives

➤ Identify the basic functions of calcium in the body.
➤ Explain the pathophysiology and etiology of calcium imbalances.
➤ Identify specific assessment findings in calcium imbalances.
➤ Identify priority nursing concerns for a client experiencing a calcium imbalance.
➤ Describe the therapeutic management of calcium imbalances.
➤ Describe the management of nursing care for a client who is experiencing a calcium imbalance.

NCLEX-RN® Test Prep

Access the NEW Web-based app that provides students with additional practice questions in preparation for the NCLEX experience.

Review at a Glance

calcitonin also called thyrocalcitonin; a calcium-lowering hormone produced by thyroid gland that lowers calcium by inhibiting bone-resorbing osteoclasts and promoting osteoblasts that lead to bone formation

calcitriol active hormone form of vitamin D; promotes absorption of calcium in intestines, decreases calcium excretion via kidneys, and acts with PTH to maintain homeostasis

calcium pump a "pump" driven by ATP that takes calcium into and out of cells; initiated by mechanical or electrical stimulus during relaxation and contraction of skeletal muscles (involves a change in membrane potential) and smooth muscle (intracellular calcium causes contraction)

Chvostek sign tapping over facial nerve just anterior to ear that causes ipsilateral facial muscle contraction or twitching; indicates a positive response and is a sign of hypocalcemia; a form of latent tetany

hypercalcemia increased total serum calcium concentration to >10.5 mg/dL

hyperparathyroidism a condition caused by excess levels of

parathyroid hormone, demonstrated by a PTH >55 pg/dL

hypocalcemia decreased total serum calcium concentration to <8.5 mg/dL; any condition that causes a decrease in PTH production may lead to hypocalcemia

hypoparathyroidism a condition caused by insufficient or absent secretion of parathyroid glands, demonstrated by a PTH level <11 pg/dL

ionized calcium represents approximately 40–50% of calcium that is free or not bound to albumin; calcium level that is physiologically useful and elicits the signs and symptoms of hypocalcemia

osteoblasts bone-forming cells that lay down new bone; responsive to PTH and are stimulated by activated vitamin D; adapt to stress on bone by strengthening bone mass; a form of osteocyte

osteoclasts cells that resorb (remove) calcium from bone during processes of bone growth and repair; derived from monocytes produced in bone marrow; monocytes travel through bloodstream and collect at sites of bone resorption, where they fuse together to become osteocytes (cells that erode old bone)

osteoporosis reduction of bone mass (or density) or presence of a fragility fracture

parathyroid hormone (PTH) hormone produced by parathyroid glands; regulates serum calcium via a negative feedback system; main role is to increase serum calcium by stimulating bone resorption, increasing renal calcium absorption, and promoting renal conversion of vitamin D to its active metabolite, calcitriol; under normal conditions, when calcium is low, PTH increases; conversely, when calcium is high, PTH decreases; normal PTH level is 11–55 pg/dL

tetany neurologic disorder marked by intermittent spasms that are usually paroxysmal and involve extremities; calls for immediate intervention

Trousseau sign inflation of a blood pressure cuff on upper arm to 20 mm Hg above client's systolic pressure for about 3 minutes leads to carpal spasm; a form of latent tetany

vitamin D a fat-soluble vitamin absorbed from food and synthesized in skin exposed to sunlight

PRETEST

1 The nurse is preparing to administer alendronate to a client with osteoporosis secondary to hypercalcemia. Place the interventions in the correct order in which the nurse should perform them.

1. Ensure that the client did not eat or drink any fluids except water.
2. Place client in an upright position.
3. Determine history of GERD or other condition predisposing the client to esophageal reflux.
4. Prepare the correct dose of the medication.
5. Instruct the client to drink a full glass of water with the medication.

2 Keeping in mind the potential electrolyte imbalances possible with DiGeorge syndrome, the nurse plans to implement which nursing intervention when caring for an infant with this diagnosis? Select all that apply.

1. Place the infant on seizure precautions.
2. Position the infant on the right side.
3. Provide additional padding in the bassinette.
4. Place the infant in a prone position.
5. Provide additional oral stimulation to the infant.

3 A client develops hypocalcemia as a result of prolonged nasogastric (NG) tube suctioning. The nurse concludes that what physiological alteration is the primary cause for hypocalcemia at this time?

1. Metabolic alkalosis
2. Fluid shifts from hypoalbuminemia
3. Hypermagnesemia
4. Metabolic acidosis

4 A client has a diagnosis of ovarian cancer and is undergoing chemotherapy. After noting that the client's serum calcium level is 11.8 mg/dL, the nurse should draw which conclusion?

1. Antineoplastic medications are the cause of this elevation in calcium.
2. The ovarian cancer may have metastasized, causing the increase in calcium.
3. The client is not eating enough dairy products as a result of decreased appetite.
4. The client is developing pancreatitis.

5 A client with hypocalcemia has been started on intravenous (IV) corticosteroids. Which findings would indicate a further decrease in calcium level in the client? Select all that apply.

1. Carpal spasm while blood pressure cuff inflated
2. Twitching of cheek muscles
3. Muscle weakness
4. Frequent urination
5. Intermittent headaches

6 When assessing a client with hypercalcemia, the nurse concludes that which findings in the neuromuscular examination are consistent with this electrolyte imbalance? Select all that apply.

1. Tetany
2. A positive Trousseau sign
3. A negative Chvostek sign
4. Muscle weakness
5. Hyperactive deep tendon reflexes

7 When caring for a client with hypercalcemia who is on a cardiac monitor, the nurse checks the cardiac rhythm strip for which typical change?

1. Development of atrial fibrillation
2. Shortening of the QT interval
3. Shortening of the PR interval
4. Peaked T wave

8 A nurse prepares to administer calcium gluconate to a client post-thyroidectomy. The nurse explains to the licensed practical/vocational nurse (LPN/LVN) that this medication is being given for which reason?

1. Because of accidental removal of the parathyroid gland
2. Because it is related to increased parathyroid hormone (PTH) release during surgery
3. To prevent complications from immobility postoperatively
4. Because of hypophosphatemia after this type of surgery

9 A client presents with reports of fatigue, headache, and increasing muscle weakness, and has blood-work drawn to evaluate the serum calcium level. The nurse anticipates medical management for an abnormal value to include which therapeutic intervention?

1. Thiazide diuretics
2. Vitamin D supplements
3. Fluid restriction
4. Increased hydration

10 The nurse evaluates that discharge teaching has been effective when the client with hypocalcemia makes which statement?

1. "I shouldn't take antacids such as Tums."
2. "I should notify my healthcare provider if I feel tingling or numbness around my mouth."
3. "I will need to cut down on the amount of protein I include in my diet each day."
4. "I will watch my urine for signs of kidney stones."

➤ *See pages 100–101 for Answers and Rationales.*

I. OVERVIEW OF CALCIUM REGULATION

    A. Calcium balance and function: major extracellular cation; mainly found in hard part of bones where it is stored; calcium concentration is kept constant by a **calcium pump** that constantly moves calcium in and out of cells

      1. Serum levels

        a. Normal total serum concentration is approximately 8.5–10.5 mg/dL

        b. Ionized calcium level is 4.0–5.0 mg/dL

        c. Slightly different laboratory reference ranges may appear due to differences in laboratory calibration; always check reference ranges with agency's laboratory norms

        d. Three forms of calcium exist in body

          1) Forty-five percent is bound to protein, mostly albumin; part of total serum calcium concentration

          2) Forty percent is **ionized calcium** (free or unbound from proteins, specifically albumin), which is physiologically active and clinically important for neuro-muscular transmission; many symptoms of low calcium are often not apparent until ionized calcium is <4.0 mg/dL; although many laboratories most commonly measure total serum calcium level, ionized calcium level is recommended for a critically ill client

          3) 15% is bound to other substances such as phosphate, citrate, or carbonate

        e. Serum protein concentration, specifically albumin, is an important determinant of calcium concentration; remember to evaluate calcium in relation to serum albumin because changes in serum protein level can cause changes in serum calcium level

        f. Certain formulas can be used to obtain a calcium level corrected for an albumin level; for example, total serum calcium will decrease or increase 0.8 mg/dL for every 1 gram/dL decrease or increase in albumin above or below 4 grams/dL

2. Functions in body
   a. Important in enzyme activation to stimulate many essential chemical reactions required for hormone secretion and the function of cell receptors
   b. Significant role in skeletal and heart muscle relaxation, activation, excitation, and contraction
   c. Exerts a sedating, or calming, effect on nerve cells
   d. Plays a major role in nerve impulse transmission as it determines speed of ionic influxes through nerve membranes
   e. Plays a role in blood clotting by activating specific steps as an enzymatic cofactor in blood coagulation (most important is conversion of prothrombin to thrombin)
   f. Assists in regulation of acid–base balance
   g. Gives firmness and rigidity to bones and teeth
   h. Maintains cell membrane permeability
   i. Essential for lactation
3. System interactions
   a. **Parathyroid hormone (PTH)** raises plasma calcium level by promoting transfer of calcium from bone to plasma
      1) PTH responds to ionized calcium level, regulates calcium concentration in ECF, and has bone-resorbing (removal of calcium from bone) effects
      2) PTH helps with intestinal absorption of calcium by activating **vitamin D** (a fat-soluble vitamin)
      3) PTH also aids in calcium reabsorption in kidneys
      4) Overall effect of PTH is to increase calcium and decrease phosphorus
      5) Under normal conditions, PTH responds to changes inionized calcium via a negative feedback system; if ionized calcium level is low, PTH will be elevated; conversely, if ionized calcium level is high, PTH will be low
      6) Normal PTH level is 11–54 pg/mL

Practice to Pass

Can you identify the system interactions that control calcium concentrations in the body?

   b. Calcium is dependent upon **calcitriol** (most active form of vitamin D)
      1) Calcitriol makes calcium and phosphate available for new bone formation
      2) Calcitriol plays a major role in preventing symptomatic **hypocalcemia** (abnormally low serum calcium level) and hypomagnesemia (decreased serum magnesium, clinically noted by increased neuromuscular irritability)
      3) Calcitriol also promotes calcium absorption from intestine (duodenum), helps PTH mobilize calcium from bone, and limits calcium excretion if client has hypocalcemia
   c. **Calcitonin**, a calcium-lowering hormone produced by thyroid gland, acts against PTH by transferring calcium from plasma to skeletal system
      1) Calcitonin is directly secreted when serum calcium level is high (**hypercalcemia**), to lower plasma calcium level
      2) Calcitonin inhibits osteoclastic activity and promotes osteoblasts that result in bone formation; **osteoclasts** resorb (remove) bone during process of growth and repair, whereas **osteoblasts** are bone-forming cells that respond to PTH, which in turn is stimulated by activated form of vitamin D
   d. Calcium interferes with iron absorption, so clients with high calcium levels may be prone to iron deficiency and need iron supplements
   e. Calcium has inverse or reciprocal relationship with phosphorus; when calcium goes up, phosphorus levels go down; conversely, when calcium levels decrease, phosphorus levels increase
4. See Table 4-1 for lifespan factors affecting calcium balance

B. **Sources of calcium**
   1. Cellular level
      a. Over 99% of body calcium is deposited in bones, but can be mobilized from bones to keep blood level constant when dietary intake is inadequate

Table 4-1	Lifespan Considerations for Health Maintenance: Calcium Balance	
Lifespan Considerations	**Common Risk Factors for Imbalances**	**Nursing Implications**
Infants	*Hypocalcemia* DiGeorge syndrome: immaturity of parathyroid glands in first few days of life *Hypercalcemia* Excessive use of cow's milk	Assess infants with DiGeorge syndrome for signs of hypocalcemia A deficit of calcium in bones; may not be able to make up later in life Newborns may exhibit flaccid muscles or failure to thrive
Children	*Hypocalcemia* DiGeorge syndrome *Hypercalcemia* Prolonged immobilization following surgery, trauma, casting Excessive intake of calcium-rich foods	Assess for signs of increased neuromuscular excitability and muscle cramps Institute seizure precautions Assess child for signs of decreased cardiac output, decreased level of consciousness, constipation, and neuromuscular impairment Child may exhibit activity intolerance and/or developmental delay Child is at increased risk for injury and spontaneous fractures Teach parents to avoid giving excessive amounts of calcium-rich foods
Adults	*Hypocalcemia* Excessive use of magnesium-based antacids Renal failure *Hypercalcemia* Thiazide diuretics	Instruct clients to avoid use of magnesium-based antacids Review common OTC names containing magnesium Instruct on foods high in calcium Encourage liberal intake of fluids Assess client for signs of renal calculi Instruct client to avoid excessive use of calcium-based antacids

        b. The <1% outside bone is located in extracellular fluid and soft tissues

        c. A total of 1–2 kg of calcium is present in an average adult

        d. Calcium pump helps to regulate flow of calcium at cellular level

        e. Thirty percent is absorbed in GI tract

        f. In kidneys, 98% of filtered calcium is reabsorbed in proximal renal tubules, and rest is excreted by kidneys; reabsorption rates of filtered calcium are high

    2. Dietary level

        a. Calcium is obtained from ingested foods; about 40% of calcium consumed is absorbed

        b. Adults should consume at least 1000–1200 mg (1–1.2 grams) of calcium daily

        c. Daily calcium requirement for infants is 270 mg, children 1–3 years need 500 mg, children 4–8 years require 800 mg, and children 9–18 years require 1300 mg

        d. Pregnant, lactating, and postmenopausal women should consume 1.2–1.5 grams of calcium daily

        e. Upper limit for calcium intake is 2.5 grams daily

        f. Foods high in dietary calcium include milk, yogurt, cheese, calcium-fortified orange juice, ice cream, canned salmon, sardines, broccoli, tofu, rhubarb, spinach, almonds, figs, and turnip greens

        g. Dietary factors that decrease calcium absorption include oxalic acids found in beets, spinach, and peanuts, phytic acids found in grains, excess phosphorus consumption, and polyphenols (tannins) found in teas (see Box 4-1 for a listing of factors affecting calcium absorption)

Box 4-1	The following factors *promote* calcium absorption:
Factors That Affect Calcium Absorption in the Body	• Vitamin D • Milk products • Adequate stomach acid • Growth hormones
	The following factors *decrease* calcium absorption:
	• Vitamin D deficiency • High intake of phosphorus, protein, and/or fiber in the diet • Phytates, oxalates, and polyphenols (tannins) • Decreased absorption with aging

II. HYPOCALCEMIA

    A. **Definition, etiology, and pathophysiology**

!   1. Serum calcium level below 8.5 mg/dL or ionized calcium below 4 mg/dL

          2. Cellular-level transport

!   a. Moves in and out of cells via a calcium pump

              b. Adds to bone by osteoblasts—bone-forming cells that lay down new bone

              c. Calcium is responsive to PTH and is stimulated by activated vitamin D

          3. Predisposing clinical conditions result from decreased physiological availability of calcium, decreased calcium intake or absorption, or increased calcium excretion (see Box 4-2 for a listing of clinical conditions that can lead to hypocalcemia)

              a. **Hypoparathyroidism**: a condition caused by insufficient or lack of secretion of PTH by parathyroid glands

                  1) Primary (or idiopathic) hypoparathyroidism (rare) is due to tumor, depressed function, or a hereditary disorder; secondary hypoparathyroidism is related to surgical removal of parathyroid glands

                  2) Postsurgical symptoms of hypocalcemia may be due to impaired blood supply to remaining parathyroid tissue or possibly by release of calcitonin from thyroid gland

Practice to Pass

What are the predisposing conditions that lead to calcium imbalance in the body?

Box 4-2	• Hypoparathyroidism
Clinical Conditions That Lead to the Development of Hypocalcemia	• Hypomagnesemia or hyperphosphatemia • Alkalotic states • Multiple blood transfusions (citrate-buffered blood products) • Medications (loop diuretics, antiepileptics, phosphates, antineoplastic agents, radiographic contrast media, corticosteroids, bisphosphonates, antacids, and heparin) • Hypoalbuminemia • Acute pancreatitis • Vitamin D deficiency • Malabsorptive states • Renal disease • Alcoholism • Gram-negative sepsis • Medullary thyroid carcinoma • Burns • Chronic diarrhea • DiGeorge syndrome • Cardiac surgery using cardiopulmonary bypass

     b. Hypomagnesemia: abnormally low magnesium levels (<1 mg/dL)
- **1)** Magnesium helps regulate mechanisms that keep serum calcium within normal; magnesium is needed for synthesis and release of parathormone, or PTH
- **2)** If magnesium is low, PTH release is impaired, lowering serum calcium
- **3)** Hypomagnesemia lowers the threshold for **tetany** (neurologic disorder marked by intermittent spasms, usually paroxysmal, and involves extremities)
- **4)** Hypomagnesemia is also seen with hypokalemia and hypocalcemia
- **5)** Many medications that decrease magnesium also cause hypocalcemia

     c. Alkalosis: an actual or relative increase in alkalinity of blood due to accumulation of bases or reduction in acid (pH >7.45)
- **1)** In alkalosis, more ionized calcium binds to albumin
- **2)** Though serum calcium may be normal, symptoms such as tetany occur due to decrease in physiologically active ionized calcium
- **3)** Tetany may result if the pH rises above 7.6; prolonged nasogastric tube (NGT) suctioning or diarrhea lead to metabolic alkalosis

     d. Massive blood transfusion: citrate is a preservative added to units of red blood cells that acts as an anticoagulant; in massive rapid transfusions, citrate can combine with ionized calcium and render this inactive, leading to a transient hypocalcemia (due to citrate toxicity)

     e. Medications that can lead to development of hypocalcemia are listed in Table 4-2

     f. Hypoalbuminemia (low serum albumin levels <3.5 grams/dL): can result in low total serum calcium concentration although ionized calcium may be normal; signs of hypocalcemia occur when ionized calcium level falls below normal; some causes are malnutrition, malabsorption syndromes, burns, and chronic renal failure

     g. Acute pancreatitis
- **1)** PTH secretion is inadequate with this disorder, thereby preventing uptake of calcium from bones to correct hypocalcemia

Table 4-2   **Medications That Can Lead to Hypocalcemia**

Medication	Action
Loop diuretics	Promote renal excretion of calcium
Phenytoin and phenobarbital	Alter hepatic metabolism of vitamin D
Citrated blood products	Citrate prevents calcium from becoming ionized, causing transient hypocalcemia
Phosphates	Have inverse relationship; increased phosphate levels lead to low calcium levels
Plicamycin, calcitonin, and etidronate disodium	Inhibit bone resorption of calcium
Antineoplastic drugs (cisplatin) and antibiotics (gentamycin and tetracyclines)	Lower magnesium levels, thus lowering calcium levels
Some radiographic contrast media, such as gallium nitrate	Inhibit bone resorption
Corticosteroids in large doses	Intestinal calcium absorption is reduced; renal calcium excretion is increased
Bisphosphonates in excessive doses	Inhibit bone resorption
Magnesium-containing antacids	Compete with calcium for absorption in the intestines
Heparin, protamine, and glucagon	Promote bone resorption and lead to **osteoporosis**, a condition resulting from a reduction in bone mass or density or presence of a fragility fracture

2) There is also a lack of pancreatic lipase from impaired fat digestion

3) Dietary calcium and calcium secreted into intestine from ECF bind to undigested fat in intestine and are excreted, which results in decreased calcium absorption and increased calcium excretion

4) May also result from secretion of calcitonin when inflamed pancreas secretes excessive glucagon

h. Hyperphosphatemia—excessive phosphorus levels (>4.5 mg/dL): phosphorus has a reciprocal relationship with calcium; is commonly seen in clients with renal failure; may also occur with excess treatment of hypercalcemia, resulting in lowering of calcium; excessive phosphorus in total parenteral nutrition (TPN) may also contribute to hypocalcemia

i. Inadequate vitamin D: due to inadequate dietary consumption, insufficient exposure to sunlight, or malabsorption states; recall that calcium absorption occurs in duodenum only in the presence of activated vitamin D

j. Malabsorption syndromes: may occur when effective intestinal surfaces are lost, making fewer available sites for calcium absorption

1) It is important to remember that calcium absorption occurs primarily in small intestine

2) Conditions such as Crohn disease; procedures such as small bowel resection, partial gastrectomy with gastrojejunostomy, and jejunoileal bypass; or excessive laxative use may interfere with calcium absorption

k. Renal disease: kidneys cannot produce activated form of vitamin D (calcitriol), which leads to reduced absorption of calcium, thus hypocalcemia; retention of phosphorus also helps to decrease calcium levels

l. Alcoholism: may lead to intestinal malabsorption, dietary deficiencies, hypoalbuminemia, pancreatitis, and hypomagnesemia, all of which contribute to decreased calcium levels

m. Neonatal hypocalcemia: due to functional immaturity of parathyroid glands during first 3 days of life; after first 3 days, hypocalcemia may be caused by milk with high phosphate content; those at high risk are those with asphyxia at birth and infants born to mothers with type 1 diabetes mellitus

n. Gram-negative sepsis: leads to a decrease in ionized calcium and as such is a true hypocalcemia; possible causes are parathyroid gland insufficiency, inadequate dietary vitamin D, or renal hydroxylase insufficiency

o. Medullary thyroid carcinoma: may produce hypocalcemia if excess calcitonin is secreted by tumor

p. Burns: fluid shifts outside the cell with burn or wound injuries and large molecules can also be lost, leading to hypoalbuminemia

B. Assessment
1. Clinical manifestations: due to increased neuromuscular irritability (see Table 4-3)
   a. Cardiovascular: decreased blood pressure and myocardial contractility leading to pulse rate and rhythm changes; ECG changes include prolonged QT interval and lengthened ST segment; cardiac arrest can occur
   b. Respiratory: laryngospasm can occur, leading to respiratory compromise and airway failure; respiratory arrest can occur
   c. Renal: low serum calcium levels are associated with renal failure; other electrolyte disturbances are seen in conjunction with clinical manifestations of renal failure
   d. Neuromuscular
   1) Positive **Trousseau sign**: inflation of blood pressure cuff on upper arm to 20 mm above the systolic BP for about 3 minutes results in carpal spasm(see Figure 4-1A)
   2) Positive **Chvostek sign**: tapping over facial nerve just anterior to ear results in ipsilateral facial muscle contracting or twitching (see Figure 4-1B)

Practice to Pass

Explain how the neurologic system is affected by hypocalcemia.

Table 4-3	Comparison of Clinical Manifestations of Hypocalcemia and Hypercalcemia	
System	**Manifestations of Hypocalcemia**	**Manifestations of Hypercalcemia**
Neuromuscular	Parasthesias, muscle spasms, tetany Positive Chvostek and Trousseau signs Hyperactive deep tendon reflexes (DTRs) Laryngospasm	Muscle weakness Increased fatigue Depressed DTRs
Gastrointestinal	Hyperactive bowel sounds Abdominal cramps Diarrhea	Hypotonic bowel sounds Nausea and vomiting Constipation Anorexia
Central nervous system	Irritability Depression Apprehension or anxiety Confusion Delusions Hallucinations Memory impairment Seizures	Headache Personality changes Acute psychosis Bizarre behavior Confusion Lethargy to coma Memory impairment
Cardiac	Hypotension Decreased myocardial contractility Prolonged QT interval Lengthened ST segment Cardiac arrest	Hypertension Heart block Shortened QT interval Shortened ST segment Cardiac arrest
Respiratory	Respiratory arrest	No major manifestations
Renal	Oliguria Anuria	Polyuria Polydipsia Renal colic and kidney stones
Hematologic	Increased bleeding and bruising	No major manifestations
Integumentary	Dry, brittle nails and hair Pathologic fractures	Bone pain Osteomalacia Pathologic fractures

Figure 4-1

A. Positive Trousseau sign.
B. Positive Chvostek sign.

Mary Ann Hogan, *Pearson Reviews & Rationales: Fluids, Electrolytes, & Acid-Base Balance with Nursing Reviews & Rationales*, 4e, © 2019, Pearson Education, Inc., New York, NY.

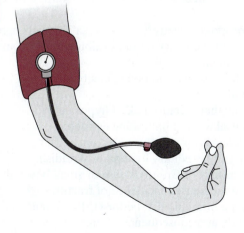

A

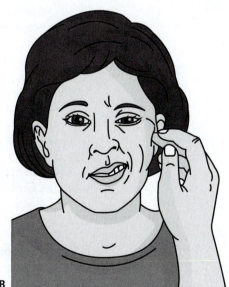

B

3) Above signs are clinical indicators of tetany; characterized by hyperactive deep tendon reflexes; seizures can occur

4) Other: paresthesias and tingling in hands and feet; muscle spasms of extremities and face; hyperactive reflexes and increased irritability and apprehension; mental status changes ranging from depression, memory impairment, delusion, and hallucinations to seizures

  e. Gastrointestinal: possible hyperactive bowel sounds and diarrhea

  f. Musculoskeletal: possible bone fractures due to demineralization; in children, chronic hypocalcemia may retard growth and cause rickets; can lead to osteomalacia and osteoporosis in adults

  g. Other systems: increased bleeding or bruising from abnormal clotting mechanisms; development of cataracts and calcification of basal ganglia; intestinal cramps; dry, brittle nails and hair; bone pain; increased bleeding or bruising may occur

2. Diagnostic and laboratory findings

  a. Plasma levels, urinary levels, and radiology measurements

    1) Total serum calcium level <8.5 mg/dL

    2) Ionized calcium level <4.0 mg/dL or <40%

    3) Twenty-four-hour urinary calcium level (reference levels): low calcium diet <150 mg/24 hours; average calcium diet 100–250 mg/24 hours; high calcium diet 250–300 mg/24 hours; useful for determining parathyroid gland disorders

    4) X-rays to detect bone fractures and thinning

    5) Bone mass density tests for signs of osteoporosis

    6) CT scan to detect tumors of parathyroid gland

  b. Associated electrolyte levels

    1) Hypomagnesemia (<1 mg/dL)

    2) Hypokalemia (<3.5 mg/dL)

    3) Hyperphosphatemia (>2.6 mg/dL)

    4) Albumin <3.5 grams/dL

    5) PTH <11 mg/dL if caused by hypoparathyroidism

    6) Elevated creatinine from renal insufficiency

    7) Elevated alkaline phosphatase

  c. Trending of results

    1) ECG tracings demonstrate characteristic changes with hypocalcemia; trending ECG changes can help to monitor client's status and response to therapeutic treatment

    2) Monitor appropriate electrolyte levels (calcium, phosphorus, magnesium, potassium) and serum chemistry findings (albumin, BUN, and creatinine levels)

    3) Monitor albumin and PTH levels

    4) Review results of x-rays and bone density tests

3. Identification of risk factors

  a. Assess for factors that increase risk of hypocalcemia

    1) Postmenopausal women not taking estrogen

    2) Post-thyroidectomy or parathyroidectomy

    3) Family history of hereditary hypoparathyroidism

    4) Clients with history of Crohn disease or small bowel dysfunction

    5) Clients with an increased incidence of fractures

    6) Clients who are immobile (or bedfast), due to inadequate calcium stores present in body as a consequence of immobility

    7) Clients who have osteoporosis and/or osteopenia

  b. Medications

    1) Obtain pertinent client history of medications that can alter calcium levels

    2) Examine client's prescription and over-the-counter (OTC) medications and supplements for possible interactions

     c. Dietary

       1) Dietary patterns that lack adequate calcium and vitamin D sources

       2) Excessive use of dietary phosphorus supplements

       3) Clients with eating disorders who use laxatives regularly

       4) Lactose-intolerant clients may be at risk for not meeting adequate calcium intake needs unless alternative-form products are used

       5) Dietary factors that limit absorption of calcium (oxalates, phytates, and tannins)

C. Priority nursing concerns: possible decrease in cardiac output, risk for seizure activity and/or tetany, possible respiratory impairment (gas exchange, respiratory arrest), possible fractures (may be associated with osteoporosis), inadequate dietary calcium intake, insufficient client knowledge of condition and management

D. Therapeutic management: treatment focuses on restoring normal levels, preventing complications, and treating underlying problems

  1. Replacement therapies

    a. Calcium gluconate 10% solution, 500 mg to 2 grams at a rate of <0.5 mL/min (10–20 mL) by slow IV push, or calcium chloride 10% solution, 500 mg to 1 gram (5–10 mL) at a rate of <1 mL/min by slow IV push in an emergency

    b. All calcium preparations can cause venous irritation, but calcium chloride causes more venous irritation and may cause sloughing of tissue, so calcium gluconate is the most commonly used preparation

    c. Administer with D_5W or normal saline (NS) and do not add to solutions containing bicarbonate because rapid precipitation may occur

    d. May give slow IV infusion of calcium gluconate until tetany has been controlled or until calcium reaches 8–9 mg/dL

    e. Daily oral doses of elemental calcium, usually 1.0–3.0 grams/day

    f. Postoperative clients may require an additional supplement with calcitriol 0.5–1.0 mcg/dL; dosage range based on cause or complication of hypocalcemia

    g. Vitamin D supplements may be prescribed: 1–3 mg/dL with supplemental calcitriol 0.25–1.0 mcg/dL if hypocalcemia from vitamin D dietary deficiency

    h. Phosphorus-binding antacids may be prescribed to increase calcium

    i. Because magnesium is needed for proper calcium function, if hypomagnesemia is present, it must be corrected by magnesium replacement; see Chapter 5 for detailed information on hypomagnesemia

    j. Thiazide diuretics may be used to decrease urinary excretion of calcium

  2. Continued monitoring of client (laboratory values and physical manifestations) to watch for efficacy of treatment

    a. Continuous ECG monitoring, especially during calcium gluconate or calcium chloride administration

    b. Continually reassess neurologic, respiratory, and cardiac status

    c. Monitor clients receiving calcium replacement who are also on digoxin for enhanced digitalis effect—check pulse

    d. Monitor clients who may experience hypocalcemia as a result of surgical intervention and/or possible endocrine dysfunction

  3. Restoration of balance (normal serum Ca^{++} level) to maintain homeostasis and prevent development of further complications

    a. Monitor serum magnesium and potassium levels in clients who are hypocalcemic because sometimes there can be concurrent electrolyte abnormalities that may require correction

    b. Monitor endocrine function and evaluate PTH status

E. Client-centered nursing care

  1. Obtain thorough nursing history and physical examination

    a. Subjective: such as symptoms, family history, previous thyroid or parathyroid surgeries

      b. Objective: such as signs of hypocalcemia, predisposing clinical conditions that are documented in health record, risk factors

      c. Medication history: medications that may cause hypocalcemia, hypomagnesemia, or hyperphosphatemia; OTC and herbal therapies that may interfere with calcium function

  2. Monitor pertinent client assessment data for potential effects related to hypocalcemia and for response to therapeutic treatment

      a. Monitor serum calcium, phosphate, magnesium, albumin, creatinine, PTH, and potassium levels and report abnormal findings to healthcare provider

      b. ECG changes and heart rate and rhythm pattern

      c. Observe for signs of tetany and document findings relative to Chvostek and Trousseau signs; check reflexes

  3. Monitor therapeutic serum digoxin levels, if applicable, because calcium replacement therapy can enhance effects of digoxin

  4. Assess for signs of dehydration that may result from diarrhea or renal insufficiency

  5. Assess I&O (intake and output): maintain intake of 2000–3000 mL/day and output of 1000–1500 mL/day; monitor daily weight

  6. Protect client from injury and maintain a safe environment, as client is likely to present with neuromuscular changes

      a. Be prepared for emergencies as a result of hypocalcemia, such as tetany, seizures, laryngospasm, and respiratory and cardiac arrest

      b. Initiate seizure precautions and maintain a quiet environment

      c. Closely observe respiratory and airway status; have emergency tracheostomy kit available and IV calcium gluconate for postoperative thyroidectomy clients (may have inadvertent removal of parathyroid gland)

      d. Observe for signs of tetany for clients receiving multiple blood transfusions

      e. Observe for signs of bleeding or increased bruising

  7. Monitor for possibility of hypercalcemia as a result of replacement therapy

F. Medication therapy

  1. Oral replacement therapy

      a. Approximately 1.5–3.0 grams/day of oral calcium gluconate is needed to raise total calcium by 1 mg/dL

      b. Calcium citrate and calcium lactates are other oral calcium salts that are more soluble and may be better absorbed in older adults; calcium is best absorbed when taken in divided doses versus all at once

      c. Calcitonin may be prescribed instead of calcium salts for postmenopausal women who cannot take estrogen; subcutaneous or IM salmon calcitonin doses are 100 IU/day or intranasally: 1 spray (200 IU) daily, alternating nostrils

      d. Vitamin D supplements may be prescribed, initially 400–1000 IU/day if dietary deficiency is present or calcitriol 0.25–0.5 mg/capsule, then maintenance

  2. Parenteral replacement therapy

      a. See section D1 for calcium formulations, dosage, and rate of administration; too rapid administration can cause bradycardia and cardiac arrest

      b. For postoperative hypocalcemia from thyroidectomy, radical neck dissection, or parathyroidectomy, an infusion of calcium gluconate may be needed in first 24–48 hours; titrate to clinical signs and calcium levels; this hypocalcemia is usually transient

  3. Dietary therapy

      a. Recommendation for older clients is 1000–1500 mg daily

      b. Encourage adequate calcium intake from the various food groups daily; encourage foods high in calcium, such as dairy products

      c. Be aware of foods that decrease absorption of calcium and possibly limit them in diet

G. **Client education**

1. Predisposing factors associated with hypocalcemia and how to reduce them

    a. Paresthesias and tingling and numbness in extremities are early warning signs of tetany

    b. Report onset of signs of tetany or seizures immediately to healthcare provider

    c. Take oral replacements as prescribed

    d. Avoid overuse of antacids or laxatives containing phosphorus

    e. Use with caution bisphosphonates for prevention of osteoporosis

    f. Importance of regular exercise

2. Dietary education

    a. Foods rich in calcium and protein

    b. Sources of vitamin D and protein are important to keep calcium level normal

    c. Use appropriate substitutes for milk and dairy products if client is lactose intolerant

    d. Avoid foods or antacids high in phosphorus

    e. Limit foods that decrease absorption of calcium in the diet

    f. Collaborate with dietitian to meet dietary goals

H. **Evaluation**

1. Total serum calcium is between 8.5 and 10.5 mg/dL; ionized calcium level is between 4.0 and 5.0 mg/dL; urine calcium within normal reference range

2. Resolution of signs and symptoms of hypocalcemia

3. Levels of magnesium, potassium, and phosphorus are within normal limits

4. PTH levels are within normal limits if caused by hypoparathyroidism

5. I&O are within normal limits; daily weight is stabilized

6. Client demonstrates ability to adhere to interventions

Practice to Pass

A client has received calcium gluconate IV push for severe hypocalcemia. How will you evaluate the therapeutic response to calcium gluconate and what nursing interventions are appropriate for this therapy?

III. HYPERCALCEMIA

A. **Definition, etiology and pathophysiology**

1. Serum calcium level above 10.5 mg/dL

2. Cellular-level transport

    a. Movement occurs via a calcium pump

    b. Removed from bone by osteoclasts that are derived from monocytes that are produced in bone marrow

    c. Monocytes travel through bloodstream and collect at sites of bone resorption, where they fuse together to become osteocytes (cells that erode old bone)

3. Predisposing clinical conditions

Practice to Pass

How would you compare the differences and similarities that occur in the central nervous system between hypocalcemia and hypercalcemia?

    a. Can result from increased calcium intake or absorption, a shift from calcium from bone to ECF, or decreased calcium excretion (see Table 4-3 for clinical manifestations of hypercalcemia); symptoms may not appear until serum calcium level is higher than 12 mg/dL

    b. See Table 4-4 for description of clinical conditions predisposing to hypercalcemia

B. **Assessment**

1. Clinical manifestations: occur because of decreased neuromuscular irritability (refer again to Table 4-3)

    a. Cardiovascular: hypertension, decreased ST segments, and shortened QT interval on ECG; cardiac dysrhythmias such as heart block and cardiac arrest

    b. Neuromuscular: depressed neuromuscular excitability as evidenced by decreased deep tendon reflexes; impairment of memory, personality changes or bizarre behavior or acute psychosis, lethargy, headache, confusion, fatigue, or coma (seizures are rare)

    c. Gastrointestinal: hypotonic bowel sounds, constipation, history of peptic ulcer disease; anorexia, nausea and vomiting; abdominal pain

Table 4-4	Clinical Conditions That Lead to the Development of Hypercalcemia
Condition	**Explanation**
Hyperparathyroidism	Increased PTH causes calcium release from bone, enhances absorption of calcium in intestines, and increases renal absorption of calcium; adenoma of parathyroid gland is most common cause
Metastatic cancer	Most common cause of hypercalcemia, especially with myeloma, pulmonary, breast, and ovarian cancers; related to increased release of calcium from bone that is destroyed; occurs locally when tumor cell products stimulate osteoclastic bone resorption or systemically stimulate bone resorption and increased calcium excretion
Use of thiazide diuretics	Potentiates action of PTH on kidneys and decreases calcium excretion; results in small to moderate increases in calcium
Sarcoidosis	Results in increased active metabolite of vitamin D made in cells with this and other granulomatous diseases
Immobility	Reduces the longitudinal stress on long bones and can lead to bone resorption occurring at a faster rate than bone formation
Paget disease	Interferes with the process of replacement of old bone with new bone; leads to fragile bones that are misshapen; often affects bones of skull, spine, pelvis, and legs
Hypophosphatemia	A phosphorus level <3.0 mg/dL; phosphorus is inversely related to calcium
Hyperthyroidism (thyrotoxicosis)	Associated with high bone turnover; excessive bone resorption
Renal tubular acidosis	Increases ionized portion of calcium
Milk-alkali syndrome	Can occur in clients with peptic ulcer disease who use milk or antacids, especially calcium carbonate (Tums or Oscal), for prolonged periods of time
Familial hypocalciuric hypercalcemia	A rare autosomal dominant disorder
Lithium therapy	Competes with calcium and other important cations affecting neurotransmitters, cell membranes, and body water
Vitamin D intoxication	Increases absorption of calcium
Steroid therapy	Increases calcium resorption from bone

    d. Renal: polyuria and polydipsia due to altered renal function; decreased ability of kidneys to concentrate urine; renal colic can occur from development of kidney stones due to excess calcium; renal failure may occur; altered voiding patterns due to polyuria and polydipsia

     e. Musculoskeletal: pathologic bone fractures; bone thinning; bone pain, impaired mobility with transfer

  2. Diagnostic and laboratory findings

    a. Plasma, urinary levels, and radiology measurements

       1) Plasma calcium level of >11 mg/dL; in malignancies, total serum calcium may be >14 mg/dL

      2) Ionized plasma calcium level of >5.0 mg/dL or >40%

      3) Twenty-four-hour urinary calcium level of >400 mg/24 hours

      4) PTH level >55 pg/dL if due to hyperparathyroidism

        5) Radiology findings that confirm presence of pathologic fractures, kidney stones, and/or bone mineral density abnormality

    b. Associated electrolyte levels: hypophosphatemia (<3.0 mg/dL)

    c. Trending of results

      1) Monitor calcium and phosphorus levels

      2) Assess for signs and symptoms of resolving hypercalcemia

      3) Monitor creatinine and BUN

   4) Monitor daily weight in response to therapeutic regimens
   5) Monitor strict I&O
   6) Monitor ECG for shortening of ST segment and QT interval
   7) Results of x-rays for bone changes and fractures; results of bone density tests
   8) Monitor for renal calculi and calcium deposits in renal parenchyma on x-ray
   9) If parathyroid tumor, surgical removal should bring PTH to normal; control of tumor from malignancy should help restore balance
3. Identification of risk factors that increase risk of hypercalcemia
   a. Cancer or known metastasis
   b. Overactive parathyroid glands (hyperparathyroidism)
   c. Renal impairment
   d. Immobility due to clinical conditions or sedentary lifestyle
   e. Excessive dietary intake of calcium-rich foods
   f. Excessive intake of antacids for gastric distress
C. Priority nursing concerns: possible decreased cardiac output and/or dysrhythmias, possible constipation; potential for injury because of neuromuscular and sensorium changes, possible alterations in fluid balance, possible need for client education to support client adherence to therapy
D. Therapeutic management
1. Decrease calcium intake
   a. Limit milk and dairy products
   b. Eliminate use of calcium carbonate antacids until calcium levels return to within normal limits
2. Promote calcium excretion
   a. Use loop diuretics, such as furosemide or bumetanide, to promote increased urine output, thus excreting more calcium
   b. Maintain hydration of 3000–4000 mL (3–4 L) of fluid/day; oral fluids should be high in acid ash, such as cranberry or prune juice
   c. Give 0.9% saline (NaCl) infusion of 300–500 mL/hour up to 6 liters as prescribed until volume status restored, then 0.45% NaCl may be used; watch for fluid overload as a consequence of therapy, especially if the client has preexisting cardiac or respiratory disease
   d. Corticosteroids such as oral prednisone to decrease GI absorption of calcium; may take 5–10 days for calcium levels to fall
   e. Chronic management of hypercalcemia is effective only with parathyroidectomy for primary hyperparathyroidism
3. Continued monitoring of client
   a. Serum calcium and phosphorus levels
   b. Continuous ECG monitoring to detect cardiac arrhythmias
   c. Strict I&O and daily weight
   d. If plicamycin is used, monitor client for tissue sloughing at IV site because drug has vesicant properties; also closely monitor renal function (drug is nephrotoxic)
   e. Monitor for side effects of corticosteroids such as hyperglycemia, weight gain, and mood changes, bearing in mind the long-term side effects
4. Restoration of balance
   a. Monitor calcium and phosphorus levels
   b. Monitor neurologic and cardiac status
   c. Monitor for balanced I&O and stable daily weight
   d. Monitor for absence of treatment-related signs of heart failure or hypocalcemia
5. Treatment of hypercalcemic crisis (see Table 4-5)
6. Dialysis: during oliguric/anuric stage, severe renal dysfunction can lead to life-threatening fluid and electrolyte imbalances

Table 4-5	Therapy for Hypercalcemic Crisis
Isotonic saline (0.9% NaCl)	May be infused at 300–500 mL/hr initially and up to 6 liters until intravascular volume restored or total calcium 8–9 mg/dL; promotes calcium excretion; loop diuretics should be used if heart failure develops
Bisphosphonates (e.g., pamidronate)	Can be given intravenously to inhibit bone resorption—90 mg in 1 liter NS or D_5W over 4 hours for severe hypercalcemia (>13.5 mg/dL), returns calcium to normal within 24–48 hours with effects lasting for weeks in most clients
Plicamycin	Can be given intravenously to inhibit bone resorption, specifically if hypercalcemia induced by metastasis; doses of 24 mcg/kg in 500 mL D_5W over 4–6 hours gradually reduce calcium
Salmon calcitonin	May temporarily lower level by 1–3 mg/dL in clients with severe hypercalcemia; starting dose is 2–8 units/kg intramuscularly or subcutaneously every 6–12 hours; effective within 2 hours after initial dose, peaks in 24–48 hours, and duration is 4–7 days
Intravenous phosphorus	Decreases calcium by increasing phosphorus: dose greater than or equal to 1500 mg over 6–8 hours in emergency situations only

E. **Client-centered care**
  1. Monitor pertinent client assessment data for potential effects of hypercalcemia and for response to therapeutic treatment
     a. Obtain a thorough nursing history
        1) Subjective (family history, history of previous cancer, history of kidney stones, postoperative parathyroidectomy)
        2) Objective (signs of hypercalcemia, predisposing conditions, risk factors)
        3) Medication history (those that may cause hypercalcemia or an excess of medications to treat hypocalcemia)
        4) OTC or herbal therapies that may lead to hypercalcemia
     b. Assess particular systems for specific findings
        1) Neurologic system for changes in level of consciousness or subtle personality changes
        2) Cardiovascular system to determine if client is on digoxin (hypercalcemia can enhance digoxin effects) and to detect presence of dysrhythmias
        3) Genitourinary system for flank and thigh pain from renal calculi and forpolyuria
        4) Gastrointestinal system for nausea and vomiting, constipation, and decreased bowel sounds
        5) Musculoskeletal system for weakness of muscles, diminished deep tendon reflexes, and observable fractures
     c. Hypercalcemic crisis is considered a medical emergency; report laboratory results immediately to healthcare provider for therapeutic treatment
     d. Monitor PTH if hypercalcemia is from primary hyperparathyroidism
     e. Frequently assess for heart failure in clients receiving hydration therapy
     f. Identify symptoms of digoxin toxicity when client has hypercalcemia and is also receiving digoxin
     g. Monitor client for signs of hypocalcemia as a result of treatment
  2. Prevent injuries and maintain safe environment
     a. Monitor for pathologic fractures in clients with long-term hypercalcemia
     b. Assist client with mobility and transfer attempts in order to prevent injury and maintain safety
  3. Administer medications as prescribed, assessing for therapeutic response and client condition during course of drug therapy

4. Assess I&O
   a. Encourage clients to drink 3–4 liters of fluid per day, especially fluids such as cranberry juice or prune juice so that calcium salts will not deposit in urine
   b. Monitor color and characteristics of urine, and observe urine for presence of calculi (stones)
   c. Obtain daily weight
5. Assess for signs of fluid overload from treatment or dehydration from polyuria
6. Dietary interventions to decrease calcium levels
   a. Limit calcium sources in diet
   b. Limit medications that provide hidden sources of calcium in diet
   c. Refer client to a dietitian as appropriate
7. If hypercalcemic state is due to malignancy, long-term treatment may be indicated
8. Encourage adherence with therapeutic regimen

F. **Medication therapy**
   1. Hydration therapy
      a. Isotonic saline (0.9% sodium chloride or NaCl) at a rate of 300–500 mL/hr, up to 6 liters, in emergency or 0.45% NaCl until serum calcium level is diluted
      b. Titrate to prevent signs of heart failure
   2. Specific drug therapies
      a. Loop diuretics: such as furosemide or bumetanide; enhance calcium excretion and prevent volume overloading during hydration
      b. Plicamycin: inhibits osteoclastic bone resorption and decreases bone turnover; used selectively with malignant hypercalcemia because of nephrotoxicity; use cautiously with impaired renal function
      c. Corticosteroids (glucocorticoids): inhibit calcium absorption in intestine, inhibit osteoclastic bone resorption and increase urinary excretion of calcium; give prednisone BID initially, then change to maintenance dose; may not reduce calcium significantly for 5–10 days so use in conjunction with other measures to decrease calcium
      d. Phosphate salts: administered orally for several days or rectally by Fleet retention enema 100 mL twice daily; limit phosphate therapy to clients with phosphate levels <3.0 mg/dL and normal renal function; a dose of elemental phosphorus may be given orally three times per day and modestly lowers serum calcium; controversy exists about use of IV phosphates
      e. Bisphosphonate drugs: retard bone turnover by inhibiting activity of osteoclasts; pamidronate is given IV over 24 hours; alendronate is an oral drug that is taken with water upon arising, 30 minutes before food or other medications (should not be taken with caffeinated products, mineral water, or orange juice)
      f. Calcitonin (salmon) is given IM or subcutaneously every 6–12 hours to temporarily lower serum calcium
      g. Gallium nitrate: inhibits bone resorption; may be given via IV over 24 hours for 5 days along with saline diuresis; do not use if creatinine <2.5 mg/dL

G. **Client education**
   1. Predisposing factors associated with hypercalcemia and how to avoid them
   2. Correct method of taking prescribed medications
   3. Notify healthcare provider if flank pain develops (risk of kidney stones)
   4. Strain urine for kidney stones if indicated (demonstrate to clients as needed)
   5. Notify healthcare professional if symptoms worsen
   6. Avoid over-the-counter antacids that contain high amounts of calcium
   7. Dietary education
      a. Discuss foods highest in calcium and offer alternative options; a low-calcium diet (<400 mg/day) is recommended if hypercalcemia due to vitamin D toxicity

Practice to Pass

A client has hypercalcemia due to milk-alkali syndrome. Which foods and antacids will you teach this client to avoid?

      b. Instruct client to increase fluid intake to 2000–3000 mL in 24 hours, especially fluids high in acid ash such as prune or cranberry juice

      c. Increase dietary fiber and fluid to prevent constipation

      d. Avoid taking large doses of vitamin D supplements

      e. Refer client to a dietitian to meet dietary goals

H. Evaluation

  1. Total serum calcium is between 8.5 and 10.5 mg/dL

  2. Serum ionized calcium is between 4.0 and 5.0 mg/dL

  3. Serum phosphorus level is between 2.5 and 4.5 mg/dL

  4. Twenty-four-hour urine calcium is within normal limits

  5. PTH is within normal limits if cause was primary hyperparathyroidism or surgery

  6. Signs of heart failure from hydration therapy are absent

  7. Serum creatinine and BUN are within normal limits

  8. Signs and symptoms of hypercalcemia resolve

  9. Absence of clinical manifestations of treatment-induced hypocalcemia

  10. There are no signs of complications of hyper- or hypocalcemia

  11. The client demonstrates adherence to therapeutic management regime

Case Study

A 54-year-old male with a diagnosis of multiple myeloma has been admitted to your unit. The client reports increasing fatigue, muscle weakness, and bone pain. Lab work indicates pancytopenia, hyperuricemia, hypercalcemia, and elevated creatinine. Bone scans and x-rays have been prescribed.

1. What do you suspect is the cause of these signs and symptoms?

2. What is the pathophysiological mechanism for the calcium imbalance?

3. What immediate medical treatment do you anticipate and why?

4. What are your priority nursing interventions?

5. How will you determine if therapy has been effective?

For suggested responses, see pages 191–192.

POSTTEST

1 A client is admitted with chronic renal failure. The nurse would use which statement to explain the need to monitor for hypocalcemia?

  1. "Your kidneys do not eliminate as much calcium, so we need to check for signs of hypocalcemia."

  2. "Your calcium level can decrease because it goes down when the creatinine in the bloodstream is high."

  3. "Signs of hypocalcemia will appear before you experience pain from renal colic."

  4. "Your kidneys are unable to produce calcitriol, which is needed to regulate calcium levels in the bloodstream."

2 A client presents with a mildly elevated calcium level. The nurse identifies which items in the nursing history as contributing factors to the abnormal calcium level? Select all that apply.

  1. Use of a thiazide diuretic

  2. Recent reports of polyuria

  3. A high-protein diet

  4. Ingesting a bisphosphonate weekly

  5. Recent immobility from a fractured hip

3 A client with hypercalcemia is receiving digoxin. The nurse plans to incorporate which item in client assessments?

1. Checking for Trousseau sign
2. Frequent pulse checks
3. Auscultation of bowel sounds
4. Inspection of skin for signs of bleeding

4 A client returns to the unit following a thyroidectomy. The nurse plans to frequently assess for which important manifestations at this time? Select all that apply.

1. Signs of laryngospasm
2. Polyuria
3. Hypertension
4. Hypoactive deep tendon reflexes
5. Facial muscle twitching

5 Which assessment findings should the nurse expect to see in a client who has a calcium level of 12.2 mg/dL? Select all that apply.

1. Hyperactive reflexes
2. Anxiety
3. Polyuria
4. Constipation
5. Bone pain

6 The nurse notes that a client's total serum calcium level is 7.9 mg/dL. Because the client has no symptoms of imbalance at this time, what interpretation should the nurse make?

1. This level reflects only the ionized calcium.
2. The client's magnesium is high, resulting in false levels of calcium.
3. Phosphorus is low, resulting in low serum calcium levels.
4. This does not reflect the ionized calcium that results in symptomatology.

7 When caring for the client with signs of severe hypocalcemia, the nurse anticipates administration of which therapeutic measure?

1. Isotonic normal saline (0.9% NaCl) as a rapid infusion
2. Calcium gluconate 10% by slow IV push
3. Intravenous phosphorus over 6–8 hours
4. Calcium chloride 10% by rapid IV push

8 A client who has a serum calcium level of 11.8 mg/dL is receiving a 0.9% sodium chloride infusion. The nurse determines that hydration has been effective after noting which client data?

1. Chvostek sign is positive.
2. Volume status has been restored.
3. Calcium level is 11.0 mg/dL.
4. Serum creatinine is elevated.

9 The nurse caring for a client with a calcium imbalance places highest priority on nursing interventions that help to manage which of the following?

1. Renal signs and symptoms
2. Cardiac changes
3. Hematological disorders
4. Neuromuscular clinical manifestations

10 The nurse determines that a client with a serum calcium level of 12 mg/dL understands client teaching when the client makes which statement?

1. "If my stomach becomes upset, I can just take more Tums."
2. "I will need to take my phosphorus supplements once a day."
3. "I will need to be on strict bedrest to help with this problem."
4. "I will need to drink many more fluids than I have been, even up to two to three liters each day."

➤ *See pages 101–103 for Answers and Rationales.*

POSTTEST

ANSWERS & RATIONALES

Pretest

1 **Answer: 1, 3, 4, 2, 5 Rationale:** Anything other than water will interfere with the absorption of alendronate. It must be given on an empty stomach with a full glass of water. This should be the first step because the drug cannot be given if the client has already eaten or had fluids other than water. Alendronate is contraindicated if client has a history of reflux disease, hiatal hernia, or esophagitis, so checking for this history should be done second before the medication is prepared. After determining that the drug can be administered, the drug should be prepared as the third step using three checks. The client must be positioned upright to take the dose as the fourth step, and remain in this position for 30 minutes following ingestion of the pill, as it can cause esophagitis. After positioning the client in an upright position, the medication must be administered with at least 8 ounces of water (last step). **Cognitive Level:** Applying **Client Need:** Pharmacological and Parenteral Therapies **Integrated Process:** Nursing Process: Implementation **Content Area:** Adult Health **Strategy:** The core concept is the proper steps that must be taken prior to administration of a medication. Recall the assessments that must be done prior to administering alendronate to ensure that it is safe to administer. It is given in such a way as to provide optimum absorption. **Reference:** Adams, M. P., Holland, N., & Urban, C. (2014). *Pharmacology for nurses: A pathophysiologic approach* (4th ed.). Upper Saddle River, NJ: Pearson, p. 737.

2 **Answer: 1, 3 Rationale:** DiGeorge syndrome is characterized by immature parathyroid glands, causing a deficiency of parathormone production, leading to hypocalcemia. Hypocalcemia leads to increased excitability of the neuromuscular system and potential seizures. For this reason, the infant should be placed on seizure precautions. Providing additional padding in the bassinette helps to protect the infant in the event of a seizure. It is unnecessary to place the infant on the right side. The infant should not be placed in a prone position. There is no need to provide additional oral stimulation to the infant. **Cognitive Level:** Analyzing **Client Need:** Reduction of Risk Potential **Integrated Process:** Nursing Process: Implementation **Content Area:** Child Health **Strategy:** To answer this question correctly, it is necessary to understand the risk of hypocalcemia with DiGeorge syndrome. Consider the risks of hypocalcemia to choose correctly. **Reference:** London, M. L., Ladewig, P. W., Davidson, M., Ball, R., Bindler, R., & Cowen, K. (2014). *Maternal and child nursing care* (4th ed.). Upper Saddle River, NJ: Pearson Education, p. 1344.

3 **Answer: 1 Rationale:** Prolonged NGT suctioning leads to metabolic alkalosis. Changes in pH will alter the level of ionized calcium. Alkalosis increases calcium binding to albumin, leading to a decrease in ionized calcium. There may be fluid shifts from hypoalbuminemia, but this would not be from NG tube suctioning. Hypomagnesemia can be a cause of hypocalcemia. Metabolic acidosis decreases calcium binding to albumin, leading to more ionized calcium. **Cognitive Level:** Applying **Client Need:** Physiological Adaptation **Integrated Process:** Nursing Process: Evaluation **Content Area:** Adult Health **Strategy:** Recognize that NG suctioning removes acidic fluids, resulting in an alkalotic state. Recall that calcium salts are bound in alkalosis and serum levels decrease to choose correctly. **Reference:** LeMone, P., Burke, K., Bauldoff, G., & Gubrud, P. (2015). *Medical surgical nursing: Clinical reasoning in patient care* (6th ed.). New York, NY: Pearson, pp. 204–207.

4 **Answer: 2 Rationale:** Many malignant tumors produce chemicals that are carried in the blood to cause release of calcium from the bones, most commonly in association with ovarian cancer, renal cell carcinoma, and breast cancer, among others. Several antineoplastic medications can lead to hypocalcemia, rather than hypercalcemia. An inadequate intake of dairy products is a dietary cause of hypocalcemia. Pancreatitis can lead to hypocalcemia, not hypercalcemia. **Cognitive Level:** Applying **Client Need:** Physiological Adaptation **Integrated Process:** Nursing Process: Evaluation **Content Area:** Adult Health **Strategy:** Recall physiology of malignancy to stimulate release of calcium from the bones to direct you to the correct option. **Reference:** LeMone, P., Burke, K., Bauldoff, G., & Gubrud, P. (2015). *Medical surgical nursing: Clinical reasoning in patient care* (6th ed.). New York, NY: Pearson, pp. 207–209.

5 **Answer: 1, 2 Rationale:** Large doses of corticosteroids decrease calcium absorption in the intestines, leading to a further decrease in serum calcium levels. A positive Chvostek sign (twitching of cheek muscles) indicates hypocalcemia and hypomagnesemia. A positive Trousseau sign (carpal spasm during BP cuff inflation) would be seen with hypocalcemia. Polyuria occurs with hypercalcemia. Muscle weakness is a symptom associated with hypercalcemia. Intermittent headaches are unrelated to hypercalcemia. **Cognitive Level:** Applying **Client Need:** Physiological Adaptation **Integrated Process:** Nursing Process: Evaluation **Content Area:** Adult Health **Strategy:** Critical words are *hypocalcemia* and *corticosteroids*. Recall the signs and symptoms of hypocalcemia to direct you to the correct options. **Reference:** LeMone, P., Burke, K., Bauldoff, G., & Gubrud, P. (2015). *Medical surgical nursing: Clinical reasoning in patient care* (6th ed.). New York, NY: Pearson, pp. 207–209.

6 **Answer: 3, 4 Rationale:** Elevated serum levels of calcium interfere with nerve conduction and muscle contraction, leading to muscle weakness. Chvostek sign (facial muscle twitching) is found in clients who have hypocalcemia, so a negative Chvostek sign helps to rule out the opposite disorder (hypocalcemia). Due to greater influx of nerve impulses that occurs with hypocalcemia (not hypercalcemia), tetany can take place. Insufficient calcium leading to hypocalcemia contributes to the carpopedal spasms indicative of Trousseau sign. Inadequate calcium (hypocalcemia) causes an increase in neuromuscular irritability, leading to hyperactive reflexes. **Cognitive Level:** Applying **Client Need:** Physiological Adaptation **Integrated Process:** Nursing Process: Assessment **Content Area:** Adult Health **Strategy:** Recall that excessive calcium results in decreased transmission at the neuromuscular junction to direct you to the correct option. **Reference:** LeMone, P., Burke, K., Bauldoff, G., & Gubrud, P. (2015). *Medical surgical nursing: Clinical reasoning in patient care* (6th ed.). New York, NY: Pearson, pp. 207–209.

7 **Answer: 2 Rationale:** Hypercalcemia causes a shortened plateau phase of the action potential, which in turn causes shortening of the QT interval. Although atrial fibrillation could occur, the nurse is more concerned about the development of heart block, secondary to the slowing of atrioventricular conduction. Because atrial ventricular conduction is slowed with hypercalcemia, the PR interval would be prolonged. Peaked T waves are associated with hyperkalemia, not hypercalcemia. **Cognitive Level:** Applying **Client Need:** Physiological Adaptation **Integrated Process:** Nursing Process: Assessment **Content Area:** Adult Health **Strategy:** This question requires knowledge of ECG interpretation and changes associated with electrolyte abnormalities. Recall ECG changes associated with high calcium levels to direct you to the correct option. **Reference:** Kee, J. (2017). *Laboratory and diagnostic tests with nursing implications* (8th ed.). New York, NY: Pearson Education, pp. 102–103.

8 **Answer: 1 Rationale:** The parathyroid glands regulate calcium. The glands lie just underneath the thyroid gland and may be accidentally removed when a thyroidectomy is done, leading to hypocalcemia. An increased release of PTH would result in increased calcium release, not a decrease. Immobility contributes to osteoporosis and calcium resorption from the bones, which leads to elevated calcium levels. Hypophosphatemia is usually seen with hypercalcemia. Calcium gluconate would not be given to treat hypercalcemia. **Cognitive Level:** Applying **Client Need:** Physiological Adaptation **Integrated Process:** Teaching and Learning **Content Area:** Adult Health **Strategy:** The critical word is *post-thyroidectomy*. Recall anatomy and function of the parathyroid gland to choose correctly. **Reference:** LeMone, P., Burke, K., Bauldoff, G., & Gubrud, P. (2015). *Medical surgical nursing: Clinical reasoning in patient care* (6th ed.). New York, NY: Pearson, pp. 204–207.

9 **Answer: 4 Rationale:** Symptoms of fatigue, headache, and increasing muscle weakness are clinical manifestations of hypercalcemia. Increased hydration is needed to reduce the serum concentration and aid in elimination. Thiazide diuretics inhibit calcium excretion and may worsen the state of hypercalcemia. Vitamin D supplements will increase absorption of vitamin D in the intestine, which could lead to an increased calcium level. Fluid restriction will cause hemoconcentration, leading to increased serum calcium. **Cognitive Level:** Analyzing **Client Need:** Physiological Adaptation **Integrated Process:** Nursing Process: Planning **Content Area:** Adult Health **Strategy:** First determine that the symptoms reflect hypercalcemia. Eliminate three options because these would all increase calcium levels even further. **Reference:** LeMone, P., Burke, K., Bauldoff, G., & Gubrud, P. (2015). *Medical surgical nursing: Clinical reasoning in patient care* (6th ed.). New York, NY: Pearson, pp. 207–209.

10 **Answer: 2 Rationale:** Numbness and tingling are signs of hypocalcemia and should be reported to the healthcare provider. The antacid Tums (calcium carbonate) is a good source of calcium and does not need to be avoided. Protein should be encouraged rather than restricted in the presence of hypocalcemia. Kidney stones occur more frequently in the presence of hypercalcemia because of higher solute load. **Cognitive Level:** Analyzing **Client Need:** Reduction of Risk Potential **Integrated Process:** Teaching and Learning **Content Area:** Adult Health **Strategy:** Review nursing and medical interventions to increase a client's calcium level. Recall early warning signs of tetany to direct you to the correct option. **Reference:** LeMone, P., Burke, K., Bauldoff, G., & Gubrud, P. (2015). *Medical surgical nursing: Clinical reasoning in patient care* (6th ed.). New York, NY: Pearson, pp. 204–207.

Posttest

1 **Answer: 4 Rationale:** An inability to produce calcitriol explains why the client may experience hypocalcemia and therefore needs to be aware of what symptoms might occur. If the kidneys were not eliminating calcium, the client would experience hypercalcemia, not hypocalcemia. Although the creatinine goes up with renal failure, this does not explain why the calcium is low. The damaged kidneys cannot make calcitriol, which is needed to absorb calcium. Renal colic occurs secondary to elevated calcium levels. **Cognitive Level:** Applying **Client Need:** Reduction of Risk Potential **Integrated Process:** Communication and Documentation **Content Area:** Adult Health **Strategy:** The critical term is *chronic renal failure*. Recall physiology of renal failure to direct you to the correct option. **Reference:** LeMone, P., Burke, K., Bauldoff, G., & Gubrud, P. (2015). *Medical surgical nursing: Clinical reasoning in patient care* (6th ed.). New York, NY: Pearson, pp. 204–207.

2 **Answer: 1, 5 Rationale:** Thiazide diuretics cause reabsorption of calcium in the distal tubule, which can contribute to hypercalcemia is some clients. Immobility reduces the

ANSWERS & RATIONALES

longitudinal stress on long bones and can lead to bone resorption occurring at a faster rate than bone formation. Polyuria is a clinical manifestation of hypercalcemia, not a contributing factor. Eating a high-protein diet can contribute to the development of hypocalcemia, not hypercalcemia. Bisphosphonates are used in the treatment of osteoporosis and hypercalcemia. They prevent bone resorption of calcium, thereby helping to lower serum calcium levels and prevent further breakdown of the bone matrix. **Cognitive Level:** Analyzing **Client Need:** Reduction of Risk Potential **Integrated Process:** Nursing Process: Assessment **Content Area:** Adult Health **Strategy:** Systematically evaluate each option for factors that would promote intake or retention of calcium. Note the question has more than one correct answer, so evaluate each option as a true–false statement. **Reference:** LeMone, P., Burke, K., Bauldoff, G., & Gubrud, P. (2015). *Medical surgical nursing: Clinical reasoning in patient care* (6th ed.). New York, NY: Pearson, pp. 207–209.

3 **Answer: 2 Rationale:** Because the elevation of serum calcium levels can affect cardiac conduction, the client is at increased risk for digoxin toxicity, and the heart rate should be checked more frequently to detect dysrhythmias. A Trousseau sign is checked when calcium levels are low, not elevated. Although hypercalcemia can cause a decrease in peristalsis and constipation, this is not related to the use of digoxin. The use of digoxin would not place the client at risk for bleeding; this is more of a concern when hypocalcemia is present. **Cognitive Level:** Applying **Client Need:** Reduction of Risk Potential **Integrated Process:** Nursing Process: Assessment **Content Area:** Adult Health **Strategy:** The core concept is that the client is on digoxin; recall the role of calcium in cardiac contractility and the action of digoxin to direct you to the correct option. **Reference:** LeMone, P., Burke, K., Bauldoff, G., & Gubrud, P. (2015). *Medical surgical nursing: Clinical reasoning in patient care* (6th ed.). New York, NY: Pearson, pp. 207–209.

4 **Answer: 1, 5 Rationale:** Hypocalcemia frequently results from accidental removal or destruction of parathyroid tissue or its blood supply during surgery. Clinical manifestations of tetany include laryngospasm postoperatively. Facial muscle twitching indicates Chvostek sign, indicating hypocalcemia. Polyuria can accompany hypercalcemia because the excess solute excreted draws water with it. Hypertension has many causes but hypocalcemia is not among them. Hypoactive deep tendon reflexes occur with hypercalcemia. **Cognitive Level:** Applying **Client Need:** Reduction of Risk Potential **Integrated Process:** Nursing Process: Assessment **Content Area:** Adult Health **Strategy:** Recall the parathyroid glands can be accidentally removed during surgery, resulting in hypocalcemia. Differentiate between signs of hypocalcemia and hypercalcemia to choose correctly. **Reference:** LeMone, P., Burke, K., Bauldoff, G., & Gubrud, P. (2015). *Medical surgical nursing: Clinical reasoning in patient care* (6th ed.). New York, NY: Pearson, pp. 204–207.

5 **Answer: 3, 4, 5 Rationale:** A serum calcium level of 12.2 mg/dL reflects hypercalcemia. Altered renal function is seen with hypercalcemia, causing a decreased ability of the kidneys to concentrate urine, as evidenced by the polyuria. With decreased neuromuscular irritability in hypercalcemia, contractions of the intestinal muscles are decreased, contributing to slowing of peristalsis and constipation. Osteoporosis and bone thinning can occur with hypercalcemia as calcium is resorbed from the bone, leading to bone pain. The excess calcium in cell membranes reduces transmission of neuromuscular impulses, leading to hypoactive reflexes. Clinical manifestations of hypercalcemia are secondary to decreased neuromuscular irritability. Anxiety would be seen with hypocalcemia, which causes increased neuromuscular irritability. **Cognitive Level:** Applying **Client Need:** Physiological Adaptation **Integrated Process:** Nursing Process: Assessment **Content Area:** Adult Health **Strategy:** First recognize that the calcium level is elevated, indicating hypercalcemia. Recall the effect of elevated calcium levels on the neuromuscular, renal, and skeletal systems to choose correctly. **Reference:** LeMone, P., Burke, K., Bauldoff, G., & Gubrud, P. (2015). *Medical surgical nursing: Clinical reasoning in patient care* (6th ed.). New York, NY: Pearson, pp. 204–207.

6 **Answer: 4 Rationale:** Ionized calcium is the portion of the serum calcium that is not bound to protein and is physiologically active and clinically important. The level indicated is the total serum calcium level, which is a combination of ionized calcium, which is free and unbound, and nonionized calcium, which is bound to protein and not physiologically active. Low magnesium levels are associated with low calcium levels, not high magnesium levels. When serum calcium levels are low, the phosphorus level is usually reciprocal, and would be elevated. **Cognitive Level:** Analyzing **Client Need:** Physiological Adaptation **Integrated Process:** Nursing Process: Assessment **Content Area:** Adult Health **Strategy:** The question requires correlation of a hypocalcemic lab value to its cause. Recall factors that influence serum calcium levels to direct you to the correct answer. **Reference:** LeMone, P., Burke, K., Bauldoff, G., & Gubrud, P. (2015). *Medical surgical nursing: Clinical reasoning in patient care* (6th ed.). New York, NY: Pearson, pp. 204–207.

7 **Answer: 2 Rationale:** Calcium gluconate is an appropriate treatment for correction of severe hypocalcemia. Saline infusions are given to treat hypercalcemia, not hypocalcemia. When serum calcium levels are low, phosphorus levels are usually high, as calcium and phosphorus have a reciprocal relationship. Phosphorus would not be given to treat low calcium levels. Although calcium chloride can be given to treat severe hypocalcemia, it is given slowly, not by rapid IV push. **Cognitive Level:** Applying **Client Need:** Pharmacological and Parenteral Therapies **Integrated Process:** Nursing Process: Planning **Content Area:** Adult Health **Strategy:** Critical words are *severe hypocalcemia*. Eliminate two options because they would be given to increase calcium. Eliminate a third option, recognizing that calcium should never be given rapidly. **Reference:** LeMone, P., Burke, K., Bauldoff, G., & Gubrud, P. (2015). *Medical surgical nursing: Clinical reasoning in patient care* (6th ed.). New York, NY: Pearson, pp. 204–207.

8 **Answer: 2 Rationale:** Hypercalcemia causes polyuria, which can lead to volume depletion. Restoration of volume status would be an indicator that the hydration has been effective. A positive Chvostek sign would be indicative of hypocalcemia, indicating the infusion has overcorrected the calcium imbalance. A calcium level of 11.0 mg/dL is still elevated, indicating that the infusion has not corrected the imbalance. An elevated creatinine level reflects impaired renal function and would not be used to measure effectiveness of the therapy. **Cognitive Level:** Analyzing **Client Need:** Pharmacological and Parenteral Therapies **Integrated Process:** Nursing Process: Evaluation **Content Area:** Adult Health **Strategy:** This question requires you to look for the absence of signs indicative of hypercalcemia and restoration of fluid hydration. Evaluate each option and its association with fluid and electrolyte balance to make a selection. **Reference:** LeMone, P., Burke, K., Bauldoff, G., & Gubrud, P. (2015). *Medical surgical nursing: Clinical reasoning in patient care* (6th ed.). New York, NY: Pearson, pp. 207–209.

9 **Answer: 4 Rationale:** Although all systems are impacted by calcium imbalance, the major clinical manifestations of calcium imbalance are due to either increased or decreased neuromuscular irritability. Renal signs such as polyuria are likely to be present only with hypercalemia. Cardiac changes are not as frequently seen with calcium imbalance, unless the imbalance is severe. Although the clotting cascade is influenced by calcium, the term *hematologic disorders* is too vague to be correct. **Cognitive Level:** Applying **Client Need:** Reduction of Risk Potential **Integrated Process:** Nursing Process: Implementation **Content Area:** Adult Health **Strategy:** Note that the question does not specify if calcium is decreased or elevated. Recall the major system affected by calcium to choose correctly. **Reference:** LeMone, P., Burke, K., Bauldoff, G., & Gubrud, P. (2015). *Medical surgical nursing: Clinical reasoning in patient care* (6th ed.). New York, NY: Pearson, pp. 202–209.

10 **Answer: 4 Rationale:** The client with hypercalcemia (above 10.5 mg/dL) should increase fluid intake to 2–3 liters a day. Hydration leads to increased calcium excretion and prevents the development of kidney stones. Tums contain calcium carbonate, which contributes to further increases in the already elevated calcium level. Although phosphorus supplements can help to increase the phosphorus levels and decrease the elevated calcium level, they need to be taken three to four times a day. Strict bedrest leads to increased calcium from osteoclastic activity. **Cognitive Level:** Analyzing **Client Need:** Reduction of Risk Potential **Integrated Process:** Teaching and Learning **Content Area:** Adult Health **Strategy:** Recall the treatment modalities for hypercalcemia to answer this question. Eliminate two options that actually increase calcium levels and recall the role of fluids to choose correctly. **Reference:** LeMone, P., Burke, K., Bauldoff, G., & Gubrud, P. (2015). *Medical surgical nursing: Clinical reasoning in patient care* (6th ed.). New York, NY: Pearson, pp. 207–209.

References

Adams, M. P., Holland, N., & Urban, C. (2017). *Pharmacology for nurses: A pathophysiologic approach* (5th ed.). New York, NY: Pearson.

Ball, J., Bindler, R., & Cowen, K. (2014). *Child health nursing: Partnering with children and families* (3rd ed.). Upper Saddle River, NJ: Pearson.

Berman, A., Snyder, S., & Frandsen, G. (2016). *Kozier & Erb's fundamentals of nursing: Concepts, process, and practice* (10th ed.). New York, NY: Pearson.

Ignatavicius, D., & Workman, M. (2016). *Medical-surgical nursing: Patient-centered collaborative care* (8th ed.). Philadelphia, PA: Elsevier Saunders.

Kee, J. L. (2017). *Pearson handbook of laboratory and diagnostic tests* (8th ed.). New York, NY: Pearson.

LeMone, P., Burke, K., Bauldoff, G., & Gubrud, P. (2015). *Medical surgical nursing: Clinical reasoning in patient care* (6th ed.). New York, NY: Pearson.

London, M., Ladewig, P., Davidson, M., Ball, J., Bindler, R., & Cowen, K. (2017). *Maternal and child nursing care* (5th ed.). New York, NY: Pearson Education.

ANSWERS & RATIONALES

5 Magnesium Balance and Imbalances

Chapter Outline

Overview of Magnesium
Regulation

Hypomagnesemia

Hypermagnesemia

 NCLEX-RN® Test Prep

Access the NEW Web-based app
that provides students with additional
practice questions in preparation
for the NCLEX experience.

Objectives

➤ Identify the basic functions of magnesium in the body.
➤ Explain the pathophysiology and etiology of magnesium
imbalances.
➤ Identify specific assessment findings in magnesium imbalances.
➤ Identify priority nursing concerns for a client experiencing a
magnesium imbalance.
➤ Describe the therapeutic management of magnesium imbalances.
➤ Describe the management of nursing care for a client who is
experiencing a magnesium imbalance.

Review at a Glance

hypermagnesemia an excess of
magnesium in blood, with a serum level
of greater than 2.1 mEq/L

hypomagnesemia a deficit of magnesium in blood, with a serum level of
less than 1.4 mEq/L

magnesium second most abundant
cation in body, found mainly in bone and
within cells

1 The nurse would expect a client to have a high serum level of magnesium after seeing which health problem listed in the medical history?

1. Malabsorption
2. Anemia
3. Overuse of laxatives
4. Excessive alcohol intake

2 The nurse should assess for which classic manifestation in a client with a magnesium level of 2.9 mEq/L?

1. Diarrhea
2. Hyperreflexia
3. Hypertension
4. Diminished deep tendon reflexes

3 The nurse is educating the client who has a magnesium level of 1.2 mEq/L. What information is most important for the nurse to include in discussions with the client?

1. Avoiding hazardous activities
2. Weekly laboratory evaluation
3. Dietary counseling
4. Moderate alcohol consumption

4 A mother of a child seen in the clinic reports she has been giving the child enemas to treat frequent bouts of constipation. To determine whether the child is at risk of developing hypermagnesemia, the nurse places priority on asking which question?

1. "When did you last give the child an enema?"
2. "What type of enema are you giving your child?"
3. "When did the child last have a bowel movement?"
4. "Why do think your child is constipated?"

5 A client with chronic renal failure has a magnesium level of 2.8 mEq/L. When reviewing the client's dietary history, the nurse identifies which frequently eaten foods as a possible cause of this laboratory value? Select all that apply.

1. Hot chocolate
2. Apples
3. Pork sausage
4. Spinach salad
5. Swiss cheese

6 A client admitted with a history of alcoholism has a magnesium level of 1.2 mEq/L. The nurse should also plan to check the results of serum laboratory studies for which alteration?

1. Elevated potassium
2. Elevated phosphorus
3. Decreased sodium
4. Decreased calcium

7 The nurse who is teaching a review of basic nutrition is discussing the effects of various electrolytes and minerals in the body. In describing the action of magnesium, the nurse would explain that it has which effect because it diminishes acetylcholine?

1. Nerve stimulant
2. Muscle relaxant
3. Vitamin metabolizer
4. Stimulant for release of blood glucose

8 Following bowel resection surgery, a client's magnesium level is 1.0 mEq/L. Which assessment finding should the nurse report to the healthcare provider immediately?

1. Hyperactive reflexes
2. Nausea
3. Anorexia
4. Abdominal pain

PRETEST

9 The nurse is teaching a client with hypomagnesemia to take 600 mg of magnesium oxide with each meal. How many tablets would the nurse administer for the dose if each tablet contains 400 mg? Record your answer rounding to one decimal place.

Fill in your answer below.

_____ tablets

. . . .

10 When caring for a client with a magnesium level of 1.1 mEq/L secondary to malabsorption, the nurse encourages the client to increase intake of which type of food?

1. Poultry
2. Tomatoes
3. Dairy products
4. Nuts

➤ *See pages 114–116 for Answers and Rationales*

I. OVERVIEW OF MAGNESIUM REGULATION

A. Magnesium balance and function: second most abundant cation in human body; absorbed in small intestine; conserved by kidneys during times of inadequate dietary intake and excreted by kidneys during times of excessive intake

1. Serum levels
   a. Normal plasma levels of **magnesium** range from 1.5 to 2.1 mEq/L
   b. Maintenance of magnesium levels in body is mostly a function of dietary intake
   c. Serum concentration of magnesium does not parallel tissue concentration; body stores may be more adequately measured by urinary magnesium excretion

2. Functions in the body
   a. Plays a major role in at least 300 fundamental enzymatic reactions
   b. Powers sodium-potassium pump
   c. Aids in converting adenosine triphosphate (ATP) to adenosine diphosphate (ADP) for energy release
   d. Transmits electrical impulses across nerves and muscles; important for skeletal muscle relaxation following contraction
   e. Maintains normal heart rhythm
   f. Involved in nucleic acid metabolism
   g. Needed for thiamine activity and for calcium and vitamin B_{12} absorption and utilization
   h. May be involved in stabilization of DNA and RNA
   i. Relaxes smooth muscles of bronchi and bronchioles
   j. Fights tooth decay by binding calcium to tooth enamel
   k. Decreased magnesium levels may contribute to secondary decreases in potassium, calcium, and phosphate levels
   l. Involved in fatty acid oxidation and is a cofactor in carbohydrate metabolism and protein synthesis
   m. Decreases or blocks release of acetylcholine, thereby acting as a smooth muscle relaxant

3. System interactions
   a. Plays a central role in secretion and action of insulin, thereby controlling blood glucose
   b. Necessary for release of parathyroid hormone (PTH) and plays a role in preeclampsia
   c. PTH and aldosterone indirectly affect magnesium reabsorption or excretion in kidneys
   d. High amounts of calcium and poorly digested fats and phosphates interfere with magnesium absorption due to binding mechanism in small intestine

4. See Table 5-1 for lifespan factors affecting magnesium balance

Table 5-1	Lifespan Considerations for Health Maintenance: Magnesium Balance	
Lifespan Considerations	**Common Risk Factors for Imbalances**	**Nursing Implications**
Infants	*Hypomagnesemia* Chronic diarrhea Malabsorption syndromes Failure to thrive Short bowel syndrome	Teach parents to include magnesium (Mg^{++})–rich foods in diet when diarrhea is present Teach parents to monitor infant for muscle twitching and increases in deep tendon reflexes (DTRs)
Children	*Hypomagnesemia* Cardiac surgery Multiple blood transfusions DKA: Mg^{++} lost in urine Prolonged nasogastric suction Cystic fibrosis: Mg^{++} bound to fatty stools and excreted	Assess child for muscle cramping and twitching, hyperactive DTRs, and neuromuscular changes Teach parents to encourage foods high in Mg^{++}
Adults	*Hypermagnesemia* Chronic renal failure: Mg^{++} not excreted *Hypomagnesemia* Acute pancreatitis: Mg^{++} binds to fats Chronic alcoholism and malnutrition: lack of dietary intake of Mg^{++}	Teach client to be alert to signs of hypermagnesemia Teach client to be alert to signs of hypomagnesemia Encourage intake of Mg^{++}-rich foods

B. Sources of magnesium

    1. Cellular level

        a. More than 50% of magnesium is found in bone

        b. Much of remaining magnesium in body is intracellular (approximately 45%), with residual amount present in extracellular spaces

        c. Most magnesium within cells is found in mitochondria and only 5–10% is free in cytosol

        d. Potassium, magnesium, and calcium are tied together intracellularly to maintain a neutral electrical charge; therefore, an altered level of any of these would ultimately affect the others

    2. Dietary level

        a. Average diet contains between 168 and 720 mg of magnesium per day

        b. Recommended allowance for magnesium is 300–350 mg for young men and women with an extra 150 mg per day during pregnancy and lactation; another way to calculate magnesium need is to base it on 4.5 mg per kilogram of body weight

        c. Sources of dietary magnesium; see Box 5-1 for foods high in magnesium

II. *HYPOMAGNESEMIA*

    A. Definition, etiology, and pathophysiology

        1. A serum magnesium level below 1.5 mEq/L

        2. Cellular level

            a. Hypomagnesemia usually occurs with nutritional or metabolic abnormalities; can occur because of reduced absorption, increased renal loss, or redistribution of body magnesium

            b. Approximately 50% of dietary magnesium is usually absorbed; absorption is inhibited by phytates, oxalates, and fat

        3. Predisposing clinical conditions

            a. Chronic alcoholism is the most common cause

            b. Decreased magnesium intake may be due to dietary factors or prolonged intravenous therapy without magnesium supplementation; in parenteral nutrition

Box 5-1	• Dark green leafy vegetables, such as raw spinach
Foods High in Magnesium	• Nuts and seeds
	• Fish such as mackerel, pollock, tuna, and others
	• Beans and lentils
	• Whole grains
	• Brown rice
	• Fruits such as avocadoes, bananas, and dried fruits
	• Dark chocolate or cocoa

Practice to Pass

By what mechanism does hypokalemia occur with hypomagnesemia?

therapy, magnesium moves into cells from bloodstream, leading to low serum magnesium levels

  c. Decreased absorption may be caused by inflammatory bowel disease, small bowel resection (less surface available to absorb), GI cancer, chronic pancreatitis, or medications such as gentamicin (aminoglycoside antibiotic), or cisplatin (antineoplastic agent)

  d. Increased intestinal (lower GI) losses may occur because of prolonged diarrhea, draining intestinal fistulas, and ileostomy

  e. Increased renal excretion may result from diuretic use (furosemide or ethacrynic acid), hyperaldosteronism that leads to volume expansion, diabetes that leads to osmotic diuresis, and medications such as aminoglycoside antibiotics, amphotericin B, and cyclosporine

  f. Losses can also occur because of burns and debridement therapy, sepsis, or alkalosis

B. Assessment

  1. Clinical manifestations

  a. Do not usually occur until serum level drops below 1 mEq/L

   b. Muscle twitching, tremors; hyperreactive reflexes occur because of effect of magnesium on neuromuscular function and hypocalcemic effect

   c. Laryngeal stridor (a life-threatening symptom) can occur

  d. Cardiovascular manifestations include supraventricular tachycardia and ventricular dysrhythmias (premature ventricular contractions and ventricular fibrillation) and increased susceptibility to digoxin toxicity (possibly enhanced by concurrent hypokalemia)

  e. Electrocardiogram (ECG) changes include diminished voltage of P wave; T waves that are broad, flat, or inverted; ST segments that are depressed; and QT intervals that are prolonged; a prominent U wave may be present

  f. Following cardiac surgery in children, watch for ventricular tachycardia and Torsades de Pointes (see Figures 5-1 and 5-2)

  g. Central nervous system manifestations include mood changes, such as apathy, depression, and confusion

  h. GI manifestations include nausea and vomiting, diarrhea, and anorexia, which occur because of concurrent hypokalemia

  i. Growth failure in children can occur

  j. Severe deficiency can lead to seizures, hallucinations, or tetany

  k. Signs and symptoms are somewhat similar to those of hypokalemia or hypocalcemia because they are all cations; positive Chvostek sign and Trousseau sign can occur

  2. Diagnostic and laboratory findings

  a. Plasma magnesium levels <1.5 mEq/L

  b. Associated electrolyte levels: concurrent decreases in calcium, potassium, and phosphate levels

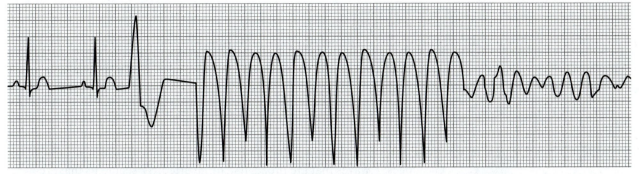

P Wave: Two normal P waves present; PR Interval: Not discernable during dysrhythmia; QRS Complex: Wide and distorted during dysrhythmia; QT Interval: Not discernable during dysrhythmia; Heart Rate: Atrial: Not discernable, Ventricular: Rapid; Rhythm: Both regular and irregular; Ectopic Beats: PVCs, ventricular tachycardia/fibrillation.

Figure 5-1

Ventricular tachycardia deteriorating into ventricular fibrillation.

Source: Osborn, Kathleen S.; Wraa, Cheryl E.; Watson, Annita, *Medical Surgical Nursing: Preparation For Practice*, Combined Volume, 1st Ed., ©2010. Reprinted and Electronically reproduced by permission of Pearson Education, Inc., Upper Saddle River, New Jersey.

    c. Trending of results
        1) Because most magnesium is stored in cells, plasma levels may be normal despite an overall body depletion of magnesium
        2) Hypomagnesemia should be considered with reference to presenting clinical manifestations or presence of other electrolyte imbalances, such as hypocalcemia or hypokalemia
   3. Identification of risk factors: dietary insufficiency or previously identified coexisting medical conditions that lead to or exacerbate hypomagnesemia
C. Priority nursing concerns
   1. Inadequate nutrition related to decreased magnesium intake
   2. Insufficient knowledge of magnesium content in food and alternative food choices
   3. Possibility of neuromuscular manifestations
   4. Possible decreased cardiac output if ventricular dysrhythmias occur

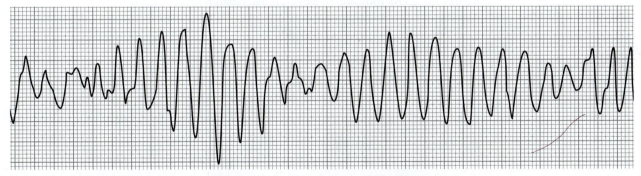

P Waves: Not discernable; PR Interval: Not discernable; QRS Complex: Wide, distorted, and varying heights; QT Interval: not discernable; Rate: Rapid; Rhythm: Both regular and irregular; Ectopic Beats: All.

Figure 5-2

Torsades de Pointes.

Source: Osborn, Kathleen S.; Wraa, Cheryl E.; Watson, Annita, *Medical Surgical Nursing: Preparation For Practice*, Combined Volume, 1st Ed., ©2010. Reprinted and Electronically reproduced by permission of Pearson Education, Inc., Upper Saddle River, New Jersey.

D. Therapeutic management
1. Replacement therapies
    a. Vary depending on presenting signs and symptoms and severity of condition
    b. May include intravenous infusion of magnesium sulfate, oral magnesium salts, and dietary interventions
2. Continued monitoring of client
    a. Serum magnesium levels and other electrolyte imbalances
    b. Neuromuscular manifestations
    c. Altered GI function
    d. Cardiovascular changes/dysrhythmias
    e. ECG changes: T waves that are broad, flat, or inverted; ST segments that are depressed; and QT intervals that are prolonged
    f. Unresolved signs and symptoms after therapy
3. Restoration of balance
    a. Promote dietary changes to increase magnesium intake
    b. Administer magnesium supplements as prescribed
    c. Provide parenteral administration if warranted
    d. Monitor a client taking digoxin because there is increased susceptibility to digoxin toxicity with hypomagnesemia

E. Client-centered nursing care
1. Identify risk factors: malabsorption and/or GI dysfunction, renal disease, diabetes, alcohol intake, and medications such as diuretics
2. Monitor clients with diabetes for hyperglycemia leading to osmotic diuresis, resulting in decreased magnesium
3. Monitor client receiving continuous IV fluid therapy, who may need addition of magnesium to solution
4. Monitor client with hyperaldosteronism because volume expansion may result in decreased magnesium
5. Monitor client taking a diuretic for increased renal excretion of magnesium
6. Institute ECG monitoring and seizure precautions
7. Monitor for stridor and/or difficulty swallowing
8. Keep bed rails raised if client is confused; take other safety precautions as needed
9. Maintain accurate intake and output (I&O) records
10. Monitor deep tendon reflexes (DTRs) in clients receiving IV magnesium solutions; depressed DTRs indicate an elevated magnesium level
11. Monitor for hypotension in clients receiving IV magnesium replacements, which could be a sign of **hypermagnesemia**

F. Medication therapy
1. Oral replacement therapy
    a. Magnesium-containing antacids
    b. Magnesium oxide 300 mg/day in divided doses
    c. Use caution because oral administration may cause diarrhea, leading to decreased absorption
2. Parenteral replacement therapy
    a. Magnesium sulfate 2 grams (16 mEq) in 50% solution IV as prescribed; infuse slowly as prescribed; rapid administration could lead to respiratory or cardiac arrest
    b. Magnesium chloride 48 mEq/day by continuous IV infusion; administer slowly as prescribed for reason described above
    c. Ensure that client maintains a urine output of at least 30 mL/hr or 120 mL every 4 hours during therapy to avoid rebound hypermagnesemia if renal insufficiency is present

Practice to Pass

What commonly used antacids are high in magnesium?

      d. Monitor deep tendon reflexes (such as patellar reflex) before each dose of paren-
teral magnesium; if reflex is present, hypermagnesemia from previous doses has
not occurred

      e. Watch for signs of rebound hypermagnesemia

   3. Dietary therapy: for mild hypomagnesemia, encourage foods high in magnesium
(refer back to Box 5-1)

G. Client education

   1. Teach awareness of predisposing factors, including:

      a. Diabetes mellitus

      b. Anorexia and nausea and vomiting

      c. Chronic diarrhea or chronic aluminum-based laxative abuse

      d. Alcoholism

      e. Hyperaldosteronism

      f. Renal tubular disorders

      g. Chronic diuretic therapy

      h. Hypokalemia or hypocalcemia

      i. Metabolic alkalosis

   2. Dietary education

      a. Review foods high in magnesium

      b. Increase intake of hard water or mineral water as these are high in magnesium

      c. Recommend 300–350 mg magnesium intake daily with an extra 150 mg for preg-
nant or lactating women

      d. Collaborate with dietitian as necessary

H. Evaluation

   1. Serum magnesium, calcium, and other electrolyte levels are within normal limits

   2. Client remains safe and free from injury

   3. Manifestations of hypomagnesemia resolve

III. HYPERMAGNESEMIA

A. Definition, etiology, and pathophysiology

   1. A serum magnesium level above 2.1 mEq/L

   2. Cellular level: usually due to iatrogenic causes

      a. Decreased renal excretion of magnesium, such as with decreased urine output or
renal failure

      b. Increased magnesium intake, such as with overuse of magnesium-containing ant-
acids, cathartics, or enemas; total parenteral nutrition; or hemodialysis using hard
water dialysate

   3. Predisposing clinical conditions

      a. Untreated diabetic ketoacidosis (glucose carries cations across cell membranes)

      b. Adrenal insufficiency (Addison disease): causes fluid and electrolyte shifts

      c. Magnesium treatment in preeclampsia of pregnancy

      d. Lithium ingestion

      e. Volume depletion

B. Assessment

   1. Clinical manifestations

      a. Neuromuscular symptoms are most common, including decreased deep ten-
don reflexes and depressed neuromuscular activity; similar to those seen in
hyperkalemia

      b. Cardiovascular manifestations include hypotension, bradycardia, bradydysrhyth-
mias, flushing and sensation of warmth, possible cardiac arrest

      c. ECG may show prolonged PR interval, widened QRS complex, and elevated T wave

Practice to Pass

What foods would you
recommend to a client
who needs to increase
magnesium intake?

Box 5-2	Antacids	Laxatives
Medications Containing Magnesium	• Maalox • Riopan • Milk of Magnesia • Mylanta • Gaviscon • Gelusil • Rolaids	• Milk of Magnesia • SloMag • MagOx • Epsom salt • Maalox • Magnesium citrate

Practice to Pass

What cardiovascular symptoms may occur with hypermagnesemia?

    d. CNS depression may include somnolence, weakness and lethargy, respiratory depression, and coma

  2. Diagnostic and laboratory findings

    a. Plasma magnesium levels are >2.1 mEq/L

    b. Associated electrolyte levels: none

    c. Trending of results: degree of elevation of magnesium is proportionate to severity of symptoms

C. Priority nursing concerns

  1. Possible decreased cardiac output if cardiac conduction abnormalities are present

  2. Possibility of injury because of neuromuscular changes

  3. Possible threat to respiratory sufficiency

  4. Insufficient knowledge of causes of elevated magnesium levels

D. Therapeutic management

  1. Decrease magnesium intake; withdraw all magnesium-containing agents including antacids and laxatives (see Box 5-2)

  2. Promote magnesium excretion using diuretics (in stable renal function)

  3. Continued monitoring of client

    a. Overhydration, magnesium toxicity

    b. Cardiac status and ECG changes

    c. Symptoms of CNS depression

    d. Respiratory status and changes

  4. Restoration of balance

    a. Correct diabetic ketoacidosis by administration of insulin and IV dextrose to halt cellular catabolism

    b. Provide rehydration to promote increased urinary output and magnesium excretion

    c. Emergency treatment includes IV calcium gluconate to antagonize effect of magnesium and counteract cardiac and respiratory symptoms

    d. Dialysis: in clients with renal failure, dialysis may be used for magnesium removal; if hemodialysis is not feasible, peritoneal dialysis is an option

E. Client-centered care

  1. Monitor I&O

  2. Identify risk factors such as antacid use, laxative use, diabetic instability, and renal failure

  3. Monitor for potential complications

  4. Promote client safety

Practice to Pass

What role does calcium gluconate have in the treatment of hypermagnesemia?

F. Medication therapy

  1. Parenteral administration

    a. IV calcium gluconate 10% for emergency situations

    b. IV diuretics to promote urinary excretion

  2. Specific drug therapies: as above, in addition to rehydration to increase urine output

G. Client education
1. Awareness of predisposing factors
   a. Avoid medications and supplements high in magnesium
   b. Risks of chronic antacid and enema use
   c. Diabetic control measures
   d. Signs and symptoms of high or low magnesium levels
2. Dietary education: avoid high-magnesium foods (refer back to Box 5-1)

H. Evaluation
1. Manifestations of hypermagnesemia resolve and serum levels return to normal
2. Client verbalizes an understanding of importance of diet, follow-up visits, and laboratory testing

Case Study

A 32-year-old female tells the nurse she feels her heart is racing and she has been getting frequent cramps in her legs and hands for the past week or so. She has had no recent illness or injury. She has no known allergies and denies any medication or drug use. Her review of systems is negative except for constipation. Intake information for this visit is as follows: height 5'8", weight 120 lbs, BP 110/72, pulse 98, respirations 18.

1. What data from the above may indicate a risk factor for hypomagnesemia?
2. What other subjective data should be gathered?
3. What diagnostic evaluation measures would be helpful?
4. What collaborative measures should be considered?
5. What instructions would you give this client to avoid fluctuating magnesium levels?

For suggested responses, see page 192.

POSTTEST

1. When caring for a client receiving intravenous (IV) replacement of magnesium sulfate, the nurse should plan to monitor the client for which potential complication?
   1. Rebound hypermagnesemia
   2. Abdominal cramping
   3. Tachypnea
   4. Headaches

2. The nurse should plan to assess a client for hypotension and diminished deep tendon reflexes when laboratory values reflect which level of magnesium?
   1. 1.2 mEq/L
   2. 1.4 mEq/L
   3. 2.1 mEq/L
   4. 2.8 mEq/L

3. The nurse would recommend to a client who has hypomagnesemia that the client should increase intake of which foods? Select all that apply.
   1. Rice
   2. Seafood
   3. Legumes
   4. Fresh fruit
   5. Whole grains

4 The nurse anticipates that which treatment would be used for a client who has a magnesium level of 2.9 mEq/L?
1. Magnesium oxide
2. Furosemide
3. Calcium carbonate
4. Fluid restriction

5 The nurse anticipates that which client is at risk for hypermagnesemia?
1. A 16-year-old female with anorexia nervosa
2. A 57-year-old male with chronic alcohol abuse
3. A 47-year-old female with a history of partial gastrectomy
4. A 62-year-old male with chronic renal failure

6 The nurse explains to a new nurse orientee that a hyperglycemic diabetic client may experience magnesium imbalances secondary to the osmotic diuresis that occurs. The nurse instructs the orientee to observe the client for which finding?
1. Elevated liver enzymes
2. Muscle twitching
3. Bradycardia
4. Hypotension

7 The nurse should assess for which common side effect when administering oral magnesium to a client?
1. Decreased appetite
2. Decreased urine output
3. Increased thirst
4. Diarrhea

8 The nurse should assess for signs of hypomagnesemia in which clients? Select all that apply.
1. A client with a history of laxative abuse
2. A client who is noncompliant with diuretic therapy
3. A client who takes magnesium-containing antacids
4. A client who is taking gentamicin
5. A client with a history of alcohol abuse

9 A client is admitted with new-onset renal failure. The nurse should observe for which clinical manifestation of hypermagnesemia? Select all that apply.
1. Tachycardia
2. Decreased deep tendon reflexes
3. Decreased respirations
4. Hypertension
5. Weakness and lethargy

10 After treating hypomagnesemia with replacement therapy, a repeat serum magnesium level is 4.0 mEq/L. The nurse anticipates receiving a prescription for which medication?
1. Dextrose
2. Calcium gluconate
3. Potassium chloride
4. Sodium chloride

➤ *See pages 116–118 for Answers and Rationales.*

ANSWERS & RATIONALES

Pretest

1 **Answer: 3 Rationale:** Many laxatives are magnesium-based compounds. Overuse could result in increased absorption of magnesium and decreased kidney excretion. Malabsorption would more likely lead to a low magnesium level. Anemia is unrelated to the client's magnesium level. Excessive alcohol use could lead to inadequate nutrition and hypomagnesemia. **Cognitive Level:** Applying **Client Need:** Physiological Adaptation **Integrated Process:** Nursing Process: Diagnosis **Content Area:** Adult Health **Strategy:** The question requires you to correlate a high magnesium level to a cause. Eliminate factors that lower serum magnesium. Recall content of many laxatives to choose correctly. **Reference:** LeMone, P., Burke, K., Bauldoff, G., & Gubrud, P. (2015). *Medical surgical nursing: Clinical reasoning in patient care* (6th ed.). New York, NY: Pearson, pp. 210–211.

2 **Answer: 4 Rationale:** Deep tendon reflexes (DTRs) may be diminished or absent when magnesium levels are high (normal 1.5–2.1 mEq/L). This is because magnesium diminishes acetylcholine activity at the myoneural junction, thus impairing impulse transmission. Diarrhea is not a sign of hypermagnesemia. Hyperreflexia is the opposite problem of diminished deep tendon reflexes, and would be more likely to occur with hypomagnesemia. Hypotension rather than hypertension can occur with hypermagnesemia. **Cognitive Level:** Analyzing **Client Need:** Reduction of Risk Potential **Integrated Process:** Nursing Process: Assessment **Content Area:** Adult Health **Strategy:** First recognize that the magnesium level is elevated. The critical word is *manifestations* and the core concept is *hypermagnesemia*. Recall the role of magnesium in regulating the neuromuscular conduction to direct you to the correct option. **Reference:** LeMone, P., Burke, K., Bauldoff, G., & Gubrud, P. (2015). *Medical surgical nursing: Clinical reasoning in patient care* (6th ed.). New York, NY: Pearson, pp. 210–211.

3 **Answer: 3 Rationale:** A magnesium level of 1.2 mEq/L reflects hypomagnesemia. The client needs diet counseling to learn what foods are high in magnesium so they can be increased in the diet. Although clients should always avoid hazardous activities and reflexes may be hyperactive, this is not the most important action for the nurse to take. Weekly laboratory evaluations would not be sufficient to monitor the magnesium level. The client needs to have measures that will increase the magnesium and then have the level rechecked. A magnesium level of 1.2 mEq/L reflects hypomagnesemia. Alcohol intake may interfere with adequate intake of dietary sources of magnesium and would not be suggested. **Cognitive Level:** Analyzing **Client Need:** Reduction of Risk Potential **Integrated Process:** Teaching and Learning **Content Area:** Adult Health **Strategy:** First recognize that the magnesium level is low and recall that food supplies the electrolytes needed by the body. Use this concept to focus on diet counseling as the correct option. **Reference:** LeMone, P., Burke, K., Bauldoff, G., & Gubrud, P. (2015). *Medical surgical nursing: Clinical reasoning in patient care* (6th ed.). New York, NY: Pearson, pp. 209–210.

4 **Answer: 2 Rationale:** It is important to determine what type of enema the mother is using. Epsom salt contains magnesium and, if used excessively, it can be absorbed through the bowel, contributing to hypermagnesemia. Although it would be important to know how frequently the child is being given enemas, the nurse wants to determine if the child is at risk for hypermagnesemia, which would be caused by absorption of the electrolyte in the enema solution. Timing of last bowel movement will not help the nurse to know if the child has received enema solutions containing magnesium. Although a

discussion of constipation and alternatives to frequent enemas should be discussed, this is the not the best question to ask to determine if the child is at risk for hypermagnesemia. **Cognitive Level:** Applying **Client Need:** Reduction of Risk Potential **Integrated Process:** Nursing Process: Evaluation **Content Area:** Child Health **Strategy:** The critical words are *child, enema,* and *hypermagnesemia*. Recall the dangers of excessive use of enemas and cause of hypermagnesemia to choose correctly. **Reference:** London, M., Ladewig, P., Davidson, M., Ball, J., Bindler, R., & Cowen, K. (2017). *Maternal and child nursing care* (5th ed.). New York, NY: Pearson Education, pp. 1232–1260.

5 **Answer: 1, 4 Rationale:** A magnesium level of 2.8 is elevated (normal 1.5–2.1 mEq/L), most likely as a result of inadequate renal secretion secondary to chronic renal failure. Foods high in magnesium include whole grains, legumes, oranges, bananas, green leafy vegetables, and chocolate. Apples, pork sausage, and Swiss cheese are not rich sources of magnesium. **Cognitive Level:** Applying **Client Need:** Reduction of Risk Potential **Integrated Process:** Nursing Process: Assessment **Content Area:** Adult Health **Strategy:** First recognize that the magnesium level is elevated. Recall foods high in magnesium to choose correctly. **Reference:** Dudek, S. (2013). *Nutrition essentials for nursing practice* (7th ed.). Philadelphia: Lippincott Williams & Wilkins, pp. 128, 131.

6 **Answer: 4 Rationale:** Decreased magnesium levels also contribute to reductions in potassium, calcium, and phosphate because these electrolytes are also involved in cellular metabolism and are frequently low in the client with alcoholism. An elevated potassium level would not be an expected finding. An elevated phosphorus level would be expected most often in a client with renal disease such as renal failure. A decreased sodium level is an unrelated finding. **Cognitive Level:** Applying **Client Need:** Reduction of Risk Potential **Integrated Process:** Nursing Process: Planning **Content Area:** Adult Health **Strategy:** First recognize that the magnesium level is decreased. Then recall which electrolyte may be abnormal in the presence of low magnesium to direct you to choose decreased calcium. **Reference:** LeMone, P., Burke, K., Bauldoff, G., & Gubrud, P. (2015). *Medical surgical nursing: Clinical reasoning in patient care* (6th ed.). New York, NY: Pearson, pp. 209–210.

7 **Answer: 2 Rationale:** Transmission of impulses is decreased through magnesium's regulation of acetylcholine in the neuromuscular synapse, producing muscle relaxation. Because magnesium acts to regulate and diminish acetylcholine, neuromuscular transmissions are decreased, not stimulated. Acetylcholine is not involved in vitamin metabolism. Magnesium and acetylcholine are not involved in blood glucose regulation. **Cognitive Level:** Comprehension **Client Need:** Physiological Adaptation **Integrated Process:** Teaching and Learning **Content Area:** Adult Health **Strategy:** This question requires you to translate the chemical action of magnesium to its

ANSWERS & RATIONALES

ANSWERS & RATIONALES

physiological effect in the body. Recall the action of acetylcholine on neuromuscular function to help you choose correctly. **Reference:** LeMone, P., Burke, K., Bauldoff, G., & Gubrud, P. (2015). *Medical surgical nursing: Clinical reasoning in patient care* (6th ed.). New York, NY: Pearson, pp. 209–210.

8 Answer: 1 Rationale: A magnesium level of 1.0 mEq/L reflects hypomagnesemia (normal 1.5–2.1 mEq/L), which can lead to tetany if levels continue to decrease. Hyperactive reflexes are early signs of tetany. Although the client's nausea needs to be addressed, it may be related to effects of the anesthesia, postoperative medications, or an electrolyte imbalance, and is not of as high a priority as hyperactive reflexes. Anorexia may be related to the client's postoperative status and is of lesser priority. Although it needs to be addressed, abdominal pain is an expected finding in the client who has just had a bowel resection. **Cognitive Level:** Analyzing **Client Need:** Reduction of Risk Potential **Integrated Process:** Nursing Process: Diagnosis **Content Area:** Adult Health **Strategy:** Recognize the critical level of the magnesium. Recall that this imbalance can lead to seizures to direct you to hyperactive reflexes. **Reference:** LeMone, P., Burke, K., Bauldoff, G., & Gubrud, P. (2015). *Medical surgical nursing: Clinical reasoning in patient care* (6th ed.). New York, NY: Pearson, pp. 209–210.

9 Answer: 1.5 Rationale: The question is set up with the desired dose as the numerator and the dose on hand as the denominator. Multiply that by the quantity (which is one tablet) to obtain the correct result. 600/400 × 1 tab = 1.5 = 1.5 tabs. **Cognitive Level:** Applying **Client Need:** Physiological Integrity:Pharmacological and Parenteral Therapies **Integrated Process:** Nursing Process: Implementation **Content Area:** Adult Health **Strategy:** Recognize that only 400 mg is contained in each pill. Divide the desired amount (600 mg) over what you have (400 mg) to calculate the correct dose. **Reference:** Olsen, J., Giangrasso, A., Shrimpton, D., & Dillon, P. (2016). *Medical dosage calculations* (11th ed.). New York, NY: Pearson, p. 105.

10 Answer: 4 Rationale: Sources of magnesium in the diet include green leafy vegetables, nuts, legumes, whole grains, seafood, bananas, oranges, and chocolate. Poultry is not high in magnesium. Tomatoes are lower in magnesium than green leafy vegetables. Dairy products are not rich in magnesium. **Cognitive Level:** Application **Client Need:** Reduction of Risk Potential **Integrated Process:** Nursing Process: Implementation **Content Area:** Adult Health **Strategy:** Specific knowledge of the mineral content of various types of foods is needed to answer the question. Recall foods high in magnesium to choose correctly. **Reference:** LeMone, P., Burke, K., Bauldoff, G., & Gubrud, P. (2015). *Medical surgical nursing: Clinical reasoning in patient care* (6th ed.). New York, NY: Pearson, pp. 209–210.

Posttest

1 Answer: 1 Rationale: Replacement of any electrolyte solution can lead to elevated levels of that electrolyte if the infusion is given too quickly or excessive replacement is given. Abdominal cramping and diarrhea are seen more often with oral magnesium replacements. Replacement of magnesium can lead to hypermagnesemia, which would be reflected by respiratory depression, not tachypnea. Replacement of magnesium can lead to hypermagnesemia; headaches are not associated with this imbalance. **Cognitive Level:** Applying **Client Need:** Physiological Adaptation **Integrated Process:** Nursing Process: Planning **Content Area:** Adult Health **Strategy:** The critical words in the question are *IV*, *magnesium sulfate*, and *complication*. Recall the need to infuse magnesium slowly to prevent rapid increases in plasma levels to direct you to the correct option. **Reference:** LeMone, P., Burke, K., Bauldoff, G., & Gubrud, P. (2015). *Medical surgical nursing: Clinical reasoning in patient care* (6th ed.). New York, NY: Pearson, pp. 210–211.

2 Answer: 4 Rationale: A level of 2.8 mEq/L is elevated. Symptoms of hypermagnesemia include hypotension, bradycardia and heart block, decreased or absent deep tendon reflexes, and muscle weakness. A magnesium level of 1.2 mEq/L is below normal and symptoms would include hypertension, bradycardia, and increased deep tendon reflexes. A magnesium level of 1.4 mEq/L is below normal, and symptoms would include hypertension, prolonged PR and QT intervals, and increased deep tendon reflexes. A level of 2.1 mEq/L is within normal limits. **Cognitive Level:** Analyzing **Client Need:** Physiological Adaptation **Integrated Process:** Nursing Process: Assessment **Content Area:** Adult Health **Strategy:** The critical words are *hypotension* and *diminished deep tendon reflexes*. Recall that these are symptoms associated with hypermagnesemia to choose correctly. **Reference:** LeMone, P., Burke, K., Bauldoff, G., & Gubrud, P. (2015). *Medical surgical nursing: Clinical reasoning in patient care* (6th ed.). New York, NY: Pearson, pp. 210–211.

3 Answer: 2, 3, 5 Rationale: Legumes, seafood, and whole grains are high in magnesium. Rice and fresh fruit contain either low or trace amounts of magnesium. **Cognitive Level:** Applying **Client Need:** Physiological Adaptation **Integrated Process:** Teaching and Learning **Content Area:** Foundational Sciences **Strategy:** This question requires specific knowledge to make the correct choices. Recall food sources high in magnesium to choose correctly. **Reference:** Dudek, S. (2013). *Nutrition essentials for nursing practice* (7th ed.). Philadelphia: Lippincott Williams & Wilkins, pp. 128–131.

4 Answer: 2 Rationale: Treatment for hypermagnesemia is to promote urinary excretion of magnesium to decrease serum levels, so a diuretic may be indicated. Laxatives may contain magnesium, and a magnesium-containing laxative could worsen the imbalance. Antacids often contain magnesium, which could worsen the imbalance. Fluid restriction would be contraindicated because it would prevent flushing of excess magnesium from the body. **Cognitive Level:** Analyzing **Client Need:** Reduction of Risk Potential **Integrated Process:** Nursing Process: Planning **Content Area:** Adult Health **Strategy:** First determine that the magnesium level is elevated. Eliminate the magnesium source, the option that would inhibit magnesium excretion, and the option that is not useful. **Reference:** LeMone, P., Burke, K., Bauldoff, G., & Gubrud, P. (2015). *Medical surgical nursing*: *Clinical reasoning in patient care* (6th ed.). New York, NY: Pearson, pp. 209–210.

5 **Answer: 4 Rationale:** Clients with chronic renal failure have difficulty excreting magnesium and are at risk to develop hypermagnesemia. Clients with anorexia restrict intake of nutrients and so would be at risk to develop hypomagnesemia. Clients with chronically high alcohol intake often do not have adequate dietary intake of foods high in magnesium. Hypomagnesemia is often seen in these clients. A partial gastrectomy may cause faster gastric emptying and transit through the small intestine, which would reduce absorption of magnesium. **Cognitive Level:** Analyzing **Client Need:** Physiological Adaptation **Integrated Process:** Nursing Process: Assessment **Content Area:** Adult Health **Strategy:** Critical words are *hypermagnesemia* and *risk*. Eliminate two options because intake of magnesium is reduced in these conditions. Recall that magnesium is absorbed in the small intestine to eliminate a third option. **Reference:** LeMone, P., Burke, K., Bauldoff, G., & Gubrud, P. (2015). *Medical surgical nursing*: *Clinical reasoning in patient care* (6th ed.). New York, NY: Pearson, pp. 210–211.

6 **Answer: 2 Rationale:** The osmotic diuresis that occurs with hyperglycemia can lead to urinary losses of magnesium and hypomagnesemia. Symptoms include hyperactive reflexes and neuromuscular irritability (muscle twitching), cardiac dysrhythmias, mood changes, depression, and confusion. Elevated liver enzymes are not seen with hypomagnesemia. Bradycardia would be seen with hypermagnesemia. Hypotension can occur with hypermagnesemia. **Cognitive Level:** Analyzing **Client Need:** Physiological Adaptation **Integrated Process:** Teaching and Learning **Content Area:** Adult Health **Strategy:** First recognize the electrolyte imbalance that will occur in hypomagnesemia, secondary to hyperglycemia, producing a hyperosmotic state in the blood leading to diuresis. Recall signs of low magnesium to be directed to the correct option. **Reference:** LeMone, P., Burke, K., Bauldoff, G., & Gubrud, P. (2015). *Medical surgical nursing*: *Clinical reasoning in patient care* (6th ed.). New York, NY: Pearson, pp. 209–210.

7 **Answer: 4 Rationale:** Oral magnesium supplements frequently cause diarrhea, which can decrease the absorption of the magnesium. Oral magnesium supplements should not cause a decrease in appetite. Oral magnesium supplements do not reduce urine output. Oral magnesium supplements do not result in increased thirst. **Cognitive Level:** Applying **Client Need:** Pharmacological and Parenteral Therapies **Integrated Process:** Nursing Process: Assessment **Content Area:** Adult Health **Strategy:** The critical word is *oral*. Recall magnesium is a common ingredient in laxatives to direct you to the correct option. **Reference:** LeMone, P., Burke, K., Bauldoff, G., & Gubrud, P. (2015). *Medical surgical nursing*: *Clinical reasoning in patient care* (6th ed.). New York, NY: Pearson, pp. 209–210.

8 **Answer: 4, 5 Rationale:** A side effect of gentamicin is hypomagnesemia because of excretion through the kidneys. Clients who have a history of alcohol abuse often do not consume sufficient nutrients with magnesium and experience hypomagnesemia. Many laxatives contain magnesium, which will be absorbed in the small intestines and could lead to hypermagnesemia. Loop diuretics can contribute to magnesium losses, but if a client is noncompliant with diuretic therapy, the risk for magnesium loss is reduced. Use of magnesium antacids would place the client at risk for hypermagnesemia. **Cognitive Level:** Analyzing **Client Need:** Physiological Adaptation **Integrated Process:** Nursing Process: Assessment **Content Area:** Adult Health **Strategy:** Eliminate laxative abuse and antacid use because these conditions would contribute to an increase of magnesium. Eliminate noncompliance with diuretic therapy because this would reduce the amount of magnesium lost in the urine. **Reference:** LeMone, P., Burke, K., Bauldoff, G., & Gubrud, P. (2015). *Medical surgical nursing*: *Clinical reasoning in patient care* (6th ed.). New York, NY: Pearson, pp. 209–210.

9 **Answer: 2, 3, 5 Rationale:** Depressed deep tendon reflexes are among the most common clinical manifestations of hypermagnesemia. Decreased respirations can occur with hypermagnesemia. Weakness and lethargy can occur with hypermagnesemia because of neuromuscular depressant effects. The client is at risk for bradycardia rather than tachycardia. The client is at risk for hypotension rather than hypertension. **Cognitive Level:** Applying **Client Need:** Reduction of Risk Potential **Integrated Process:** Nursing Process: Assessment **Content Area:** Adult Health **Strategy:** Recall magnesium's role in the regulation of acetylcholine at the neuromuscular junction to direct you to the correct options. **Reference:** LeMone, P., Burke, K., Bauldoff, G., & Gubrud, P. (2015). *Medical surgical nursing*: *Clinical reasoning in patient care* (6th ed.). New York, NY: Pearson, pp. 209–210.

10 **Answer: 2 Rationale:** A magnesium level of 4.0 mEq/L is elevated. Calcium gluconate is the antagonist given to counteract the effect of excess magnesium on cardiac and muscular tissues. Dextrose would not help to counteract the effects of the elevated magnesium level.

ANSWERS & RATIONALES

Potassium chloride is not given to treat high magnesium levels. Sodium chloride is a salt and is not useful in treating elevated magnesium levels. **Cognitive Level:** Analyzing **Client Need:** Reduction of Risk Potential **Integrated Process:** Nursing Process: Planning **Content Area:** Adult Health **Strategy:** Recognize that the magnesium level is dangerously elevated. Recall the need to antagonize the cardiac and muscular effects of excessive magnesium to choose correctly. **Reference:** LeMone, P., Burke, K., Bauldoff, G., & Gubrud, P. (2015). *Medical surgical nursing: Clinical reasoning in patient care* (6th ed.). New York, NY: Pearson, pp. 209–210.

References

Adams, M., Holland, L., & Urban, C. (2017). *Pharmacology for nurses: A pathophysiologic approach* (5th ed.). New York, NY: Pearson.

Ball, J., Bindler, R., & Cowen, K. (2014). *Child health nursing: Partnering with children and families* (3rd ed.). Upper Saddle River, NJ: Pearson.

Berman, A., Snyder, S., & Frandsen, G. (2016). *Fundamentals of nursing: Concepts, process, and practice* (10th ed.). New York, NY: Pearson.

Ignatavicius, D., & Workman, M. (2015). *Medical-surgical nursing: Patient-centered collaborative care* (8th ed.). Philadelphia, PA: Elsevier Saunders.

Kee, J. L. (2017). *Pearson's handbook of laboratory and diagnostic tests* (8th ed.). New York, NY: Pearson.

LeMone, P., Burke, K., Bauldoff, G., & Gubrud, P. (2015). *Medical surgical nursing: Clinical reasoning in patient care* (6th ed.). New York, NY: Pearson.

London, M., Ladewig, P., Davidson, M., Ball, J., Bindler, R., & Cowen, K. (2017). *Maternal and child nursing care* (5th ed.). New York, NY: Pearson.

Osborne, K. S., Wraa, C. E., & Watson, A. B. (2010). *Medical surgical nursing: Preparation for practice.* Upper Saddle River, NJ: Pearson Education.

Phosphorus Balance and Imbalances

6

Chapter Outline

Overview of Phosphorus
  Regulation

Hypophosphatemia

Hyperphosphatemia

Objectives

➤ Identify the basic functions of phosphorus in the body.
➤ Explain the pathophysiology and etiology of phosphorus imbalances.
➤ Identify specific assessment findings and diagnostic tests as they relate to phosphorus imbalances.
➤ Identify priority nursing concerns for phosphorus imbalances.
➤ Describe the therapeutic management of phosphorus imbalances.
➤ Describe the management of nursing care for a client who is experiencing a phosphorus imbalance.

NCLEX-RN® Test Prep

Access the NEW Web-based app that provides students with additional practice questions in preparation for the NCLEX experience.

Review at a Glance

2,3-diphosphoglycerate (2,3-DPG) a substance found in red blood cells that facilitates delivery of oxygen to tissues

adenosine triphosphate (ATP) a compound stored in muscle containing three phosphorus groups that produces energy when split

hyperphosphatemia serum phosphate level greater than 4.5 mg/dL

hypophosphatemia serum phosphate level less than 2.5 mg/dL

metastatic calcification precipitate of calcium phosphate in soft tissues, joints, and arteries as a complication of hyperphosphatemia

parathyroid hormone (PTH or parathormone) secreted by parathyroid gland to regulate calcium and phosphorus metabolism

phospholipids a lipid substance containing phosphorus and fatty acids

phosphorus/phosphate a nonmetallic element usually found in combination with other elements; terms are often used interchangeably

refeeding syndrome a state of hypophosphatemia that can occur when infusing high levels of calories into clients who have anorexia or are malnourished from any cause

renal osteodystrophy an alteration of bone morphology in clients with chronic kidney disease (CKD); a means of measuring the skeletal component of CKD

tetany a nervous system disorder marked by intermittent tonic spasms that are usually paroxysmal and involve extremities

total parenteral nutrition (TPN) intravenous provision of total nutritional needs for a client unable to take appropriate amounts of food by enteral route; administered via a central venous access device

vitamin D a fat-soluble vitamin essential for calcium and phosphorus absorption from small intestine and metabolism

PRETEST

1. A 6-month-old infant has a phosphorus level of 5.0 mEq/L. To help determine the cause of this level, the nurse should ask the infant's parent which question?

1. "Has the baby had a lot of diarrhea lately?"
2. "What kind of milk do you feed the baby?"
3. "Is the baby eating a lot of solid foods?"
4. "Has the baby been vomiting a lot lately?"

2. When checking serum phosphorus levels on a pediatric client with hypophosphatemia, the nurse anticipates finding which information?

1. Levels will be highest in the early morning.
2. Normal levels are slightly higher secondary to rapid skeletal growth.
3. A decrease will be seen initially after starting replacement therapy.
4. An arterial sample must be obtained to provide the most accurate level.

3. When checking a client's laboratory values, the nurse notes the phosphate level is 1.7 mg/dL. The nurse should also check laboratory values for evidence of which of the following?

1. An elevated platelet count
2. A decrease in hemoglobin level
3. A decrease in calcium level
4. An elevated magnesium level

4. The nurse would assess for manifestations of hypophosphatemia in a client who has which predisposing clinical conditions? Select all that apply.

1. Superficial thickness burns
2. Diabetic ketoacidosis
3. Hypermagnesemia
4. Oliguria
5. Chronic alcohol abuse

5. The nurse would plan to include the need for which foods in the diet when providing discharge teaching for a client with a phosphorus level of 1.5 mg/dL? Select all that apply.

1. Green leafy vegetables
2. White breads
3. Citrus fruits
4. Eggs
5. Liver

6. A client has just been started on total parenteral nutrition (TPN) for severe malnutrition. The nurse determines refeeding syndrome has occurred after noting which laboratory test result?

1. Magnesium 2.5 mg/dL
2. Calcium 9.8 mg/dL
3. Phosphorus 1.2 mg/dL
4. Potassium 4.2 mEq/L

7. Which finding in a client's history would alert the nurse to assess for signs and symptoms of hypophosphatemia?

1. Withdrawal from alcohol
2. Oliguric phase of acute tubular necrosis
3. Short-term gastric suction
4. Occasional use of aluminum-containing antacids

8. Which concurrent electrolyte imbalance should the nurse anticipate while caring for a client with a phosphate level of 4.9 mg/dL?

1. Hyperkalemia
2. Hyponatremia
3. Hypocalcemia
4. Hypermagnesemia

9 A client has developed a serum phosphorus level of 5.0 mg/dL secondary to cytotoxic drug therapy. Because of the concurrent hyperuricemia that occurs with this therapy, the nurse anticipates administration of which medication?

1. Aluminum hydroxide
2. Allopurinol
3. Acetazolamide
4. Albiglutide

10 When providing discharge teaching for a client who requires a diet high in phosphates, the nurse should include which statement?

1. "High levels of phosphates are found in food additives."
2. "Increase your vitamin A intake to enhance phosphorus absorption."
3. "Aluminum-based antacids increase phosphorus absorption."
4. "Soy and soy products are excellent sources of phosphorus."

➤ *See pages 132–133 for Answers and Rationales.*

I. OVERVIEW OF PHOSPHORUS REGULATION

A. Phosphorus balance

1. Serum levels
   a. Normal serum **phosphate** levels range from 2.5 to 4.5 mg/dL (1.7 to 2.6 mEq/L) in adults, 4.5 to 5.5 mg/dL in children, and 3.5 to 8.6 mg/dL in newborns
   b. Levels are higher in children because of their higher rate of skeletal growth
   c. Newborns have almost twice the adult level of **phosphorus**
   d. Most phosphorus (P^+) exists in the body as phosphate ions (PO_4^2)
   e. Phosphorus is the second most abundant mineral in body
      1) 85% is combined with calcium in teeth and bones, also in skeletal muscle
      2) 14% is found in intracellular fluid (ICF)
      3) 1% is found in extracellular fluid (ECF) and viscera
   f. Phosphorus is the primary anion in ICF
   g. Ionized calcium and phosphorus exist in a reciprocal balance in blood

2. Functions in body
   a. Essential for muscle function, red blood cells, and nervous system function; plays a part in metabolism of carbohydrates, fats, and proteins
   b. Plays a crucial role in formation of teeth and bones
   c. Plays a part in cellular metabolism of DNA and **adenosine triphosphate (ATP)**, a compound stored in muscle that contains three phosphorus groups and produces energy when split
   d. Assists in regulating calcium levels
   e. Aids renal regulation of acids and bases through its role in phosphate buffer system
   f. Found in cell membranes as **phospholipids** that help maintain cell membrane integrity
   g. Required for release of oxygen from hemoglobin in form of **2,3-diphosphoglycerate (2,3-DPG)**

3. System interactions
   a. Serum levels vary during day related to glucose intake, insulin administration, and hyperventilation, which increases cellular uptake of phosphorus
   b. Phosphorus assists in maintaining acid–base balance

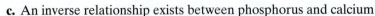

Practice to Pass

The school nurse is putting together a bulletin board that highlights foods high in various nutrients to use as a teaching tool for children and school visitors, including parents. What types of foods would the nurse identify on the display as being rich in phosphorus?

c. An inverse relationship exists between phosphorus and calcium
   1) When calcium levels increase, phosphorus levels decrease; thus, calcium influences phosphorus regulation
   2) When phosphorus levels increase, calcium levels decrease; thus, calcium levels are influenced by phosphorus
d. Phosphorus imbalances are often related to therapeutic interventions for other disorders
4. See Table 6–1 for lifespan factors affecting phosphorus balance

B. Sources of phosphorus
1. Cellular level
   a. Major anion of intracellular fluid; found also in extracellular fluid
   b. Kidneys are responsible for 90% of phosphate excretion
   c. Normal phosphate balance requires an efficient renal conservation mechanism
   d. During times of low phosphate intake, kidneys retain more phosphorus
2. Dietary level
   a. Adequate intake is ensured by consumption of a balanced diet
   b. Average dietary intake ranges from 800 to 1600 mg/dL and is consistent with recommended daily intake
   c. See Box 6–1 for a listing of foods high in phosphorus
   d. Absorption via active and passive transport in duodenum and jejunum
   e. Absorption influenced by **vitamin D**, a fat-soluble vitamin, and **parathyroid hormone (PTH)**, a hormone secreted by parathyroid gland that regulates calcium and phosphorus levels
   f. Absorption inhibited by glucocorticoids, high magnesium diet, hypothyroidism, and aluminum-containing antacids
   g. Increased consumption of foods that contain food additives will result in increased ingestion of phosphates (see Box 6–2 for a list of examples of phosphorus-containing additives found in many processed foods)

Table 6–1	Lifespan Considerations for Health Maintenance: Phosphorus Balance	
Lifespan Considerations	**Common Risk Factors for Imbalances**	**Nursing Implications**
Infants	*Hyperphosphatemia* Use of cows' milk instead of formula or human milk	Assess infant for signs of hyperphosphatemia
Children	*Hypophosphatemia or hyperphosphatemia* Phosphorus is not a common imbalance in children, but imbalances may be seen in relation to calcium imbalances	Check for low phosphorus levels when child has hypercalcemia Check for high phosphorus levels when hypocalcemia is present
Adults	*Hyperphosphatemia* Renal failure Excessive use of phosphorus-containing enemas or laxatives	Assess for signs of hyperphosphatemia Assess client for signs of renal osteodystrophy Instruct client to restrict intake of foods high in phosphorus and processed foods
	Hypophosphatemia Excessive use of phosphate-binding antacids	Instruct clients on dangers of excessive use of phosphorus-containing enemas Instruct clients to avoid excessive use of aluminum-containing antacids

Box 6–1	• Red meat
Foods High in Phosphorus	• Organ meats (brain, liver, kidney)
	• Fish
	• Poultry
	• Eggs
	• Milk and milk products
	• Legumes
	• Whole grains
	• Nuts

Box 6–2	• Sodium phosphate: a texturizer
Phosphorus-Containing Additives Found in Many Processed Foods	• Aluminum phosphate: used in bread to improve texture
	• Calcium phosphate: a conditioner for bread dough
	• Potassium phosphate dibasic: an emulsifier and gelling agent
	• Ammonium phosphate: adjusts pH
	• Phosphate oxychloride liquid: a starch-modifying agent
	• Phosphoric acid: a pH adjuster used in beer and cheese
	• Potassium phosphate monobasic: a sequestering agent used in ice cream mixes
	• Sodium phosphate dibasic and monobasic: an emulsifier

II. *HYPOPHOSPHATEMIA*

   A. Definition, etiology, and pathophysiology
   1. Definition: a serum phosphorus level below 2.5 mg/dL (1.7 mEq/L)
   2. Cellular level
      a. Can result from transient shifts of phosphorus into cells, as in respiratory or metabolic acidosis
      b. Increased release of PTH leads to a decrease in serum phosphorus level
      c. Mobilization of calcium from other sources may reduce phosphorus levels
      d. Renal excretion of phosphorus may be increased
      e. Administration of highly concentrated glucose solutions leads to insulin release, which promotes movement of glucose and phosphorus into cells, known as **refeeding syndrome**; this secondarily causes hypophosphatemia
   3. See Table 6–2 for a list of predisposing clinical conditions

   B. Assessment
   1. Clinical manifestations
      a. Signs begin to appear when serum phosphorus levels drop below 2.0 mg/dL
      b. Hematologic effects
         1) Anemia from increased fragility of red blood cells from low ATP levels
         2) Altered granulocyte functioning
         3) Bruising and bleeding from platelet dysfunction and destruction
      c. Central nervous system depressant effects
         1) Slurred speech
         2) Confusion, apprehension
         3) Seizures
         4) Coma
      d. Neuromuscular effects
         1) Polyneuropathy
         2) Muscle weakness, including respiratory muscle weakness (may be seen as difficulty weaning from ventilator, if used)

Table 6–2	Predisposing Clinical Conditions for Hypophosphatemia
Mechanism of Hypophosphatemia	**Associated Clinical Conditions**
Loss of phosphorus	Increased intestinal losses from prolonged use of aluminum- and magnesium-containing antacids, which bind to phosphorus
	Severe vomiting and diarrhea; phosphorus is absorbed in the small intestine in the presence of vitamin D
	Prolonged gastric suction
	Increased renal excretion from hyperparathyroidism, hypomagnesemia, hypokalemia, thiazide diuretic therapy, diuretic phase of acute tubular necrosis, renal tubular disorders, polyuria, and glycosuria from uncontrolled diabetic ketoacidosis
	Hypercalcemia (may cause phosphaturia through stimulation of parathyroid hormone release)
	Medications: corticosteroids; androgens; aluminum component of some antacids combines with phosphorus, which lowers phosphorus levels; drugs containing large amounts of calcium can also lower phosphorus levels
Phosphorus utilization	A depletion of ATP, which impairs a cell's energy supply, and a decrease in 2,3-DPG level in RBCs; this in turn reduces release of oxygen from hemoglobin, keeping it bound and less available to tissues
	Refeeding syndrome, which may carry a high mortality rate
	Diabetic ketoacidosis
	Administering TPN without adequate amounts of phosphorus
	Extracellular fluid volume expansion (a side effect)
	Respiratory alkalosis (may stimulate glycolysis— the breakdown of glucose—which stimulates movement of phosphorus into cells)
	Severe burns, possibly from hyperventilation and acceleration of glycolysis
Inadequate phosphorus intake or absorption	Decreased intestinal absorption from vitamin D deficiency, malabsorption disorders, and starvation
	Alcoholism and severe alcohol abuse (especially during withdrawal) related to poor nutritional intake, vomiting, diarrhea, and use of antacids
	Poor dietary intake, malnutrition, and hypomagnesemia
	May be found more frequently in clients in critical care units because of nutritional deficiencies

    e. Cardiovascular effects
        1) Reports of chest pain
        2) Dysrhythmias related to decreased oxygenation
        3) Reduced stroke volume from decreased myocardial contractility
    f. Respiratory effects
        1) Alkalosis from an increased rate/depth of breathing in response to hypoxemia
        2) Respiratory muscle fatigue leading to respiratory failure
    g. Gastrointestinal effects
        1) Hypoactive bowel sounds
        2) Anorexia, dysphagia, vomiting
        3) Gastric atony and ileus related to reduced gastric motility
  2. Diagnostic and laboratory findings
    a. Plasma levels
        1) Mild hypophosphatemia: serum values of 1.0–2.5 mg/dL
        2) Severe hypophosphatemia: <1.0 mg/dL

          b. Associated electrolyte levels
             1) Serum magnesium: may be decreased because of increased renal excretion of magnesium
             2) Serum calcium: may be elevated because of inverse relationship of calcium and phosphorus
             3) Arterial blood gases: may show respiratory or metabolic acidosis
          c. Trending of results
             1) Monitor laboratory values over time to determine effectiveness of therapy
             2) In prolonged hypophosphatemia, osteomalacia and pseudofractures may occur
          d. X-rays may show skeletal changes of osteomalacia
      3. Identification of risk factors
          a. Alcohol withdrawal
          b. Malnourished clients
          c. Reduced ability to eat normally
          d. Total parenteral nutrition (TPN) administration, in which total nutritional needs are provided intravenously through a central venous access device for a client unable to take sufficient nutrients by enteral route
          e. Diabetic and uremic clients

C. Priority nursing concerns
      1. Bone pain
      2. Possible fractures because of shifting of phosphorus out of bone tissue
      3. Possible reduced gas exchange if respiratory muscles are weak
      4. Possible reduction in cardiac output
      5. Heightened risk for falls because of sensory or neuromuscular dysfunction

D. Therapeutic management
      1. Replacement therapies
          a. Administer phosphorus via oral supplements or intravenous (IV) route
          b. Avoid use of phosphorus-binding antacids (those that contain aluminum)
          c. Adjust subsequent doses of replacement medication based on clinical presentation and serum phosphate levels
      2. Continued monitoring of client
          a. Check serum levels periodically in clients at risk
          b. Assess diabetic clients for ketoacidosis
          c. Anticipate problems in clients who have a long history of antacid use; determine which products the client uses
          d. Be alert to clients who have difficulty speaking
          e. Note weakening respiratory efforts
          f. Monitor mechanically ventilated client for increased incidence of hypophosphatemia from respiratory alkalosis
          g. Monitor for chest pain and cardiac dysrhythmias
          h. Assess serial hand grasps for increasing weakness
          i. Monitor for client reports of joint stiffness and arthralgia
          j. Investigate episodes of bleeding and/or bruising
          k. Watch for hypophosphatemia with the start of anabolism after prolonged periods of catabolism
          l. Monitor for other associated fluid and electrolyte imbalances, especially in clients with nausea and vomiting and/or diarrhea

E. Restoration of balance
      1. Achieved through oral, enteral, or parenteral replacement
      2. Normal phosphate levels should be achieved in 7–10 days

F. Client-centered nursing care
      1. Identify client populations at risk, especially those who are malnourished, receiving TPN, or receiving calories via enteral (tube) feedings

---

Practice to Pass

What neuromuscular manifestations should be assessed for in a client at risk for developing hypophosphatemia?

2. Identify and eliminate causes of hypophosphatemia
3. Consult with healthcare provider to obtain appropriate prescription for supplementation
4. Assess and document level of consciousness and neurologic status with each set of vital signs (VS)
5. Inform client/significant other that altered sensorium is temporary and will improve as phosphorus levels improve
6. Use reality therapy by encouraging presence of family members and use of clock and calendar at the bedside
7. Incorporate seizure precautions into care
8. Have an appropriate-size airway readily available
9. Assist client in activities of daily living and ambulating
10. Monitor breath sounds for crackles, wheezes, and shortness of breath
11. Monitor for elevated blood pressure, increased heart rate, and increased temperature
12. If a wound infection is suspected, culture wound(s) and any drain sites
13. Use meticulous aseptic technique when giving care
14. Promote oral hygiene and skin care
15. Medicate for pain as indicated
16. Assess serum phosphate levels and trends; watch for concurrent development of hypercalcemia in presence of hypophosphatemia
17. Monitor for possible hyperphosphatemia after initiation of therapy
18. Assess dietary intake and output (I&O) and include when possible client's food preferences in diet

G. Medication therapy

1. Oral replacement therapy
   a. Monobasic potassium and sodium phosphates; potassium and sodium phosphates
      1) Well absorbed following oral administration; vitamin D may enhance absorption
      2) Enters ECF and is then transported to sites of action
      3) Excreted mainly by kidneys; acidifies urine
      4) Contraindicated in hyperkalemia, hyperphosphatemia, hypocalcemia, severe renal impairment, and untreated Addison disease
      5) Diarrhea is most frequent side effect
      6) Oxalates (in spinach and rhubarb) and phytates (in bran and whole grains) may reduce absorption of phosphates by binding them in GI tract
      7) Monitor serum phosphate, potassium, sodium, and calcium levels prior to and periodically throughout therapy
   b. Phosphate/biphosphate
      1) Osmotically active bowel preparation and oral preparation used for its laxative effect
      2) Enema contains 7 grams sodium phosphate and 19 grams sodium biphosphate; oral preparation contains 18 grams sodium phosphate and 48 grams sodium biphosphate
      3) Up to 20% of rectally administered sodium and phosphate may be absorbed
      4) Excreted by kidneys
      5) Side effects include cramping, nausea
      6) May cause increased serum sodium and phosphorus levels, decreased serum calcium levels, and acidosis
      7) Oral preparations should be thoroughly dissolved in a full glass of water and administered after meals to minimize gastric irritation and laxative effect and to enhance palatability
      8) Do not administer simultaneously with antacids containing aluminum, magnesium, or calcium

9) Advise clients to maintain a high fluid intake to decrease risk of developing kidney stones

10) Instruct client to promptly report diarrhea, weakness, fatigue, muscle cramps, unexplained weight gain, swelling of lower extremities, shortness of breath, and unusual thirst or tremors

2. Parenteral replacement therapy

    a. Usually reserved for severe hypophosphatemia (<1 mg/dL)

    b. Potassium phosphate (KPO_4) or sodium phosphate ($NaPO_4$) used

    c. May be added to TPN solutions

    d. When giving KPO_4, do not exceed 10 mEq/hr; give slowly over 2–6 hours

    e. Complications of IV therapy may include:

        1) Tetany from hypocalcemia

        2) Calcium and phosphorus in tissues may combine and form deposits

        3) Hypotension from too rapid an infusion rate

    f. Monitor infusion site for signs of infiltration, which may lead to tissue necrosis or sloughing

3. Dietary therapy

    a. Daily requirements are 0.15 mM/kg/day or 10 mM/day; if under stress, requirements increase to 30–45 mM/day

    b. Phosphorus is plentiful in a normal diet

    c. Refer to Box 6–1 again for a listing of foods that tend to be high in phosphorus

H. Client education

1. Teach client and family to recognize signs and symptoms of hypophosphatemia

2. Discuss importance of avoiding phosphorus-binding antacids, such as aluminum hydroxide

3. Discuss with client pertinent conditions that cause hypophosphatemia

4. Carry out dietary education and provide a list of foods high in phosphorus

I. Evaluation

1. Client regains a serum phosphorus value within normal range

2. Client can identify signs and symptoms of hypophosphatemia

3. Client exhibits no evidence of injury caused by neurosensory changes

4. Client exhibits adequate gas exchange: respiratory rate of 12–20 breaths/minute, normal depth and pattern, and oxygen saturation (SaO_2) level of at least 92%

5. Within 24 hours of initiating therapy, client exhibits purposeful movement and has full range of motion and muscle strength

6. Client has no signs or symptoms of heart failure and VS are within normal limits

Practice to Pass

What are the important elements of care during administration of potassium phosphate in intravenous fluids for a client who has hypophosphatemia?

III. *HYPERPHOSPHATEMIA*

A. Definition, etiology, and pathophysiology

1. Definition: a serum phosphorus level above 4.5 mg/dL (2.6 mEq/L)

2. See Table 6–3 for etiology and pathophysiology of hyperphosphatemia

B. Assessment

1. Clinical manifestations

    a. Most signs relate to the development of hypocalcemia or soft tissue calcification

    b. Numbness and tingling around mouth and in fingertips, muscle spasms, and tetany from increased phosphorus and corresponding decreased calcium

    c. Signs of **metastatic calcification** (precipitation of calcium phosphate in soft tissues, joints, and arteries) may include oliguria, corneal haziness, and conjunctivitis

    d. ECG changes and conduction disturbance, tachycardia

    e. Anorexia, nausea and vomiting

    f. Muscle weakness, hyperreflexia, tetany, flaccid paralysis

Table 6–3 **Etiology and Pathophysiology of Hyperphosphatemia**

Mechanism of Hyperphosphatemia	Associated Clinical Conditions
Cellular release of phosphorus (phosphate shifts from cells into extracellular fluid)	Respiratory or lactic acidosis or diabetic ketoacidosis because of movement of phosphorus out of cells
	Tumor lysis syndrome, which occurs with neoplastic diseases (leukemia, lymphoma) when treated with cytotoxic agents
	Rhabdomyolysis (breakdown of striated muscle), which releases phosphorus from cells because of tissue trauma, viral infections, heat stroke, increased metabolism, and catabolic states
	Chemotherapy for malignant tumors
	Massive transfusions because phosphorus can leak from cells during storage of blood
Phosphorus retention	Decreasing glomerular filtration rates (renal insufficiency, acute and chronic renal failure, chronic glomerulonephritis), which prevent adequate excretion of phosphates
	Decreased urinary losses unrelated to decreased renal function such as in hypoparathyroidism or volume depletion
	Hypocalcemia from antacids, diuretic agents, or steroids
	Hypoparathyroidism (primary or secondary), which causes a decrease in calcium and increased renal absorption of phosphorus
	Can occur with other conditions that cause cellular destruction and release of phosphorus into extracellular fluid
	Excess human growth hormone
	Hyperthyroidism, hypoparathyroidism
	Prolonged or excessive administration of heparin, tetracycline, pituitary extract, and salicylates
Excessive intake	Excessive intake of phosphorus or its supplements
	Infants fed cow's milk instead of human milk (940 mg of phosphorus in cow's milk compared to 150 mg in an equal amount of human milk)
	Vitamin D excess or increased GI absorption
	Large milk intake for the treatment of peptic ulcers
	Overzealous administration of oral or IV phosphorus supplements

2. Diagnostic and laboratory findings
   a. Serum phosphorus plasma levels are greater than 4.5 mg/dL (2.6 mEq/L)
   b. In clients with chronic renal failure (CRF), phosphorus values may be kept slightly higher (4–6 mg/dL) to ensure adequate levels of 2,3-DPG and thereby minimize effects of chronic anemia on oxygen delivery to tissues
   c. With increased phosphorus levels, serum calcium levels drop and hypocalcemia develops
      1) Hypocalcemia is more likely to occur in sudden, severe hyperphosphatemia (such as after IV administration of phosphates)
      2) Hypocalcemia may also occur in a client with CRF
   d. Chronic hyperphosphatemia in a client with CRF may contribute to development of **renal osteodystrophy**, which may be assessed by skeletal x-rays
   e. Calcification formation and precipitation in soft tissues may be anticipated if the product of the serum calcium level multiplied by the serum phosphorus level yields a number higher than 70 mg/dL (normal product is about 30–40 mg/dL)
3. Identification of clients at risk
   a. Infants being fed cow's milk
   b. Clients using phosphates in an enema solution or regular laxative
   c. Clients in end-stage renal failure

Practice to Pass

What clinical manifestations may be seen in a client diagnosed with hyperphosphatemia?

C. Priority nursing concerns

   1. Insufficient knowledge about purpose of phosphate-binding medications and importance of reducing gastrointestinal (GI) phosphorus absorption to control hyperphosphatemia and prevent long-term complications

   2. Possible injury associated with calcium phosphate precipitation in soft tissues (corneas, lungs, kidneys, gastric mucosa, heart, blood vessels) and periarticular regions of large joints (hips, shoulders, elbows) and development of hypocalcemic tetany

D. Therapeutic management

   1. Decrease phosphorus intake in diet or in prescribed or over-the-counter drugs

   2. Promote phosphorus excretion

      a. Increase GI and renal excretion of phosphorus

      b. Perform renal dialysis in clients with renal failure

      c. Maintain fluid volume to ensure adequate BP to enhance phosphorus excretion, particularly in clients receiving cytotoxic medications

   3. Possibly limit calcium supplements and products containing vitamin D according to healthcare provider recommendation until phosphorus levels approach normal

   4. In clients with renal failure, serum phosphate values may be kept higher to ensure adequate levels of 2,3-DPG to improve tissue oxygenation

E. Client-centered nursing care

   1. Monitor serum phosphorus and calcium levels

   2. Calculate calcium-phosphorus product and consult healthcare provider for abnormally high results

   3. Identify clients at risk and treat underlying cause

   4. Continue to monitor client for increasing hypocalcemia

      a. Monitor for numbness and tingling of fingers and around mouth (*circumoral*), and for hyperactive reflexes and muscle cramps

      b. Consult healthcare provider promptly if symptoms of hypocalcemia (such as positive Trousseau or Chvostek sign) develop to avoid tetany

   5. Monitor VS

   6. Monitor I&O; keep clients well hydrated; pay particular attention to the types of fluids being ingested (avoid carbonated beverages, which are high in phosphates); monitor urine output to be sure that it is adequate for phosphate excretion; check serum BUN and creatinine levels

   7. Consult healthcare provider if client develops indications of soft tissue (metastatic) calcification (oliguria, corneal haziness, conjunctivitis, irregular heart rate, papular eruptions)

   8. Administer IV and oral phosphorus supplements cautiously in clients with normal phosphorus levels to avoid hyperphosphatemia; monitor serum phosphate levels periodically throughout administration

   9. Avoid use of phosphate-containing enemas, especially in children and those with slowed bowel-emptying times

  10. Encourage client to avoid intake of foods that are high in phosphorus content (refer back to Box 6–1) and to increase intake of vegetables, which tend to be lower in phosphorus than some food groups

F. Medication therapy

   1. Avoid phosphate-containing laxatives and enemas, such as Fleet's Phospho-soda

   2. Phosphate binders, such as sevelamer, are available in liquid, tablet, and capsule forms; administer with meals to enhance binding of phosphate contained in food

   3. Aluminum-containing antacids bind phosphates in GI tract; be aware that aluminum-based products cause constipation and may lead to dementia if used over prolonged periods of time; examples include aluminum carbonate and aluminum hydroxide

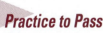

Practice to Pass

What are the three main types of phosphate binders that may be used to treat hyperphosphatemia?

> ⚠ **4.** Calcium carbonate is useful as a supplement for clients with CRF because this will help to counteract hypocalcemia, which accompanies hyperphosphatemia
>
> ⚠ **5.** In clients with hyperphosphatemia from use of cytotoxic drugs, allopurinol decreases uric acid production, which prevents formation of uric acid calculi in kidney and uric acid nephropathy (high uric acid levels can also occur with use of cytotoxic drugs)

G. Client education

1. Symptoms of hyperphosphatemia may be minimal; therefore, the client needs to be aware of methods to prevent long-term complications

⚠ **2.** Teach client purpose of phosphate binders and to take them as prescribed with or after meals to maximize their effectiveness; use bulk-building supplements or stool softeners as prescribed to combat constipating effects of some phosphate binders, especially those with an aluminum base

⚠ **3.** Avoid over-the-counter phosphorus medications such as laxatives, enemas, and vitamin-mineral supplements

4. Identify signs and symptoms of hyperphosphatemia

5. Read food and medication labels to identify phosphorus and phosphate inclusions

6. Avoid or limit foods high in phosphorus, as previously described, and avoid carbonated beverages, which have low nutrient value and are also high in phosphates

H. Evaluation

1. Client describes symptoms of hyperphosphatemia and preventative measures

2. Client creates a 3-day meal plan using foods low in or without phosphorus

3. Client verbalizes how to take medication therapy properly

POSTTEST

Case Study

Mr. G. is a 56-year-old client with newly diagnosed chronic renal failure as a complication of diabetes mellitus. He will be beginning therapy with hemodialysis. He is married and lives at home with his wife; he has three grown children who do not live in the area. You have been assigned as his case manager and need to coordinate plans for his treatment and for client and family education.

1. Do you expect Mr. G. to have hypophosphatemia or hyperphosphatemia? What is the rationale for your choice?

2. How will you explain the etiology of this electrolyte imbalance to Mr. G?

3. What dietary modifications need to be made in order to keep serum phosphorus levels under control?

4. What role will dialysis play in managing phosphorus levels?

5. What medication therapy teaching do you anticipate will be needed?

For suggested responses, see page 192.

POSTTEST

❶ The nurse uses which concept about phosphate levels in a newborn when implementing client care?

1. Phosphate levels are consistent throughout the day.
2. Phosphate levels in newborns are nearly twice the adult level.
3. Normal serum phosphate levels range from 1.5 to 2.0 mg/dL.
4. Phosphorus is the most abundant mineral in the body.

2 When caring for a client with a phosphorus level of 1.8 mg/dL, the nurse plans interventions to promote which of the following?

1. Conservation of energy
2. Increased renal perfusion
3. Decrease in peristalsis
4. Deep and rapid breathing

. . . .

3 A client experiencing hypophosphatemia has been started on sodium phosphate. The nurse instructs the client that it is acceptable to take the medication with which foods? Select all that apply.

1. Whole grains
2. Milk
3. Orange juice
4. Chicken
5. Spinach

. . . .

4 The nurse would assess for manifestations of hypophosphatemia in a client who has which predisposing clinical condition?

1. Severe vomiting and diarrhea
2. Occasional use of magnesium-containing antacids
3. Infusion of balanced total parenteral nutrition (TPN) solutions
4. Vitamin D excess

. . . .

5 When caring for a client with a serum phosphorus level of 1.9 mg/dL, the nurse should be alert to which sign?

1. Hyperactive bowel sounds
2. Dysrhythmias caused by decreased oxygenation
3. Increased muscle tone
4. Polycythemia

. . . .

6 When caring for a client with a phosphorus level of 5.2 mg/dL, the nurse should anticipate reports of which symptom?

1. Circumoral numbness
2. Hunger
3. Chest pain
4. Thirst

. . . .

7 A client with chronic renal failure (CRF) has been started on sevelamer to treat hyperphosphatemia. To enhance medication effectiveness, the nurse plans to administer it in which way?

1. On an empty stomach
2. Thirty minutes before a meal
3. With meals
4. Two hours after a meal

. . . .

8 When administering an infusion of potassium phosphate, the nurse should use an infusion pump so that phosphorus replacement does not exceed _____ mEq per hour.

Fill in your answer below:
_____ mEq/hr

. . . .

9 The nurse determines that a client with a phosphorus level of 4.9 mg/dL demonstrates an understanding of dietary instructions when the client limits intake of which food item?

1. Pork chops
2. White rice
3. Sirloin steak
4. Green peas

. . . .

10 The nurse identifies that a client who chronically uses which type of over-the-counter products is at greatest risk for developing hyperphosphatemia?

1. Enemas
2. Cough preparations
3. Cold preparations
4. Bedtime sleeping aids

➤ *See pages 133–135 for Answers and Rationales.*

POSTTEST

ANSWERS & RATIONALES

Pretest

1 **Answer: 2 Rationale:** Infant levels of phosphorus are higher than an adult's level due to the rapid turnover of bone, but a level of 5.0 mEq/L is elevated for an infant. The nurse needs to determine what is contributing to the elevated level. Asking about type of milk is important because, although infant formulas and breast milk would not cause an elevated level, cow's milk is naturally high in phosphorus. Asking about diarrhea is not helpful. Solid foods contain ordinary amounts of phosphorus. Asking about vomiting would not target the cause of hyperphosphatemia. **Cognitive Level:** Applying **Client Need:** Physiological Adaptation **Integrated Process:** Nursing Process: Evaluation **Content Area:** Child Health **Strategy:** First recognize that the phosphorus level is elevated. Recall causes of elevated phosphorus to delete the options for vomiting and diarrhea. Recall sources of phosphorus to choose the correct option. **Reference:** Davidson, M., London, M., & Ladewig, P. (2016). *Olds' maternal-newborn nursing and women's health across the lifespan* (10th ed.). New York, NY: Pearson, pp. 729–730.

2 **Answer: 2 Rationale:** Children have higher phosphate levels than adults because of their more rapid bone development rate. Serum phosphate levels vary throughout the day. Replacement therapy would result in an increase in phosphorus level. A venous sample, not arterial, is taken. **Cognitive Level:** Applying **Client Need:** Physiological Adaptation **Integrated Process:** Nursing Process: Diagnosis **Content Area:** Child Health **Strategy:** First recognize that this is a pediatric client, and pediatric phosphorus levels would normally be higher. Eliminate arterial sampling as arterial blood gases are the only common lab drawn arterially. After starting phosphorus replacement, the levels should rise. **Reference:** Kee, J. L. (2017). *Pearson's handbook of laboratory and diagnostic tests* (8th ed.). New York, NY: Pearson, pp. 321–322.

3 **Answer: 2 Rationale:** A phosphate level of 1.7 mg/dL reflects hypophosphatemia. Phosphorus is needed for formation of the red blood cell enzyme 2,3-DPG, and so a deficiency of phosphorus can lead to anemia, reflected by a decrease in hemoglobin level. Because phosphorus is needed for many cellular enzyme reactions necessary for red blood cell and platelet synthesis, the platelet count may be decreased, not increased. Calcium and phosphorus levels have a reciprocal relationship and so an elevation of calcium would be expected. Low magnesium levels, not elevated, are associated with a low phosphorus level. **Cognitive Level:** Analyzing **Client Need:** Reduction of Risk Potential **Integrated Process:** Nursing Process: Assessment **Content Area:** Adult Health

Strategy: First recognize the level reflects hypophosphatemia. Recall the role of phosphorus in red blood cell production to direct you to the correct option. **Reference:** LeMone, P., Burke, K., Bauldoff, G., & Gubrud, P. (2015). *Medical surgical nursing: Clinical reasoning in patient care* (6th ed.). New York, NY: Pearson, pp. 211–212.

4 **Answer: 2, 5 Rationale:** Because of the elevated glucose levels seen with diabetic ketoacidosis, osmotic diuresis causes a loss of phosphorus. Clients with chronic alcohol abuse often have poor dietary intake of foods high in phosphorus, contributing to hypophosphatemia. There is not a shift of fluids or significant cellular damage occurring with superficial thickness burns that would affect phosphorus levels. Hypomagnesemia would be seen with hypophosphatemia due to renal excretion of phosphorus. A decrease in urine output would contribute to less renal excretion of phosphorus, and the level would increase, not decrease. **Cognitive Level:** Applying **Client Need:** Physiological Adaptation **Integrated Process:** Nursing Process: Assessment **Content Area:** Adult Health **Strategy:** Critical words are *hypophosphatemia* and *predisposing clinical conditions*. Analyze each option recalling phosphorus is lost in the urine. Recognize that polyuria seen with acidosis will contribute to phosphorus loss to choose diabetic ketoacidosis, and poor intake of phosphorus causes decreased serum levels to choose the option for history of alcoholism. **Reference:** LeMone, P., Burke, K., Bauldoff, G., & Gubrud, P. (2015). *Medical surgical nursing: Clinical reasoning in patient care* (6th ed.). New York, NY: Pearson, pp. 211–212.

5 **Answer: 4, 5 Rationale:** Although phosphorus is found in a large number of food items, it is found in higher amounts in eggs and dairy products. Organ meats such as liver are especially rich in phosphorus. Green leafy vegetables are healthy food choices but are not excessively high in phosphorus. Citrus fruits are not high in phosphorus. Whole grain breads, rather than white bread, would be higher in phosphorus. **Cognitive Level:** Applying **Client Need:** Physiological Adaptation **Integrated Process:** Teaching and Learning **Content Area:** Adult Health **Strategy:** Recall foods high in phosphorus to choose correctly. **Reference:** LeMone, P., Burke, K., Bauldoff, G., & Gubrud, P. (2015). *Medical surgical nursing: Clinical reasoning in patient care* (6th ed.). New York, NY: Pearson, p. 212.

6 **Answer: 3 Rationale:** Phosphorus is used in the metabolism of TPN, causing a shift of phosphorus into the cells and lowering serum phosphorus levels, reflected by the low level of 1.2 mg/dL. Because of the many enzyme reactions needed for the metabolism of TPN, magnesium is used and levels drop with refeeding syndrome. A magnesium level of 2.5 mg is at the upper end of normal. Calcium levels sometimes drop with refeeding syndrome secondary to cellular shifts. A calcium level of 9.8 mg/dL is normal. A potassium level of 4.2 is normal. Potassium levels may decrease as cellular shifts occur with the metabolism of TPN. **Cognitive Level:** Analyzing **Client Need:** Physiological Adaptation **Integrated Process:** Nursing Process: Evaluation **Content Area:** Adult Health **Strategy:** First recall the purpose and content of TPN. Recall that electrolytes are used for enzyme reactions and metabolism and recognize which value is low to choose the correct option. **Reference:** LeMone, P., Burke, K., Bauldoff, G., & Gubrud, P. (2015). *Medical surgical nursing: Clinical reasoning in patient care* (6th ed.). New York, NY: Pearson, pp. 211–212.

7 **Answer: 1 Rationale:** Poor nutritional intake, vomiting, diarrhea, and overuse of antacids are related to alcoholism and alcohol abuse, and can lead to hypophosphatemia. During the oliguric phase, renal excretion of phosphorus would be diminished, contributing to elevated serum levels of phosphorus. Clients with prolonged (not short-term) gastric suction are more likely to experience hypophosphatemia. Prolonged or continuous use of aluminum-containing antacids (not occasional use) leads to hypophosphatemia. **Cognitive Level:** Analyzing **Client Need:** Physiological Adaptation **Integrated Process:** Nursing Process: Assessment **Content Area:** Adult Health **Strategy:** Recognize that some of the options have conditions that would contribute to a low phosphorus level, but identify withdrawal from alcohol as having the greatest risk. **Reference:** LeMone, P., Burke, K., Bauldoff, G., & Gubrud, P. (2015). *Medical surgical nursing: Clinical reasoning in patient care* (6th ed.). New York, NY: Pearson, pp. 211–212.

8 **Answer: 3 Rationale:** A phosphate level of 4.9 mg/dL reflects an elevated phosphorus level. Because a reciprocal relationship occurs with calcium, hypocalcemia is expected. Hypocalcemia would be expected, not hyperkalemia. Because a reciprocal relationship occurs with calcium, hypocalcemia would be expected rather than hyponatremia. Magnesium would not be affected. **Cognitive Level:** Analyzing **Client Need:** Physiological Adaptation **Integrated Process:** Nursing Process: Assessment **Content Area:** Adult Health **Strategy:** Recall the relationship between calcium and phosphorus to direct you to the correct option. **Reference:** LeMone, P., Burke, K., Bauldoff, G., & Gubrud, P. (2015). *Medical surgical nursing: Clinical reasoning in patient care* (6th ed.). New York, NY: Pearson, p. 212.

9 **Answer: 2 Rationale:** In clients with hyperphosphatemia (normal 2.5–4.5 mg/dL) from use of cytotoxic drugs, allopurinol may be ordered to decrease uric acid production, which prevents the formation of uric acid calculi in the kidney and uric acid nephropathy. Although aluminum hydroxide might be given to treat the elevated phosphorus level, the question asks which drug will be given to treat the elevated uric acid.

Acetazolamide is a carbonic anhydrase inhibitor, which is a type of diuretic used to treat glaucoma. Albiglutide is an antidiabetic agent. **Cognitive Level:** Applying **Client Need:** Pharmacological and Parenteral Therapies **Integrated Process:** Nursing Process: Diagnosis **Content Area:** Adult Health **Strategy:** Note that there are two conditions in the question—hyperphosphatemia and hyperuricemia—but the question addresses treatment of the latter only. Use knowledge of pharmacology and the process of elimination to make a selection. **Reference:** Wilson, B., Shannon, M., & Stang, K. (2016). *Pearson nurse's drug guide 2016.* New York, NY: Pearson, pp. 13, 34, 45, 59.

10 **Answer: 1 Rationale:** Many types of food additives and preservatives contain phosphorus and would be acceptable for the client who needs to increase dietary phosphorus. Vitamin A does not have an effect on phosphorus absorption. Aluminum binds to phosphorus and would be contraindicated for the client needing to increase phosphorus levels. Soy-based foods are not a good source of phosphorus. Phosphorus is found in dairy products, meats, whole grains, and nuts. **Cognitive Level:** Applying **Client Need:** Health Promotion and Maintenance **Integrated Process:** Teaching and Learning **Content Area:** Adult Health **Strategy:** Key words are *discharge teaching* and *diet high in phosphates*. Recall knowledge of phosphorus sources to direct you to the correct option. **Reference:** LeMone, P., Burke, K., Bauldoff, G., & Gubrud, P. (2015). *Medical surgical nursing: Clinical reasoning in patient care* (6th ed.). New York, NY: Pearson, pp. 211–212.

Posttest

1 **Answer: 2 Rationale:** Newborn levels of phosphate can range from 4.0 to 7.0 mg/dL. Phosphate levels differ throughout the day. Normal serum phosphate levels range from 2.5 to 4.5 mg/dL. Phosphate is the second most abundant mineral in the body. **Cognitive Level:** Applying **Client Need:** Reduction of Risk Potential **Integrated Process:** Nursing Process: Diagnosis **Content Area:** Child Health **Strategy:** The critical word is *newborn*. Recognize the three incorrect statements to eliminate them. **Reference:** Kee, J. L. (2017). *Pearson's handbook of laboratory and diagnostic tests* (8th ed.). New York, NY: Pearson, pp. 321–322.

2 **Answer: 1 Rationale:** Phosphorus is needed for adenosine triphosphate (ATP) production, which in turn is used for cellular energy. A level of 1.8 mg/dL reflects a low level of phosphorus, indicating a deficit will present for energy production in the body. Increased renal perfusion would contribute to increased secretion of phosphorus. Peristalsis is already decreased in hypophosphatemia; measures should be taken to prevent constipation. Hypophosphatemia can lead to hypoxemia and increased deep and rapid breathing.

ANSWERS & RATIONALES

Measures should be taken to reduce energy expenditure and prevent respiratory distress. **Cognitive Level:** Analyzing **Client Need:** Reduction of Risk Potential **Integrated Process:** Nursing Process: Planning **Content Area:** Adult Health **Strategy:** Recall that the normal phosphorus level is 2.5–4.5 mg/dL and then choose an intervention that will help with hypophosphatemia. **Reference:** LeMone, P., Burke, K., Bauldoff, G., & Gubrud, P. (2015). *Medical surgical nursing: Clinical reasoning in patient care* (6th ed.). New York, NY: Pearson, pp. 211–212.

3 **Answer: 2, 3, 4 Rationale:** Oxalate (in spinach and rhubarb) and phytates (found in bran and whole grains) can interfere with the absorption of phosphate by binding with them in the intestines. Milk, orange juice, and chicken do not pose this problem for absorption of phosphate. **Cognitive Level:** Applying **Client Need:** Pharmacological and Parenteral Therapies **Integrated Process:** Nursing Process: Implementation **Content Area:** Adult Health **Strategy:** Recall that calcium and phosphorus have an inverse relationship, and phytates and oxalates inhibit phosphorus absorption. **Reference:** Adams, M., Holland, L., & Urban, C. (2017). *Pharmacology for nurses: A pathophysiologic approach* (5th ed.). New York, NY: Pearson, pp. 642–644.

4 **Answer: 1 Rationale:** Phosphorus can be lost via the gastrointestinal tract through vomiting and diarrhea. Prolonged or excessive use of aluminum- or magnesium-containing antacids can contribute to hypophosphatemia, but the occasional use should not pose a problem. A balanced infusion of TPN should contain appropriate amounts of phosphorus to prevent hypophosphatemia. When TPN is first initiated, refeeding syndrome may contribute to phosphorus utilization and low levels may be seen. A deficiency of vitamin D can lead to decreased intestinal absorption of phosphorus. **Cognitive Level:** Analyzing **Client Need:** Physiological Adaptation **Integrated Process:** Nursing Process: Assessment **Content Area:** Adult Health **Strategy:** Critical words are *predisposing clinical condition*. Note the word *severe* in the correct option and recognize phosphorus will be lost with vomiting and diarrhea. **Reference:** LeMone, P., Burke, K., Bauldoff, G., & Gubrud, P. (2015). *Medical surgical nursing: Clinical reasoning in patient care* (6th ed.). New York, NY: Pearson, pp. 211–212.

5 **Answer: 2 Rationale:** Hypophosphatemia results in decreased adenosine triphosphate (ATP) production, decreasing enzyme levels of 2,3-DPG, which in turn keeps oxygen bound to hemoglobin and less available to the tissues. Clients with hypophosphatemia will experience hypoactive bowel sounds, muscle weakness, paresthesias, and anemia due to red blood cell (RBC) fragility from low ATP levels. **Cognitive Level:** Analyzing **Client Need:** Reduction of Risk Potential **Integrated Process:** Nursing Process: Assessment **Content Area:** Adult Health **Strategy:** Recall that phosphorus is needed for ATP production and oxygenation. Recognize that these

deficiencies can contribute to irregular heart rhythms to direct you to the correct option. **Reference:** LeMone, P., Burke, K., Bauldoff, G., & Gubrud, P. (2015). *Medical surgical nursing: Clinical reasoning in patient care* (6th ed.). New York, NY: Pearson, pp. 211–212.

6 **Answer: 1 Rationale:** A phosphorus level of 5.2 mg/dL reflects hyperphosphatemia, which is usually accompanied by hypocalcemia. Numbness and tingling around the mouth and in the fingertips is associated with hypocalcemia. Anorexia and nausea and vomiting are associated with hyperphosphatemia. Chest pain may be seen with hypophosphatemia associated with a decline in 2,3-DPG levels, reducing the release of oxygen to the tissues. Thirst is not a sign of this imbalance. **Cognitive Level:** Applying **Client Need:** Physiological Adaptation **Integrated Process:** Nursing Process: Assessment **Content Area:** Adult Health **Strategy:** First recognize the level reflects hyperphosphatemia. Recall that hypocalcemia is associated with hyperphosphatemia to choose correctly. **Reference:** LeMone, P., Burke, K., Bauldoff, G., & Gubrud, P. (2015). *Medical surgical nursing: Clinical reasoning in patient care* (6th ed.). New York, NY: Pearson, p. 212.

7 **Answer: 3 Rationale:** Sevelamer is a phosphate binder frequently used in patients with renal failure. In order to maximize binding of the phosphate, phosphate binders should be given with a meal or shortly after in order for the medication to have contact with the phosphate in the food. **Cognitive Level:** Applying **Client Need:** Pharmacological and Parenteral Therapies **Integrated Process:** Nursing Process: Planning **Content Area:** Adult Health **Strategy:** Note the similarities between taking sevelamer on an empty stomach and 2 hours after a meal to eliminate them. Recognize the purpose and action of the medication to direct you to the correct option. **Reference:** Adams, M., Holland, L., & Urban, C. (2017). *Pharmacology for nurses: A pathophysiologic approach* (5th ed.). New York, NY: Pearson, p. 302.

8 **Answer: 10 Rationale:** Intravenous phosphorus replacement should not exceed 10 mEq/hr in order to prevent phlebitis or potassium overload and to allow gradual return of phosphorus levels. **Cognitive Level:** Applying **Client Need:** Pharmacological and Parenteral Therapies **Integrated Process:** Nursing Process: Implementation **Content Area:** Adult Health **Strategy:** Recall safety measures related to administration of electrolytes. **Reference:** LeMone, P., Burke, K., Bauldoff, G., & Gubrud, P. (2015). *Medical surgical nursing: Clinical reasoning in patient care* (6th ed.). New York, NY: Pearson, pp. 211–212.

9 **Answer: 3 Rationale:** A phosphorus level of 4.9 mg/dL is elevated, indicating a need to restrict foods high in phosphorus, which include red meats, dairy products, eggs, poultry, organ meats, legumes, and whole grains. Sirloin steak is a red meat and high in phosphorus. Pork chops are not as high in phosphorus as the choice of sirloin steak. White rice is lower in phosphorus because it is not a whole grain. Green peas would not be excessively high in phosphorus. **Cognitive Level:** Applying **Client Need:** Physiological Adaptation **Integrated Process:** Nursing Process: Evaluation **Content Area:** Adult Health **Strategy:** Recall foods high in phosphorus to direct you to the correct option. **Reference:** LeMone, P., Burke, K., Bauldoff, G., & Gubrud, P. (2015). *Medical surgical nursing: Clinical reasoning in patient care* (6th ed.). New York, NY: Pearson, p. 212.

10 Answer: 1 Rationale: Enemas can be high in phosphorus, thus making the client at risk for hyperphosphatemia if they are frequently used. The other products listed do not necessarily have large amounts of phosphorus in them. **Cognitive Level:** Analyzing **Client Need:** Pharmacological and Parenteral Therapies **Integrated Process:** Nursing Process: Assessment **Content Area:** Adult Health **Strategy:** Analyze each option for phosphorus content, eliminating cough and cold preparations and bedtime sleeping aids because they are not high in phosphorus. **Reference:** LeMone, P., Burke, K., Bauldoff, G., & Gubrud, P. (2015). *Medical surgical nursing: Clinical reasoning in patient care* (6th ed.). New York, NY: Pearson, p. 212.

References

Adams, M., Holland, L., & Urban, C. (2017). *Pharmacology for nurses: A pathophysiologic approach* (5th ed.). New York, NY: Pearson.

Blake, J. (2016). *Nutrition and you* (4th ed.). New York, NY: Pearson.

Ball, J., Bindler, R., Cowen, K., & Shaw, M. (2014). *Principles of pediatric nursing: Caring for children* (7th ed.). New York, NY: Pearson.

Berman, A., Snyder, S., & Frandsen, G. (2016). *Fundamentals of nursing: Concepts,* *process, and practice* (10th ed.). New York, NY: Pearson.

Davidson, M., London, M., & Ladewig, P. (2016). *Olds' maternal-newborn nursing and women's health across the lifespan* (10th ed.). New York, NY: Pearson.

Kee, J. L. (2017). *Pearson's handbook of laboratory and diagnostic tests* (8th ed.). New York, NY: Pearson.

LeMone, P., Burke, K., Bauldoff, G., & Gubrud, P. (2015). *Medical surgical* *nursing: Clinical reasoning in patient care* (6th ed.). New York, NY: Pearson.

London, M., Ladewig, P., Davidson, M., Ball, J., Bindler, R., & Cowen, K. (2017). *Maternal and child nursing care* (5th ed.). New York, NY: Pearson.

Wilson, B., Shannon, M., & Stang, K. (2016). *Pearson nurse's drug guide 2016.* New York, NY: Pearson.

7 Acid–Base Balance and Imbalances

Chapter Outline

Overview of Acid–Base
  Physiology
Respiratory Acidosis

Respiratory Alkalosis
Metabolic Acidosis
Metabolic Alkalosis

Mixed Acid–Base
  Disturbances

NCLEX-RN® Test Prep

Access the NEW Web-based app
that provides students with additional
practice questions in preparation
for the NCLEX experience.

Objectives

➤ Identify the basic physiology of acid–base balance.
➤ Identify potential acid–base imbalances.
➤ Identify priority nursing concerns for acid–base imbalances.
➤ Describe the therapeutic management of acid–base imbalances.
➤ Describe the management of nursing care for a client who is
  experiencing an acid–base imbalance.

Review at a Glance

acid a substance that releases a
hydrogen (H^+) ion when dissolved in
water

base a substance that binds to a
hydrogen (H^+) ion when dissolved in
water

buffer prevents major changes in
extracellular fluid (ECF) by releasing or
accepting hydrogen (H^+) ions

compensation body process of using
its regulatory mechanisms to return pH to
normal level

HCO_3^- bicarbonate, an alkalotic
substance; a direct reflection of renal
system's ability to compensate for pH
changes

metabolic acidosis a gain of
hydrogen (H^+) ions or a loss of HCO_3^-; pH
decreases and HCO_3^- decreases

metabolic alkalosis a loss of
hydrogen (H^+) ion or a gain in HCO_3^-; pH
increases and HCO_3^- increases

mixed acid–base disorder when
two or more independent acid–base
disorders occur at same time

$PaCO_2$ measurement of CO_2 pressure
that is being exerted on the plasma and
is directly related to the amount of CO_2
being produced

PaO_2 measurement of amount of
pressure exerted by oxygen on
plasma

pH negative logarithm of H^+ ion
concentration in milliequivalents (mEq)
per liter

respiratory acidosis a condition
that occurs in response to hypoventilation; CO_2 is retained and pH is
decreased

respiratory alkalosis a decreased
level of CO_2; sometimes called a H_2CO_3
deficit; pH is elevated and $PaCO_2$ is
decreased

SaO_2 amount of oxygen attached to a
hemoglobin molecule

PRETEST

1 Arterial blood gases on a client with pneumonia indicate the client is in respiratory acidosis. Which interventions should the nurse implement to correct this acid–base imbalance? Select all that apply.

1. Restrict oral fluid intake to water only.
2. Ambulate client in hallway twice each shift.
3. Encourage frequent cough and deep breathing exercises.
4. Medicate with a nonopioid pain medication frequently for intercostal muscle pain.
5. Administer magnesium as prescribed.

2 A client receiving intravenous (IV) sodium bicarbonate for treatment of metabolic acidosis develops muscle twitching and an irregular pulse. Which action should be taken by the nurse initially?

1. Stop the infusion and notify the healthcare provider.
2. Reduce the infusion by one-half of the prescribed rate and observe client closely.
3. Monitor heart rate, blood pressure, and mental status every 15 minutes.
4. Check the client's oxygen saturation level and place client on bedrest.

3 Which arterial blood gas (ABG) result should the nurse expect to see when a client has apnea and develops acidosis?

1. pH 7.42, $PaCO_2$ 48 mm Hg, HCO_3^- 25 mEq/L
2. pH 7.29, $PaCO_2$ 62 mm Hg, HCO_3^- 23 mEq/L
3. pH 7.36, $PaCO_2$ 42 mm Hg, HCO_3^- 26 mEq/L
4. pH 7.49, $PaCO_2$ 30 mm Hg, HCO_3^- 35 mEq/L

4 The nurse concludes that which statement by a student nurse reflects correct understanding about the client's physiological attempt to restore homeostasis during acidosis?

1. "The kidneys start to work within seconds after an imbalance occurs and are very effective in restoring the body to a correct acid–base balance."
2. "The kidneys may not start to function immediately but are very effective as a buffer system to restore the acid–base balance."
3. "The kidneys are not as effective as the lungs in restoring the acid–base balance because the bicarbonate ion is not a good buffer."
4. "The kidneys are very slow to respond to any acid–base imbalance but are very effective in ridding the body of carbonic acid."

5 Which ABG result should the nurse expect to see when a client is admitted with diarrhea that has lasted for 4 days?

1. pH 7.50, $PaCO_2$ 49 mm Hg, HCO_3^- 29 mEq/L
2. pH 7.30, $PaCO_2$ 40 mm Hg, HCO_3^- 18 mEq/L
3. pH 7.40, $PaCO_2$ 38 mm Hg, HCO_3^- 26 mEq/L
4. pH 7.50, $PaCO_2$ 38 mm Hg, HCO_3^- 32 mEq/L

6 The nurse has been caring for a client who has become extremely anxious and agitated. When assessing the client, the nurse should anticipate which finding that could ultimately lead to an acid–base imbalance?

1. Rapid, deep respiratory pattern
2. Rapid, shallow respiratory pattern
3. Rapid, irregular heart rate
4. Slow, irregular heart rate

7 Which pH value on an arterial blood gas result should the nurse expect to see in an anxious client?

1. 7.45
2. 7.38
3. 7.50
4. 7.20

8 The nurse should anticipate which physiological response in a client who is attempting to compensate for a developing metabolic acidosis?

1. Heart rate will increase.
2. Urinary output will increase.
3. Respiratory rate will increase.
4. Temperature will increase.

9 The nurse assesses a client with uncontrolled type 1 diabetes mellitus (DM) for which primary acid–base imbalance?

1. Metabolic alkalosis
2. Respiratory alkalosis
3. Respiratory acidosis
4. Metabolic acidosis

10 The client with respiratory acidosis from COPD asks the nurse why continuous pulse oximetry is prescribed to monitor oxygen saturation. Which response by the nurse is best?

1. "The pulse oximeter measures your CO_2 level so ABGs need to be drawn once a day only."
2. "The pulse oximeter measures the oxygen saturation in your blood at any given time."
3. "The pulse oximeter is being used so we do not have to draw ABGs on you while you are in the hospital."
4. "The machine is used to adequately assess your ventilatory effort while you are in bed."

➤ *See pages 154–156 for Answers and Rationales.*

I. OVERVIEW OF ACID–BASE PHYSIOLOGY

A. Nature of acids and bases
1. An **acid** is a substance that releases a hydrogen (H^+) ion when dissolved in water
2. A **base** is a substance that will bind to an H^+ ion when dissolved in water
3. Weak acids do not completely separate in water; they only release some H^+ ions
4. A weak base accepts H^+ ion less easily but it is extremely valuable in preventing major alterations in extracellular fluid (ECF) pH

B. Chemical buffer systems in body
1. A **buffer** prevents major changes in ECF by releasing or accepting H^+ ions
2. Major chemical buffers are found in blood and include carbonic acid–bicarbonate buffer system, phosphate buffer system, and protein buffer system
3. Chemical buffers are present in both intracellular fluid (ICF) and ECF
4. Buffers are found in all body tissues, including bone
5. Chemical buffers act within seconds to neutralize acids and bases and keep pH within the narrow normal range of 7.35–7.45
6. Bicarbonate buffer system
   a. This system consists of a water solution that contains a weak acid, carbonic acid (H_2CO_3), and a bicarbonate salt, usually sodium bicarbonate ($NaHCO_3$)
   b. Normally body pH is maintained by keeping the ratio of bicarbonate ($\mathbf{HCO_3^-}$) to H_2CO_3 at a proportion of 20:1
      1) This ratio is changed if pH goes up or down, depending on alteration
      2) Once compensation occurs, ratio becomes stable again
   c. Bicarbonate/carbonic acid buffer system is linked to respiratory and renal systems to protect body from changes in pH

1) H_2CO_3 is the respiratory compensatory component because it can dissociate into carbon dioxide (CO_2) and water, with CO_2 being exhaled by lungs
2) HCO_3^- is the primary renal compensatory component because it can be excreted by kidneys
3) This function is illustrated by the following equation:

$$CO_2 + H_2O \leftrightarrow H_2CO_3 \leftrightarrow HCO_3^- + H^+$$

7. Phosphate buffer system buffers both ICF and ECF to maintain a normal pH
8. Protein buffer system acts in a similar manner to bicarbonate–carbonic acid buffer system because it releases or accepts H^+ readily and can exist as either an acid or a base; it is a major intracellular buffer
9. Hemoglobin–oxyhemoglobin buffer system helps to maintain pH within normal range in both arterial and venous blood, which have different amounts of CO_2

C. **Physiological buffers in body**
    1. Pulmonary regulation
        a. Lungs control respiratory carbonic acid buffer system
        b. Lungs compensate for acid–base disturbances that are primarily metabolic in nature (lactic acidosis that occurs with exercise, for example)
        c. Under control of medulla oblongata, lungs increase or decrease respiratory rate and depth in response to amount of CO_2 in ECF
        d. In an acid environment, respirations increase to blow off CO_2; in an alkaline environment, respirations slow to retain CO_2
        e. Respiratory system is extremely sensitive to changes in pH and begins compensatory efforts within seconds to minutes
            1) These mechanisms can become quickly exhausted
            2) This system is not as efficient as renal compensatory efforts
        f. Older adults have a reduced amount of gas exchange during breathing and also have less alveolar membrane so CO_2 retention and increased H^+ ions can be problematic
    2. Renal regulation
        a. Kidneys control metabolic buffer $NaHCO_3^-$ by excreting an acidic urine or an alkaline urine
        b. This system works within several hours to days, but is powerfully effective because it can eliminate either acids or bases as needed
        c. Kidneys control HCO_3^- in ECF by either reabsorbing or excreting H^+ ions
            1) Can reabsorb HCO_3^- as needed
            2) Can secrete free H^+ ions into renal tubules from peritubular capillaries
            3) Can combine ammonia (NaH_3) with hydrochloric acid (HCl) to form ammonium (NH_4Cl), which is excreted by kidneys; approximately 50% of excess H^+ can be excreted by this mechanism
        d. Kidneys can actually excrete weak acids into urine
        e. Body depends on kidneys to excrete acids from cellular metabolism; thus urine is normally acidic (average pH is 6)
        f. Renal function decreases with age so older adults do not excrete H^+ ions or synthesize HCO_3^- as efficiently; therefore, their acid–base imbalances are more difficult to correct, especially if other conditions, such as pneumonia, fever, or infection, occur
    3. **Compensation** for an acid–base imbalance occurs when body uses regulatory mechanisms to return pH to normal by transforming acids and bases within body, which will either fully compensate, partially compensate, or progress to an uncompensated state

a. A primary metabolic disturbance will cause a respiratory compensation
b. A primary respiratory disturbance will cause an acute metabolic response due to buffering system and a more chronic compensation due to renal function
c. Fully compensated means that pH remains within normal range, although other values (CO_2 and bicarbonate) may still be abnormal
d. Partial compensation means that buffers are currently working to restore homeostasis; however, pH remains abnormal
e. Decompensation refers to a worsening state of acid–base imbalance and pH remains abnormal

4. Correction of acid–base imbalance occurs when lungs and/or kidneys eliminate offending substance(s) from body; CO_2 and HCO_3^- levels are returned to normal, not just pH

D. **Measurement of acid–base status:** assessed by using arterial blood gases (ABGs) (see Table 7–1)

1. **pH:** negative logarithm of H^+ ion concentration in mEq per liter
   a. Actual concentration of H^+ ions is very small (<0.0001 mEq/liter); therefore, it has a negative logarithm
   b. Because pH is calculated as a negative value, there is an inverse relationship between pH and H^+ ion concentration; therefore, as H^+ ion concentration increases, pH decreases
   c. The normal value for pH in arterial blood is 7.35–7.45; in venous blood, pH is 7.32–7.42
   d. A pH less than 7.35 is termed *acidotic*
   e. Conversely, a pH greater than 7.45 is called *alkalotic*

2. **PaCO₂** (partial pressure of carbon dioxide): measurement of CO_2 pressure that is being exerted on plasma and is directly related to amount of CO_2 being produced
   a. Normal value of $PaCO_2$ is 35–45 mm Hg
   b. $PaCO_2$ is regulated by lungs and indicates amount of H_2CO_3 that is available to act as a buffer
   c. $PaCO_2$ is the respiratory component of an ABG
   d. Values less than 35 mm Hg are indicative of alkalosis (consistent with hyperventilation)
   e. Acidosis occurs when value rises above 45 mm Hg (consistent with hypoventilation)

3. **PaO₂** (partial pressure of oxygen): measures amount of pressure exerted by oxygen on plasma
   a. Range of normal values for PaO_2 is 80–100 mm Hg for adults under 60 years of age
   b. For every year above 60, there is an expected decrease in PaO_2 of 1 mm Hg

Table 7–1 **Arterial Blood Gas Interpretation**

Blood Gas Values	Acidosis	Normal	Alkalosis
pH	<7.35	7.35–7.45	>7.45
PaCO₂ Abnormal $PaCO_2$ with a normal HCO_3^- indicates a respiratory basis for imbalance	>45 mm Hg respiratory	35–45 mm Hg	<35 mm Hg respiratory
HCO₃⁻ Abnormal with a normal $PaCO_2$ indicates a metabolic basis for imbalance	<22 mEq/L metabolic	22–26 mEq/L	>26 mEq/L metabolic

    c. If PaO_2 drops dramatically, it indicates hypoxemia, which leads to tissue hypoxia; oxygen saturation will also decrease greatly

4. **SaO_2**: refers to percent of hemoglobin bound with oxygen; normal range is 95–100%

    a. Because most oxygen is carried on hemoglobin, the total oxygen concentration is measured using hemoglobin saturation (SaO_2)

    b. There is a relationship between PaO_2 and SaO_2 that influences binding affinity and dissociation of oxygen and hemoglobin (see Figure 7–1)

    c. Acidosis causes a "shift to the right" on oxyhemoglobin dissociation curve, which results in a decreased affinity; oxygen is more easily released to tissues

    d. Alkalosis causes a "shift to the left" on oxyhemoglobin dissociation curve, which results in an increased affinity; oxygen is held more tightly and is less available to tissues

    e. There are other factors that affect oxygen affinity, such as body temperature and transfusion of banked blood

5. Electrolyte interactions

    a. HCO_3^- (normal 22–26 mEq/L) is a direct reflection of renal system's ability to compensate for pH changes

      1) A decreased HCO_3^- level indicates acidosis

      2) Alkalosis occurs when HCO_3^- level rises above normal

    b. Base excess (BE) indicates amount of HCO_3^- available in the ECF

      1) Either a negative or positive amount of HCO_3^- is available for use

      2) Normal base excess ranges from a −3.0 to a +3.0 in adults

      3) Values above +3.0 indicate metabolic alkalosis

      4) Metabolic acidosis exists when value is below −3.0

    c. Serum anion gap (AG) represents an attempt to calculate concentrations of anions (HCO_3, chloride [Cl], proteins, phosphates, and sulfates) and cations (sodium [Na^+], potassium [K^+], magnesium [Mg^{++}], calcium [Ca^{++}])

      1) Normal range is 10–12 mEq/L

      2) Calculated value is $Na^+ - [Cl^- + HCO_3^-]$

      3) Increased AG of >16 mEq/L indicates metabolic acidosis (anion gap acidosis); always check anion gap if client has acidosis

      4) Normal AG can exist with metabolic acidosis (non-anion-gap acidosis) when there is a decrease in HCO_3^- balanced by an increase in Cl^-

      5) Serum K^+ levels are also evaluated in connection with normal AG levels

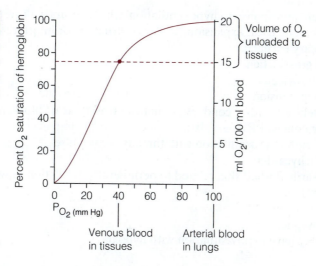

Figure 7–1

Oxygen–hemoglobin dissociation curve. The lower the PaO_2 level, the more readily hemoglobin will onload or offload oxygen.

6) Decreased AG can be seen in clients with low albumin levels or in conditions where there is an increase in unmeasured cations (multiple myeloma, lithium toxicity, or nephrotic syndrome)

d. Chloride levels are used to evaluate clients who are at risk for metabolic alkalosis

1) Urinary levels <10 mEq/L are associated with chloride-responsive metabolic alkalosis (the more commonly occurring type that is usually seen with ECF volume depletion and renal and GI losses; bicarbonate retention occurs)

2) Urinary levels >10 mEq/L are associated with chloride-resistant metabolic alkalosis (less common and is seen in clients with adrenal problems, hypertension, and Mg^{++} or K^+ depletion)

Practice to Pass

How would the nurse determine if a client was in uncompensated respiratory acidosis?

E. **Identification of simple acid–base disturbances** (refer again to Table 7–1)

1. Interpret pH
   a. Is pH less than 7.35? This indicates acidosis
   b. Is pH greater than 7.45? This indicates alkalosis

2. Identify primary cause—respiratory or metabolic
   a. Examine values for $PaCO_2$ and HCO_3^-
   b. If $PaCO_2$ is abnormal, a respiratory problem exists
   c. If HCO_3^- is abnormal, a metabolic problem exists

3. Determine presence of compensation
   a. Determine if $PaCO_2$ and HCO_3^- are decreased or increased as body attempts to maintain a 20:1 ratio of HCO_3^- to H_2CO_3
   b. Partial compensation exists when pH remains abnormal but changes start to occur in opposite system (example: pH indicates an acidotic state but HCO_3^- is increasing, indicating that body is using buffer system to bring pH back toward normal range)
   c. Full or complete compensation occurs when buffer system brings pH back to a value of 7.35–7.45, although both CO_2 and HCO_3^- values are abnormal
      1) If ABG is fully compensated and if pH is normal but less than 7.40, consider the imbalance acidosis
      2) Conversely, if pH is normal but is greater than 7.40, consider the imbalance alkalosis

II. RESPIRATORY ACIDOSIS

A. **Overview**
1. **Respiratory acidosis**: a condition in which CO_2 is retained and pH is decreased (see Table 7–2)
2. Occurs in response to hypoventilation, which occurs with respiratory depression, inadequate chest expansion, airway obstruction, or interference with alveolar–capillary exchange

B. **Clinical presentation**
1. Cardiovascular
   a. Hypotension
   b. Delayed cardiac conduction that can lead to heart block, peaked T waves, prolonged PR intervals, and widened QRS complexes
   c. Peripheral vasodilation with thready, weak pulse
   d. Tachycardia
   e. Warm, flushed skin related to peripheral vasodilation as well as to impaired gas exchange
2. Respiratory
   a. Dyspnea
   b. May have hypoventilation with hypoxia

Table 7–2	Respiratory Alterations in Acid–Base Balance	
Clinical Picture	**Acidosis**	**Alkalosis**
pH	<7.35	>7.45
$PaCO_2$	>45	<35
HCO_3^-	Elevated with compensation	Decreased with compensation
Signs and Symptoms Cardiovascular	Hypotension, heart block, peaked T waves, prolonged PR interval, weak and thready pulse, tachycardia, warm and flushed skin	Increased myocardial irritability, increased heart rate, increased sensitivity to digitalis preparations
Respiratory	Rapid and shallow respiratory pattern	Dyspnea, chest tightness
CNS	Headache, seizures, altered mental status, papilledema, decreased LOC, drowsiness, coma	Dizziness, anxiety, panic, tetany, seizures, blurred vision
Causes	Chronic obstructive pulmonary disease, sedative or barbiturate overdose, chest wall abnormalities, pneumonia, atelectasis, respiratory muscle weakness, underventilation	Hyperventilation caused by hypoxia, fear, fever, pain, exercise, anxiety, pulmonary embolus Mechanical overventilation Stimulated respiratory centers caused by septicemia, encephalitis, brain injury, salicylate poisoning, hypokalemia
Compensation	Kidneys eliminate H^+ ions and retain HCO_3^-	Kidneys conserve H^+ ions and excrete HCO_3^-

    3. Central nervous system (CNS)

       a. Headache

       b. Seizures

       c. Altered mental status, confusion, decreased level of consciousness (LOC)

       d. Papilledema

       e. Muscle twitching

       f. Drowsiness that can progress to coma

Practice to Pass

Why is the nurse concerned about hyperkalemia in the client who has respiratory acidosis?

C. Diagnostic findings

    1. pH decreased below 7.35

    2. $PaCO_2$ elevated above 45 mm Hg

    3. Hyperkalemia

D. Compensation

    1. Increased rate and depth of respirations to blow off CO_2

    2. Kidneys eliminate H^+ ions and retain HCO_3^- (urine pH less than 6)

    3. HCO_3^- levels rise when body is compensating for respiratory acidosis

E. Priority nursing concerns

    1. Effectiveness of client's gas exchange and respiratory pattern because of hypoventilation

    2. Possible altered mental status that could lead to falls or other injury

    3. Client anxiety about dyspnea or breathlessness

    4. Possible decreased cardiac output if hypoxia leads to dysrhythmias

F. Therapeutic management

    1. Treatment is directed toward correcting underlying cause and improving ventilation

    2. Implement pulmonary hygiene measures to clear respiratory tract of mucus and purulent drainage

    3. Provide adequate fluid intake to liquefy secretions

4. If indicated, administer supplemental oxygen cautiously to a client with chronic respiratory acidosis; O_2 rather than CO_2 may stimulate respirations
   a. It is important to note that clients with chronic acidosis have compensated and are adjusted to living with higher $PaCO_2$ levels
   b. Remember that CO_2 level normally stimulates respiratory drive
   c. Oxygen administration at higher levels can lead to a decreased ventilatory drive and can cause further hypoxia in a client with COPD
   d. Low-flow oxygen is an expected treatment for clients with COPD
   e. Collaborate with healthcare provider and respiratory therapist to manage chronic respiratory disease
5. Mechanical ventilation may be required to improve respiratory status; settings should be adjusted to decrease CO_2 gradually to prevent alkalosis and seizures from occurring

G. Client-centered nursing care

1. Assess respiratory rate, depth, and breath sounds; encourage coughing and deep breathing
2. Monitor client for complications and response to therapy
3. Measure apical pulse and assess for tachycardia and irregularities
4. Assess LOC
5. Monitor ECG for dysrhythmias
6. Draw serum electrolytes, especially potassium and ABGs
7. Administer oxygen as indicated and prescribed; suction as needed to clear respiratory tract of secretions that interfere with oxygenation
8. Administer medications as prescribed
9. Provide oral hygiene frequently
10. Keep side-rails up, bed at lowest level, and call bell within client's reach
11. Maintain a calm, quiet environment
12. Assess color of skin, nail beds, and mucous membranes
13. If client is confused, orient frequently to person, place, and time
14. Place in semi-Fowler to Fowler position to facilitate maximum lung expansion
15. Provide adequate fluid intake
16. Encourage pursed-lip breathing to promote CO_2 elimination as appropriate
17. Encourage frequent position changes; out of bed as tolerated

H. Medication therapy

1. Type of drugs and route of administration depend on client's baseline condition and whether disease is acute or chronic with a state of acute exacerbation
2. Medications may include:
   a. Bronchodilators to decrease bronchospasm
   b. Antibiotics to treat infections in respiratory tract
   c. Respiratory agents to decrease viscosity of pulmonary secretions, such as acetylcysteine
   d. Anticoagulants and thrombolytics to prevent or treat pulmonary emboli
3. Medications are usually administered IV in acute situations and then changed to PO as client's condition stabilizes
4. Respiratory therapists often administer medications as part of a treatment plan; they are often called on a PRN basis to assist client during acute episodes

I. Client education

1. Teach preventative measures to clients at risk
2. Teach deep breathing techniques
3. Teach signs and symptoms of infection to report to healthcare provider
4. Report signs of infections, shortness of breath, fatigue, and increased pulse rate to healthcare provider

J. Evaluation
   1. Respiratory pattern becomes deeper and rate decreases
   2. ABGs return to as near normal as possible for client
   3. Anxiety level diminishes, leading to improved work of breathing with less effort
   4. Client is oriented to person, place, and time with improved LOC
   5. Client remains free of injury or cardiac dysrhythmias

III. RESPIRATORY ALKALOSIS

A. Overview
   1. **Respiratory alkalosis**: a condition in which pH is elevated and $PaCO_2$ is decreased
   2. Occurs with hyperventilation and leads to a decreased level of CO_2; sometimes called an *H_2CO_3 deficit*
   3. Other causes can include:
      a. Respiratory center stimulation from fever, salicylate intoxication, and trauma to CNS
      b. Infection
      c. Excessive mechanical ventilation
      d. Refer back to Table 7–2

B. Clinical presentation
   1. Cardiovascular
      a. Increased myocardial irritability; palpitations
      b. Increased heart rate
      c. Increased sensitivity to digoxin
   2. Respiratory
      a. Rapid, shallow breathing
      b. Chest tightness and palpitations
   3. CNS
      a. Dizziness
      b. Lightheadedness
      c. Anxiety, panic
      d. Tetany
      e. Seizures
      f. Difficulty concentrating
      g. Blurred vision
      h. Numbness and tingling in extremities
      i. Hyperactive reflexes

C. Diagnostic findings
   1. High pH (>7.45)
   2. Low $PaCO_2$ (<35 mm Hg)
   3. Hypokalemia
   4. Hypocalcemia (as pH increases, calcium binding occurs in serum and calcium level decreases; accounts for numbness and tingling)

D. Compensation
   1. Kidneys conserve H^+ and excrete HCO_3^- (urine pH greater than 6)
   2. Low HCO_3^- indicates body is attempting to compensate

E. Priority nursing concerns
   1. Sensory-perceptual alterations or changes in thought processes because of effects on CNS
   2. Changes in breathing pattern because of hyperventilation
   3. Risk of harm to client if weakness, tetany, or seizures occur

Practice to Pass

Why would a client with uncontrolled type 1 diabetes develop metabolic acidosis, and how can this be prevented?

F. Therapeutic management
1. Treat the underlying cause
2. Have client rebreathe CO_2 by using a rebreather mask or a paper bag
3. Give oxygen therapy if client is hypoxemic
4. Medicate as appropriate and as prescribed with anti-anxiety drugs

G. Client-centered nursing care
1. Assess respiratory rate, depth, breath sounds
2. Monitor vital signs and ABGs
3. Ensure a calm, quiet environment; provide support and reassurance
4. Treat fever if this is a possible cause
5. Assist client to breathe more slowly; if needed, provide client with rebreather mask or paper bag to breathe into
6. Protect client from injury
7. Administer anti-anxiety, sedative, or analgesic medications as prescribed

H. Medication therapy
1. Sedatives or anti-anxiety agents may be used to control hyperventilation caused by anxiety
2. Analgesics may be used to control pain as a contributing factor

I. Client education
1. Teach client relaxation techniques
2. Encourage client to attend stress management classes if appropriate
3. Teach parents to keep aspirin and other salicylates out of reach of children and in an inaccessible area

J. Evaluation
1. Respiratory rate decreases
2. Numbness and tingling in extremities dissipates
3. ABGs return to normal
4. Anxiety diminishes
5. Client remains free from injury

IV. METABOLIC ACIDOSIS

A. Overview
1. **Metabolic acidosis**: an imbalance in which pH decreases and HCO_3 decreases
2. Occurs when acids other than carbonic acid accumulate in ECF or when there is a loss of HCO_3^- (see Table 7-3)
3. This condition rarely occurs spontaneously but rather is accompanied by other problems, such as GI conditions (starvation, malnutrition, and chronic diarrhea), renal (kidney failure), DKA, hyperthyroidism, trauma, shock, increased exercise, severe infection, and fever

B. Clinical presentation
1. Cardiovascular
   a. Hypotension
   b. Dysrhythmias and possible cardiac arrest
   c. Peripheral vasodilation
   d. Cool, clammy skin
2. Respiratory: deep rapid breathing pattern; possible Kussmaul respirations
3. CNS
   a. Drowsiness leading to coma
   b. Headache
   c. Confusion
   d. Lethargy and weakness

4. Gastrointestinal
   a. Nausea and vomiting
   b. Diarrhea
   c. Abdominal pain

C. Diagnostic findings
   1. pH less than 7.35
   2. HCO_3^- less than 22 mEq/L
   3. Hyperkalemia frequently seen
   4. ECG may show changes related to increased potassium levels
   5. Anion gap calculation increases; base excess decreases
   6. Increased lactate levels in sepsis/septic shock
   7. Elevated ionized (free) calcium
   8. Decreased magnesium levels

D. Compensation
   1. Lungs eliminate CO_2; kidneys conserve HCO_3^-
   2. Urine pH less than 6
   3. $PaCO_2$ decreases when compensation is occurring

E. Priority nursing concerns
   1. Possible reduced cardiac output if dysrhythmias and/or fluid volume losses are present
   2. Possible sensory-perceptual changes because of changes in neurologic functioning caused by acidosis
   3. Risk for harm or injury to client because of confusion, weakness, and drowsiness
   4. Risk for dehydration if there is excessive loss from the kidneys or gastrointestinal system

F. Therapeutic management
   1. Treatment is aimed at correcting underlying problem
   2. Provide hydration to restore water, nutrients, and electrolytes
   3. An alkalotic IV solution (sodium bicarbonate or sodium lactate) may be prescribed to correct acidosis
   4. Mechanical ventilation is used only if other treatment modalities are ineffective

G. Client-centered nursing care

   1. Monitor laboratory results such as ABGs and serum electrolytes
   2. Monitor intake and output (I&O) and daily weight; assess for edema
   3. Assess vital signs, especially respirations for rate and depth
   4. Assess LOC
   5. Assess gastrointestinal function

   6. Monitor ECG for conduction problems
   7. Protect from injury
   8. Administer medications and IV fluids as prescribed

H. Medication therapy: based on underlying cause
   1. If cause is secondary to diabetic ketoacidosis, implement hydration with normal saline, regular insulin, and potassium
   2. If diarrhea is the cause, treat with hydration and antidiarrheal agents
   3. Administer $NaHCO_3$ cautiously and only when HCO_3^- levels are very low (below 16–18 mEq/L); can cause rebound metabolic alkalosis and hypokalemia

Practice to Pass

How would the nurse prevent the client from losing H^+ ions when nasogastric suctioning is being used?

I. Client education
   1. Teach clients to seek healthcare if they have prolonged diarrhea
   2. Teach diabetic clients importance of preventing occurrences of DKA and how to manage DKA should it occur

J. Evaluation
   1. Client remains free from injury
   2. LOC returns to normal

   3. Any dysrhythmias, GI upset, or fluid volume deficits are corrected
   4. ABGs return to normal

V. METABOLIC ALKALOSIS

A. Overview
   1. **Metabolic alkalosis**: a condition in which there is an increased pH and increased HCO_3^-
   2. Occurs when there is a loss of H^+ ion (such as in vomiting or nasogastric suctioning) or an increase in HCO_3^- level (such as with ingestion of bicarbonate-based antacids)
   3. See Table 7–3

B. Clinical presentation
   1. Cardiovascular
      a. Sinus tachycardia
      b. Dysrhythmias such as atrial tachycardia or premature ventricular contractions
      c. Hypertension
   2. Respiratory: hypoventilation, possibly leading to respiratory failure
   3. CNS
      a. Dizziness
      b. Irritability or nervousness
      c. Confusion
      d. Tremors
      e. Muscle cramps
      f. Hyperreflexia
      g. Tetany; paresthesias in fingers and toes
      h. Seizures
   4. Gastrointestinal
      a. Anorexia, nausea and vomiting
      b. Paralytic ileus if hypokalemia occurs

Table 7–3   **Metabolic Alterations in Acid–Base Balance**

Clinical Picture	Acidosis	Alkalosis
pH	<7.35	>7.45
$PaCO_2$	<35 with compensation	>45 with compensation
HCO_3^-	<22	>26
Signs and Symptoms Cardiovascular	Hypotension, dysrhythmias, peripheral vasodilation, cold, clammy skin	Tachycardia, dysrhythmias secondary to hypokalemia, hypotension, premature ventricular contractions, atrial tachycardia
Respiratory	Deep, rapid respiratory pattern (Kussmaul's respirations)	Hypoventilation, respiratory failure
CNS	Drowsiness, coma, headache, confusion, lethargy, weakness, nausea and vomiting, diarrhea, abdominal pain	Dizziness, irritability, nervousness, confusion, tremors, muscle cramps, tetany, hyperreflexia, paresthesias in fingers and toes, seizures
Causes	Diabetic ketoacidosis, lactic acidosis, starvation, severe diarrhea, renal tubule acidosis, renal failure, GI fistulas, shock	Severe vomiting, excessive NG suctioning, diuretic therapy, hypokalemia, licorice, excessive $NaHCO_3$ use, excessive mineralocorticoids
Compensation	Lungs eliminate CO_2; kidneys conserve HCO_3^-	Lungs retain CO_2; kidneys excrete HCO_3^-

C. Diagnostic findings
1. pH greater than 7.45
2. HCO_3^- above 26 mEq/L
3. Hypokalemia
4. Hypocalcemia (as pH increases, calcium binding occurs and serum calcium levels decrease)
5. Hyponatremia and hypochloremia
6. Urine chloride levels reveal whether client is chloride responsive (<10 mEq/L) or chloride resistant (>10 mEq/L)
7. Base excess increases

D. Compensation
1. Lungs retain CO_2; kidneys conserve H^+ and excrete HCO_3^-
2. $PaCO_2$ increases with compensation
3. Urine pH greater than 6

E. Priority nursing concerns
1. Potential for dehydration if there is significant gastrointestinal fluid loss
2. Possible decrease in cardiac output in the presence of fluid volume losses and/or altered cardiac conduction because of hypokalemia and alkalosis
3. Risk for client injury if client experiences hypotension because of fluid volume losses
4. Possible inadequate gas exchange if client has hypoventilation

F. Therapeutic management
1. Treatment aimed at correcting underlying problem
2. Provide sufficient chloride to enhance renal absorption of sodium and excretion of HCO_3^-
3. Restore normal fluid balance

G. Client-centered nursing care
1. Assess level of consciousness, vital signs (especially respiratory rate and depth), oxygen saturation, and peripheral tissue perfusion
2. Administer medication and IV fluids as prescribed
3. Monitor I&O, daily weight
4. Protect from injury
5. Monitor ECG for conduction abnormalities
6. Monitor ABGs and serum electrolytes
7. Position to allow for maximum lung expansion (semi-Fowler to Fowler position)
8. Plan to allow for rest periods between activities
9. Administer oxygen as prescribed

H. Medication therapy
1. Normal saline–based IV fluid replacement
2. Potassium supplementation if hypokalemic
3. Histamine-2 receptor antagonists such as ranitidine or famotidine to reduce production and subsequent loss of H^+ ions in GI drainage
4. If client is chloride responsive, acetazolamide may increase bicarbonate excretion from kidneys
5. If client is chloride resistant, then correct K^+ and Mg^{++} deficits with appropriate supplementation

I. Client education
1. Teach clients to take potassium-wasting diuretics and antacids correctly
2. Teach signs and symptoms to report to healthcare provider for those at risk, especially older adults
3. Teach signs and symptoms of hypokalemia to report to healthcare provider

Practice to Pass

Why does the client with metabolic alkalosis have cardiac conduction problems that must be monitored?

J. Evaluation
1. Client remains free from injury
2. ABGs and electrolytes return to normal
3. Hypertension is corrected
4. Cardiac conduction abnormalities do not occur or are resolved
5. Client states measures to prevent problem from recurring

VI. MIXED ACID–BASE DISTURBANCES

A. Identification and treatment of primary disorder
1. A **mixed acid–base disorder** occurs when two or more independent acid–base disorders happen at same time
2. The pH is dependent on type and severity of each simple disorder
3. Respiratory acidosis and alkalosis cannot occur concurrently; it is impossible to have hyperventilation and hypoventilation at same time
4. Treatment is aimed at correcting underlying cause of each disorder
5. When identifying acid–base imbalances, mathematical formulas can be used to assess degree of expected compensation
   a. Use of these equations is usually done on an intermediate level of acid–base balance
   b. However, it is important for nurse to know that there are calculations that will identify degree of compensatory changes
6. Anion gap and urine pH values will also assist in determining which imbalance is occurring

B. Chronic and superimposed acid–base disturbances
1. Mixed metabolic acidosis and respiratory acidosis
   a. Clients with acute pulmonary edema
   b. Clients with cardiac arrest as a result of buildup of lactic acidosis and CO_2 retention due to inadequate ventilation
   c. pH values decrease and are more pronounced because of decreasing HCO_3^- level coupled with increasing CO_2 level
2. Mixed metabolic alkalosis and respiratory acidosis
   a. Seen in clients with chronic obstructive pulmonary disease (COPD) secondary to treatment with potassium-wasting diuretics, severe vomiting, or development of diarrhea
   b. Seen in clients with COPD who have a quick improvement in ventilation
   c. pH values tend to become balanced because of an increase in both HCO_3^- and PCO_2 values
3. Mixed metabolic acidosis with respiratory alkalosis
   a. Seen in clients with a rapid correction of metabolic acidosis
   b. Seen in clients with salicylate intoxication
   c. Seen in clients with Gram-negative septicemia
   d. pH values tend to become balanced because of decreases in both HCO_3^- and pCO_2
4. Mixed metabolic alkalosis and respiratory alkalosis
   a. Seen in clients postoperatively with severe hemorrhage
   b. Seen in clients who have massive transfusions
   c. Seen in clients with excessive NG drainage
   d. pH values increase and are more pronounced because of an increase in HCO_3^- coupled with a decrease in CO_2 levels
5. Mixed metabolic acidosis and metabolic alkalosis
   a. Seen in clients with gastroenteritis, vomiting, and diarrhea
   b. If imbalance is present in the same proportion, there is usually no change in values (pH, HCO_3^-, and pCO_2) even though there is hypovolemia

6. Chronic and acute respiratory acidosis
   a. Clients with chronic respiratory conditions with an acute condition superimposed can lead to increased pCO_2 levels, causing further pulmonary dysfunction and leading to serious consequences that can compromise both treatment and expected response to treatment
   b. Clients who have both a chronic and a superimposed acute respiratory acid–base imbalance should be closely monitored by a pulmonologist
   c. Respiratory therapist should be part of collaborative healthcare team managing treatment of this client

C. **Diagnostic and laboratory findings**
   1. For ABG interpretations when pH is abnormal, see Table 7–4
   2. Normal pH values
      a. Increased pCO_2 leads to respiratory acidosis with compensating metabolic alkalosis
      b. Decreased pCO_2 leads to respiratory alkalosis with compensating metabolic acidosis
   3. Changes in anion gap levels and bicarbonate levels
   4. Abnormal serum electrolyte levels can reflect changes in acid–base balance
   5. ECG results may show electrolyte disturbances
   6. CXR may show underlying cardiac or pulmonary disease
   7. Hemoglobin and hematocrit levels can indicate oxygen-carrying potential

D. **Priority nursing concerns**
   1. Possible reduced cardiac output because of dysrhythmias, fluid volume reduction, or potassium alterations
   2. Potential for client injury if there are neurologic changes caused by acid–base imbalances

E. **Therapeutic management**
   1. Treatment focuses on correcting underlying causes of disorder(s)
   2. Mixed disorders must be treated before acid–base balance can be restored
   3. A collaborative team approach (including a pulmonologist, respiratory therapist, nurses, and dietitian) is needed to assist client in restoring acid–base balance, increasing activity tolerance, and improving physiological function

F. **Client-centered nursing care**
   1. Monitor vital signs
   2. Monitor ABGs, oxygen saturation, pulmonary function tests, and CXR
   3. Protect from injury
   4. Monitor LOC
   5. Monitor ECG and laboratory results such as hemoglobin and hematocrit and serum electrolytes
   6. Ensure adequate fluid intake
   7. Implement therapeutic measures as prescribed to treat specific imbalance(s)

Table 7–4	**Abnormalities in Arterial Blood Gases**	
pH	**CO_2**	**Associated Acid–Base Imbalances**
↓	↑	Respiratory acidosis with incompletely compensating metabolic alkalosis Respiratory acidosis with coexisting metabolic acidosis
↓	↓	Metabolic acidosis with incompletely compensating respiratory alkalosis Metabolic acidosis with coexisting respiratory alkalosis
↑	↓	Respiratory alkalosis with incompletely compensating metabolic acidosis Respiratory alkalosis with coexisting metabolic alkalosis
↑	↑	Metabolic alkalosis with incompletely compensating respiratory acidosis Metabolic alkalosis with coexisting respiratory acidosis

POSTTEST

G. Medication therapy
1. Therapy is aimed at resolving underlying causes of disorders
2. Administer oxygen as prescribed using respiratory therapy guidelines
3. Specific medications are prescribed according to diagnosed condition

H. Client education
1. Clients with chronic respiratory conditions should report exacerbations to healthcare provider
2. Clients who experience fluid losses through emesis or diarrhea are at increased risk for acid–base imbalance and should notify healthcare provider if condition is not self-limiting
3. Clients with diabetes mellitus are at risk for acid–base imbalance because of alterations in glucose levels and should closely monitor these levels and use appropriate interventions to maintain within normal range
4. Clients who have renal conditions are prone to develop acid–base imbalance because of alterations in electrolyte levels; closely monitor renal status to identify potential disturbances and allow for intervention

I. Evaluation
1. Client remains free from injury
2. Mixed disorder is treated quickly and effectively
3. ABGs and any abnormal electrolyte levels return to normal
4. ECG conduction problems do not occur
5. Fluid volume is maintained
6. Level of consciousness improves
7. Client reports ways to prevent problem from reoccurring

Case Study

A 69-year-old client with chronic obstructive pulmonary disease (COPD) is admitted with an acute respiratory infection. The client has a history of hypertension, diabetes mellitus, and mild renal insufficiency. You are the nurse assigned to the care of this client.

1. What would this client's ABGs look like based on the admitting diagnosis?
2. What will you do to help improve the client's respiratory status?
3. Why is this client's $PaCO_2$ different than a client who does not have COPD?
4. What teaching does this client require in order to prevent development of metabolic alkalosis?
5. Are there any other acid–base imbalances for which this client is at risk because of the client's medical history?

For suggested responses, see pages 192–193.

POSTTEST

1 A client is admitted to the hospital with an exacerbation of COPD. Arterial blood gas (ABG) results are pH 7.30, $PaCO_2$ 51, and HCO_3^- 25. How should the nurse interpret these results?

1. Respiratory acidosis, uncompensated
2. Respiratory alkalosis partially compensated
3. Respiratory acidosis, compensated
4. Metabolic acidosis, compensated

2 A client admitted to the emergency department (ED) with chest injuries following a motor vehicle accident reports that it hurts to breathe. The client's respiratory rate is 12 and respirations are very shallow. The nurse should anticipate which arterial blood gas (ABG) results?

1. pH 7.42, $PaCO_2$ 41 mm Hg, HCO_3^- 23 mEq/L, SaO_2 96%
2. pH 7.31, $PaCO_2$ 49 mm Hg, HCO_3^- 24 mEq/L, SaO_2 87%
3. pH 7.49, $PaCO_2$ 36 mm Hg, HCO_3^- 30 mEq/L, SaO_2 89%
4. pH 7.38, $PaCO_2$ 38 mm Hg, HCO_3^- 22 mEq/L, SaO_2 90%

3 What action should the nurse take initially to avoid acid–base imbalance when a client becomes anxious and starts to hyperventilate?

1. Tell the client to stop breathing so fast because he may pass out.
2. Give the client a sedative to decrease anxiety and stop hyperventilation.
3. Give the client a paper bag to breathe into and coach client about breathing.
4. Notify the healthcare provider to obtain prescriptions for preventive measures.

4 The nurse should closely monitor a client with chronic renal failure for which primary acid–base imbalance?

1. Metabolic acidosis
2. Metabolic alkalosis
3. Respiratory acidosis
4. Respiratory alkalosis

5 A 36-year-old female is admitted with vomiting and dehydration after having the flu for 3 days. Arterial blood gas (ABG) results are pH 7.46, $PaCO_2$ 50, HCO_3^- 33, SaO_2 95%. What should these values indicate to the nurse?

1. Metabolic acidosis, uncompensated
2. Respiratory acidosis, compensated
3. Metabolic alkalosis, partially compensated
4. Metabolic alkalosis, uncompensated

6 A client in a full cardiac arrest is admitted to the emergency department (ED). Arterial blood gases (ABGs) indicate a respiratory acidosis. How should the nurse respond to correct this condition?

1. Administer $NaHCO_3$ to correct the acidosis.
2. Administer epinephrine to get a heart rate so acidosis can be corrected.
3. Ventilate client to "blow off" excess CO_2.
4. Defibrillate the client to restore a normal rhythm.

7 The nurse should identify which clients as being at risk for developing metabolic alkalosis? Select all that apply.

1. A client who has a nasogastric tube (NGT) to continuous suction
2. A client who has had diarrhea for 2 days
3. A client who is admitted with salicylate toxicity
4. A client who takes antacids frequently for heartburn
5. A client who is admitted with asthmatic bronchitis

8 The arterial blood gas (ABG) results of a 68-year-old client admitted with pneumonia are pH 7.46, $PaCO_2$ 30, HCO_3^- 19, SaO_2 72. How should the nurse interpret these results?

1. Respiratory acidosis, uncompensated
2. Respiratory alkalosis, partially compensated
3. Respiratory alkalosis, uncompensated
4. Metabolic alkalosis, partially compensated

9 A 71-year-old client develops hypertension, tachycardia, and increased respirations 2 days after surgery. Arterial blood gas (ABG) results are pH 7.29, $PaCO_2$ 52, HCO_3^- 24, SaO_2 95%. The nurse interprets that these results indicate which state of acid–base imbalance?

1. Respiratory acidosis, uncompensated
2. Respiratory acidosis, partially compensated
3. Metabolic acidosis, uncompensated
4. Metabolic acidosis, partially compensated

10 A 57-year-old client is admitted with a diagnosis of acute myocardial infarction. Arterial blood gas (ABG) results are pH 7.36, $PaCO_2$ 29, HCO_3^- 20, SaO_2 100%. The nurse should draw which conclusion about this client's status?

1. Well oxygenated with uncompensated respiratory alkalosis
2. Hypoxemic with compensated respiratory acidosis
3. Well oxygenated with compensated metabolic acidosis
4. Hypoxemic with compensated metabolic acidosis

➤ *See pages 156–157 for Answers and Rationales.*

ANSWERS & RATIONALES

Pretest

1 **Answer: 2, 3, 4 Rationale:** It would be helpful to ambulate the client, which will promote lung expansion and improve gas exchange. The respiratory acidosis in this client is secondary to retention of carbon dioxide. Cough and deep breathing exercises will stimulate expectoration of secretions, allowing for improved gas exchange. Fluids will help to liquefy secretions and do not need to be restricted to water. Medicating the client frequently with narcotics may decrease respiratory drive, but a non-narcotic medication may enable the client to breathe deeply. Magnesium has no effect on acid–base. **Cognitive Level:** Applying **Client Need:** Reduction of Risk Potential **Integrated Process:** Nursing Process: Implementation **Content Area:** Adult Health **Strategy:** Recall causes of respiratory acidosis are related to retention of carbon dioxide. Determine that coughing and deep breathing, ambulating, and fluids provide measures to best promote improved gas exchange in the lungs. **Reference:** LeMone, P., Burke, K., Bauldoff, G., & Gubrud, P. (2015). *Medical surgical nursing: Clinical reasoning in patient care* (6th ed.). New York, NY: Pearson, pp. 223–225.

2 **Answer: 1 Rationale:** Symptoms of alkalosis include irritability, confusion, cyanosis, irregular pulse, slow respirations, and muscle twitching. These symptoms warrant discontinuing the medication and notifying the primary healthcare provider because the client may have received excessive sodium bicarbonate. Reducing the infusion rate by half does not protect the client from further effects from alkalosis. Monitoring the client should be done on an ongoing basis after taking actions to safeguard the client. Checking

oxygen saturation and initiating bedrest should be done after taking actions to safeguard the client. **Cognitive Level:** Analyzing **Client Need:** Pharmacological and Parenteral Therapies **Integrated Process:** Nursing Process: Implementation **Content Area:** Adult Health **Strategy:** The critical word is *initially*, indicating all or some of the options are correct, but one takes first priority. Recognize the client is experiencing metabolic alkalosis and the severity of this to choose the correct option. **Reference:** LeMone, P., Burke, K., Bauldoff, G., & Gubrud, P. (2015). *Medical surgical nursing: Clinical reasoning in patient care* (6th ed.). New York, NY: Pearson, pp. 221–223.

3 **Answer: 2 Rationale:** Apnea and hypoventilation result in rising carbon dioxide levels, which leads to acidosis. The ABG would likely reflect respiratory acidosis without compensation, as reflected by a pH of less than 7.35, an elevated $PaCO_2$, and an HCO_3^- that is within normal limits. A pH of 7.42 with a $PaCO_2$ of 48 mm Hg and a HCO_3^- level of 25 mEq/L represents a normal ABG. A pH of 7.36 with a $PaCO_2$ of 42 mm Hg and a HCO_3^- level of 26 mEq/L represents a normal ABG. A pH of 7.52 with a $PaCO_2$ of 30 mm Hg and a HCO_3^- level of 35 mEq/L represents a mixed respiratory and metabolic alkalosis. **Cognitive Level:** Analyzing **Client Need:** Physiological Adaptation **Integrated Process:** Nursing Process: Assessment **Content Area:** Adult Health **Strategy:** Critical words are *apnea* and *acidosis*, indicating the cause will be respiratory in nature. Look for the ABG with a pH indicating acidosis to direct you to the correct option. **Reference:** LeMone, P., Burke, K., Bauldoff, G., & Gubrud, P. (2015). *Medical surgical nursing: Clinical reasoning in patient care* (6th ed.). New York, NY: Pearson, pp. 221–222, 225–226.

4 **Answer: 2 Rationale:** The kidneys respond more slowly to acid–base imbalances but are more effective than the lungs or blood buffers in restoring acid–base balance to the extracellular fluid. The primary response to acidosis is with lung compensation. The blood buffers, not the kidneys, start to work within seconds. The kidneys are more effective than the lungs because they can eliminate either acids or bases of various types. The kidneys eliminate more than carbonic acid. **Cognitive Level:** Understanding **Client Need:** Physiological Adaptation **Integrated Process:** Communication and Documentation **Content Area:** Adult Health **Strategy:** Note some of the options are only partially correct. Recall the role of the kidney in maintaining acid–base balance to choose the correct option. **Reference:** LeMone, P., Burke, K., Bauldoff, G., & Gubrud, P. (2015). *Medical surgical nursing: Clinical reasoning in patient care* (6th ed.). New York, NY: Pearson, pp. 214–215.

5 **Answer: 2 Rationale:** Diarrhea leads to loss of bicarbonate from the intestinal tract. This can cause metabolic acidosis. With metabolic acidosis, the pH is low and the HCO_3^- is also decreased. A pH of 7.50 with a $PaCO_2$ 49 mm Hg and a HCO_3^- level of 29 mEq/L is consistent with metabolic alkalosis with only partial compensation. A pH of 7.40 with a $PaCO_2$ of 38 mmHg and a HCO_3^- level of 26 mEq/L is consistent with a normal blood gas. A pH of 7.50 with a $PaCO_2$ of 38 mmHg and a HCO_3^- level of 32 mEq/L is consistent with uncompensated metabolic alkalosis. **Cognitive Level:** Analyzing **Client Need:** Physiological Adaptation **Integrated Process:** Nursing Process: Assessment **Content Area:** Adult Health **Strategy:** The critical word is *diarrhea*. Recall this leads to a loss of alkaline fluids, which will cause acidosis to direct you to the choice with a pH of less than 7.35 and a low HCO_3^- level. **Reference:** LeMone, P., Burke, K., Bauldoff, G., & Gubrud, P. (2015). *Medical surgical nursing: Clinical reasoning in patient care* (6th ed.). New York, NY: Pearson, pp. 215, 218–221.

6 **Answer: 2 Rationale:** Clients who are extremely anxious tend to hyperventilate and have a rapid, shallow respiratory pattern. A rapid, deep respiratory pattern can occur when the client has respiratory compensation for an underlying metabolic acidosis. Anxiety could lead to a rapid heart rate but it would be regular rather than irregular. A slow irregular heart rate indicates an underlying disturbance of cardiac rhythm and is not characteristic of hyperventilation. **Cognitive Level:** Applying **Client Need:** Physiological Adaptation **Integrated Process:** Nursing Process: Assessment **Content Area:** Adult Health **Strategy:** Critical words are *anxious* and *agitated*. Visualize this client when considering options. Eliminate the options that are related to pulse and not breathing. Recall breathing patterns seen in anxious clients to choose the correct option. **Reference:** LeMone, P., Burke, K., Bauldoff, G., & Gubrud, P. (2015). *Medical surgical*

nursing: Clinical reasoning in patient care (6th ed.). New York, NY: Pearson, pp. 221–222.

7 **Answer: 3 Rationale:** An anxious client often hyperventilates, leading to loss of carbon dioxide and alkalosis. A pH of 7.50 indicates an alkalotic state. A pH of 7.45 is at the high end of the normal range (7.35–7.45). A pH of 7.38 is normal. A pH of 7.20 is extremely acidotic and would be unexpected in a client who is anxious. **Cognitive Level:** Applying **Client Need:** Physiological Adaptation **Integrated Process:** Nursing Process: Assessment **Content Area:** Adult Health **Strategy:** The critical word is *anxious*. Recall anxiety will cause an increase in respiratory rate with loss of carbon dioxide, resulting in alkalosis. **Reference:** LeMone, P., Burke, K., Bauldoff, G., & Gubrud, P. (2015). *Medical surgical nursing: Clinical reasoning in patient care* (6th ed.). New York, NY: Pearson, pp. 221–222.

8 **Answer: 3 Rationale:** A client with metabolic acidosis will have an increase in respiratory rate and depth to eliminate excess carbon dioxide in an attempt to compensate for the acidosis. An increase in heart rate can occur from a variety of physiological or psychological stressors, but does not compensate for metabolic acidosis. An increase in urine output could be for a variety of reasons, including overhydration and diuretic therapy as examples. Temperature elevation can occur with a variety of conditions, such as infection, but is not a compensatory change when there is metabolic acidosis. Increases in heart rate, temperature, and urinary output are all metabolic responses that are not directly associated with maintaining acid–base balance. Initial compensation with metabolic acidosis will be via the lungs. **Cognitive Level:** Applying **Client Need:** Physiological Adaptation **Integrated Process:** Nursing Process: Assessment **Content Area:** Adult Health **Strategy:** Recall the respiratory system will try to compensate for acidosis by blowing off carbon dioxide and water to direct you to the correct option. **Reference:** LeMone, P., Burke, K., Bauldoff, G., & Gubrud, P. (2015). *Medical surgical nursing: Clinical reasoning in patient care* (6th ed.). New York, NY: Pearson, pp. 218–221.

9 **Answer: 4 Rationale:** A client with uncontrolled type 1 diabetes mellitus is at risk for developing metabolic acidosis, secondary to accumulation of ketones when fatty acids are broken down for energy. Metabolic alkalosis would not be expected. Respiratory alkalosis could occur in response to the client's metabolic acidosis, but the respiratory alkalosis is not the primary disturbance. A client with uncontrolled diabetes mellitus is at risk for acidosis, but the cause is metabolic in nature, not respiratory. **Cognitive Level:** Applying **Client Need:** Physiological Adaptation **Integrated Process:** Nursing Process: Assessment **Content Area:** Adult Health **Strategy:** Recognize this condition leads to ketoacidosis with retention of metabolic acids to direct you to the correct option. **Reference:** LeMone, P., Burke, K., Bauldoff, G., & Gubrud, P. (2015). *Medical surgical nursing: Clinical reasoning in patient care* (6th ed.). New York, NY: Pearson, pp. 218–221.

10 Answer: 2 Rationale: The pulse oximeter does measure oxygen saturation. The pulse oximeter measures the amount of oxygen, not carbon dioxide, in the blood. The pulse oximeter does not replace the need to monitor ABGs, although it provides a good indication of the client's oxygenation status. The pulse oximeter does not measure the ventilator effort of the client. **Cognitive Level:** Applying **Client Need:** Physiological Adaptation **Integrated Process:** Nursing Process: Implementation **Content Area:** Adult Health **Strategy:** Critical words are *COPD* and *pulse oximeter*. Recall the function and purpose of the latter to choose the correct option. **Reference:** Berman, A., Snyder, S., & Frandsen, G. (2016). *Fundamentals of nursing: Concepts, process, and practice* (10th ed.). New York, NY: Pearson, pp. 507–508.

Posttest

1 Answer: 1 Rationale: A pH of 7.30 indicates acidosis. A $PaCO_2$ of 51 indicates a respiratory acidosis is occurring. Because the $PaCO_2$ is elevated with a normal HCO_3^-, an uncompensated respiratory acidosis is occurring. The client is not experiencing respiratory alkalosis. The respiratory acidosis is not compensated because the pH is still outside of the normal range. The client is not experiencing metabolic acidosis because the HCO_3^- level is not low. **Cognitive Level:** Analyzing **Client Need:** Reduction of Risk Potential **Integrated Process:** Nursing Process: Assessment **Content Area:** Adult Health **Strategy:** First determine that the pH indicates acidosis and then examine CO_2 to determine that the cause is respiratory. Because bicarbonate is normal with uncompensated acidosis, choose that option. **Reference:** LeMone, P., Burke, K., Bauldoff, G., & Gubrud, P. (2015). *Medical surgical nursing: Clinical reasoning in patient care* (6th ed.). New York, NY: Pearson, pp. 223–225.

2 Answer: 2 Rationale: A client with a chest injury is likely to hypoventilate (have a shallow respiratory pattern) as a result of pain due to associated trauma. It is unknown at this time whether there are any internal injuries that could affect the client's oxygen saturation. This type of respiratory pattern is associated with respiratory acidosis. A pH of 7.42, $PaCO_2$ 41 mm Hg, and HCO_3^- 23 mEq/L represents a normal ABG. A pH of 7.49, $PaCO_2$ 36 mm Hg, and HCO_3^- 30 mEq/L represents an uncompensated metabolic alkalosis. A pH of 7.38, $PaCO_2$ 38 mm Hg, and HCO_3^- 22 mEq/L represents a normal ABG. **Cognitive Level:** Analyzing **Client Need:** Reduction of Risk Potential **Integrated Process:** Nursing Process: Assessment **Content Area:** Adult Health **Strategy:** Before looking at the options, recognize the client is at greatest risk for respiratory acidosis. Eliminate the options

where the pH is normal or it reflects alkalosis. **Reference:** LeMone, P., Burke, K., Bauldoff, G., & Gubrud, P. (2015). *Medical surgical nursing: Clinical reasoning in patient care* (6th ed.). New York, NY: Pearson, pp. 223–225.

3 Answer: 3 Rationale: Giving the client a paper bag to breathe into helps to prevent the CO_2 from dropping lower as the client rebreathes the gas that has been exhaled into the bag. Just telling the client to stop breathing fast does nothing to assist the client and could make the client become more anxious and breathe even faster. A sedative may be indicated to help the client relax and slow down respirations, but this is not the best initial action. The healthcare provider may need to be notified if the client needs further assistance, but this is not the best initial action for the nurse to take. **Cognitive Level:** Applying **Client Need:** Reduction of Risk Potential **Integrated Process:** Nursing Process: Implementation **Content Area:** Adult Health **Strategy:** Critical words are *initially* and *hyperventilate*. Recognize some of the options are partially correct, but choose the option that offers a readily available solution that can be tried before the other options may be needed. **Reference:** LeMone, P., Burke, K., Bauldoff, G., & Gubrud, P. (2015). *Medical surgical nursing: Clinical reasoning in patient care* (6th ed.). New York, NY: Pearson, pp. 225–226.

4 Answer: 1 Rationale: Because the diseased kidneys are unable to reabsorb bicarbonate and excrete excess hydrogen ions, the client with renal failure develops metabolic acidosis. Metabolic alkalosis is the opposite problem of the one the client is experiencing. The client does have acidosis but it is not respiratory in nature. The client does not have respiratory alkalosis. **Cognitive Level:** Applying **Client Need:** Physiological Adaptation **Integrated Process:** Nursing Process: Assessment **Content Area:** Adult Health **Strategy:** Recall the kidneys' role in maintaining acid–base balance and recall the major imbalance that occurs as a result of renal failure. **Reference:** LeMone, P., Burke, K., Bauldoff, G., & Gubrud, P. (2015). *Medical surgical nursing: Clinical reasoning in patient care* (6th ed.). New York, NY: Pearson, pp. 218–221.

5 Answer: 3 Rationale: The pH indicates a slight alkalosis, and the HCO_3^- is elevated, indicating a metabolic basis. The $PaCO_2$ is slightly elevated, indicating that partial compensation is occurring. The pH and HCO_3^- would be low with a normal $PaCO_2$ if there was uncompensated metabolic acidosis. The pH would be within normal limits (but nearer the acidotic end of the range), accompanied by a high CO_2 and high HCO_3^- if there was compensated respiratory acidosis. The pH and HCO_3^- would be high with a normal $PaCO_2$ if there was uncompensated metabolic alkalosis. **Cognitive Level:** Analyzing **Client Need:** Physiological Adaptation **Integrated Process:** Nursing Process: Assessment **Content Area:** Adult Health **Strategy:** First determine that the pH reflects slight alkalosis. Note the increased bicarbonate level

ANSWERS & RATIONALES

reflects that the cause is metabolic, and because the CO_2 is elevated, the pH is partially compensated. **Reference:** LeMone, P., Burke, K., Bauldoff, G., & Gubrud, P. (2015). *Medical surgical nursing: Clinical reasoning in patient care* (6th ed.). New York, NY: Pearson, pp. 221–222.

6 **Answer: 3 Rationale:** Because the cause of the acidosis is respiratory, the client needs to be ventilated in order to oxygenate the client and facilitate removal of the retained carbon dioxide. $NaHCO_3$ may need to be administered, but this is more helpful to correct metabolic acidosis, and the cause of the client's acidosis is respiratory. Epinephrine may need to be administered but the respiratory acidosis will need to be corrected through ventilation. Defibrillation may be needed depending on the client's cardiac rhythm, but this does not address the respiratory acidosis. **Cognitive Level:** Applying **Client Need:** Reduction of Risk Potential **Integrated Process:** Nursing Process: Implementation **Content Area:** Adult Health **Strategy:** The focus of the question is respiratory acidosis, so choose the option that directly assists in reversing this problem. **Reference:** LeMone, P., Burke, K., Bauldoff, G., & Gubrud, P. (2015). *Medical surgical nursing: Clinical reasoning in patient care* (6th ed.). New York, NY: Pearson, pp. 223–225.

7 **Answer: 1, 4 Rationale:** Loss of acidic contents of the stomach via NG drainage can lead to alkalosis. Frequent use of antacids (which neutralize gastric acid) can lead to an alkalotic state. Diarrhea leads to a loss of alkalotic fluids, predisposing the client to metabolic acidosis. Salicylate toxicity results in metabolic acidosis. The client with asthmatic bronchitis may be at risk for hypoventilation, leading to respiratory acidosis. **Cognitive Level:** Applying **Client Need:** Physiological Adaptation **Integrated Process:** Nursing Process: Diagnosis **Content Area:** Adult Health **Strategy:** Recall conditions that contribute to a loss of acidic body fluids and a gain of alkaline substances to direct you to the correct options. **Reference:** LeMone, P., Burke, K., Bauldoff, G., & Gubrud, P. (2015). *Medical surgical nursing: Clinical reasoning in patient care* (6th ed.). New York, NY: Pearson, pp. 225–226.

8 **Answer: 2 Rationale:** The slightly elevated pH (alkalosis), the low $PaCO_2$ (respiratory origin), and the low HCO_3^- indicate compensation is starting but is not yet fully complete because the pH is still abnormal. In addition, SaO_2 level is decreased significantly, which is not consistent with aging alone. An uncompensated respiratory acidosis would be seen on ABGs as a low pH and a high CO_2, with a normal HCO_3^-. An uncompensated respiratory alkalosis would be seen on ABGs as a high pH and a low CO_2, with a normal HCO_3^-. A partially compensated metabolic alkalosis would be seen on ABGs as a high pH and a high HCO_3^-, with a CO_2 level that has begun to rise above normal limits. **Cognitive Level:** Analyzing **Client Need:** Physiological Adaptation **Integrated Process:** Nursing Process: Assessment **Content Area:** Adult

Health **Strategy:** First determine that the pH is alkalotic. Then recognize the CO_2 is low to determine the cause is respiratory. Choose the option in which bicarbonate reflects some compensation. **Reference:** LeMone, P., Burke, K., Bauldoff, G., & Gubrud, P. (2015). *Medical surgical nursing: Clinical reasoning in patient care* (6th ed.). New York, NY: Pearson, pp. 225–226.

9 **Answer: 1 Rationale:** The pH is low (acidosis) and the $PaCO_2$ is high (respiratory origin). The HCO_3^- is normal, indicating that compensation has not occurred. The client is experiencing hyperventilation, but blood gases reveal a respiratory acidosis, probably because of prior hypoventilation. If there was a partially compensated respiratory acidosis, the pH would still be low, but the $PaCO_2$ and HCO_3^- levels would both be elevated. If there was an uncompensated metabolic acidosis, the pH and the HCO_3^- level would be low while the $PaCO_2$ level would be normal. If there was a partially compensated metabolic acidosis, the pH would still be low, but the $PaCO_2$ and HCO_3^- levels would both be low. **Cognitive Level:** Analyzing **Client Need:** Physiological Adaptation **Integrated Process:** Nursing Process: Assessment **Content Area:** Adult Health **Strategy:** First determine that the pH indicates acidosis. Next analyze the CO_2 to determine that the cause is respiratory. **Reference:** LeMone, P., Burke, K., Bauldoff, G., & Gubrud, P. (2015). *Medical surgical nursing: Clinical reasoning in patient care* (6th ed.). New York, NY: Pearson, pp. 223–225.

10 **Answer: 3 Rationale:** The pH is normal (but is nearer to the acidotic end), while the $PaCO_2$ is low (compensation has occurred) and the HCO_3^- is low (indicating metabolic origin). The oxygen saturation of 100% indicates the blood is well oxygenated. Because the pH is within normal limits and the $PaCO_2$ and HCO_3^- are low, the client has a compensated metabolic acidosis. If there was uncompensated respiratory alkalosis, the pH would be high, the $PaCO_2$ would be low, and the HCO_3^- would be normal. If there was a compensated respiratory acidosis accompanied by hypoxemia, the pH would be low, $PaCO_2$ would be high, HCO_3^- would be high, and oxygen saturation would be low. If there was a compensated metabolic acidosis accompanied by hypoxemia, the pH would be low, $PaCO_2$ would be low, HCO_3^- would be low, and oxygen saturation would be low. **Cognitive Level:** Analyzing **Client Need:** Physiological Adaptation **Integrated Process:** Nursing Process: Assessment **Content Area:** Adult Health **Strategy:** This question requires you to identify ABG results and the quality of oxygenation. Because the oxygen level is 100%, eliminate options indicating hypoxemia. Recognize the pH is within normal limits to choose a compensated condition. **Reference:** LeMone, P., Burke, K., Bauldoff, G., & Gubrud, P. (2015). *Medical surgical nursing: Clinical reasoning in patient care* (6th ed.). New York, NY: Pearson, pp. 218–221.

ANSWERS & RATIONALES

References

Berman, A., Snyder, S., & Frandsen, G. (2016). *Fundamentals of nursing: Concepts, process, and practice* (10th ed.). New York, NY: Pearson.

Holland, L., Adams, M., & Brice, J. (2018). *Core concepts in pharmacology* (5th ed.). New York, NY: Pearson.

Kee, J. L. (2017). *Pearson's handbook of laboratory and diagnostic tests* (8th ed.). New York, NY: Pearson.

LeMone, P., Burke, K., Bauldoff, G., & Gubrud, P. (2015). *Medical surgical nursing: Clinical reasoning in patient care* (6th ed.). New York, NY: Pearson.

Sole, M. L., Klein, O. G., & Moseley, M. J. (2016). *Introduction to critical care nursing* (7th ed.). St. Louis, MO: Elsevier Saunders.

Replacement Therapies for Fluid and Electrolyte Imbalances

8

Chapter Outline

Fluid Therapies

Diagnostic and Laboratory Findings

Selection of Fluid and Electrolyte Therapies

Objectives

➤ Describe concepts related to hydration therapy.

➤ Describe assessment data and diagnostic testing used to evaluate fluid balance.

➤ Identify specific solutions used for the treatment of fluid imbalance.

➤ Identify priority nursing concerns for clients receiving fluid and electrolyte replacement therapy.

➤ Describe the therapeutic management of a client receiving fluid replacement therapy.

➤ Describe the management of nursing care for a client receiving fluid replacement therapy.

NCLEX-RN® Test Prep

Access the NEW Web-based app that provides students with additional practice questions in preparation for the NCLEX experience.

Review at a Glance

ABO blood typing blood-typing system that identifies naturally occurring antigens and antibodies located on membrane of red blood cells (RBCs); helps to identify correct recipient and donor for administration of blood products

anaphylaxis a severe, potentially life-threatening allergic reaction accompanied by itching, urticaria, bronchospasm, laryngeal edema, hypotension, and vascular collapse

autologous transfusion represents donation of blood by an individual for use during perioperative period or for use as a salvage method during perioperative phase

colloid a high-molecular-weight substance that pulls fluids out of intracellular and interstitial spaces and expands intravascular volume

crystalloid a solution containing small molecules that can pass through a semipermeable membrane; may be hypotonic, isotonic, or hypertonic

fresh frozen plasma (FFP) liquid plasma portion of whole blood that contains all coagulation factors

granulocytes consist of basophils, eosinophils, and neutrophils (with platelets or platelet-poor) used to treat acquired neutropenia or severe infections unresponsive to conventional antibiotic therapy

hemolytic transfusion reaction most serious and potentially life-threatening reaction usually stemming from administration of ABO or Rh-incompatible blood and resulting in chills, low back pain, hemoglobinuria, renal failure, and shock

homologous transfusion donation of blood for other clients or for own use (designated homologous transfusion); also called *allogenic transfusion*

human leukocyte antigen (HLA) alloimmunization process by which an individual exposed to HLA antigens via nonleukocyte-depleted blood develops antibodies to those antigens that limit effectiveness of future granulocyte or possibly platelet transfusions

irradiated blood blood that is exposed to radiation to kill cells that might initiate transfusion graft versus host disease (TGVHD) in an immunocompromised individual

leukocyte-depleted blood packed red blood cells and

PRETEST

platelets that have been filtered to remove leukocytes to decrease incidence of transfusion-related febrile reactions, CMV transmission, and HLA alloimmunization

leukopheresis process by which leukocytes are extracted from withdrawn blood, which is then retransfused into donor

packed red blood cells (PRBCs) a blood product that provides same number

of RBCs as whole blood but with most plasma removed

transfusion graft versus host disease (TGVHD) condition in which donor lymphocytes attack an immuno-compromised individual, resulting in an erythematous (sunburn) rash, liver dysfunction, and pancytopenia

type and cross match process by which recipient's blood is typed to

determine ABO blood group and Rh factor and recipient's serum is mixed with donor RBCs to check for antibodies to donor's minor antigens

type and screen process whereby blood antigens and antibodies are determined but no blood product is physically held for client

PRETEST

1 A trauma victim admitted to the emergency department (ED) is hemorrhaging, in shock, and has lost a significant percentage of blood volume. Because there is no time to perform a cross match, which actions should the nurse take immediately? Select all that apply.

1. Transfuse type AB, Rh-positive blood.
2. Transfuse albumin to expand the remaining plasma volume.
3. Transfuse type O, Rh-negative blood.
4. Transfuse platelets to restore adequate clotting ability.
5. Establish an intravenous line.

2 A client with gastrointestinal (GI) bleeding suddenly develops diaphoresis with a rapid and thready pulse, and the blood pressure is difficult to auscultate. Which intravenous (IV) fluid should the nurse anticipate the healthcare provider will prescribe immediately?

1. Dextrose in water (D_5W)
2. 0.9% sodium chloride (normal saline)
3. 0.45% sodium chloride (½ normal saline)
4. Dextrose 5% in 0.45% sodium chloride (D_5½NS)

3 A client with pretransfusion hemoglobin and hematocrit values of 9 grams and 27%, respectively, received two units of packed red blood cells (PRBCs) on the evening shift. The nurse should determine the transfusions were effective when repeat laboratory tests indicate which results?

1. 11 grams, 33%
2. 12 grams, 36%
3. 13 grams, 30%
4. 15 grams, 39%

4 A client receiving 25% albumin has developed tachycardia, moist crackles, shortness of breath, and jugular vein distension. The nurse interprets these symptoms as indicating which of the following?

1. Fluid deficit (dehydration)
2. Fluid overload
3. Hypoalbuminemia
4. Impaired peripheral tissue perfusion

5 The nurse is caring for a client experiencing severe abdominal ascites secondary to cirrhosis. What assessment finding should be used by the nurse as an indication that an infusion of albumin has been effective?

1. A decrease in abdominal girth
2. A decrease in blood pressure
3. An increase in pulse
4. An increase in weight

6 Which set of changes in laboratory values should the nurse anticipate after administering isotonic intravenous fluids to a client experiencing hypertonic dehydration?

1. Increased serum osmolality, increased blood urea nitrogen (BUN), and decreased hematocrit (HCT)
2. Decreased serum osmolality, decreased BUN, and decreased HCT
3. Increased serum osmolality, increased BUN, and increased HCT
4. Decreased serum osmolality, decreased BUN, and increased HCT

7 A client with a history of congestive heart failure (CHF) has been carefully rehydrated with normal saline (0.9% sodium chloride) for isotonic dehydration related to overzealous diuresis. Which client statement indicates that the nurse's discharge teaching has been effective?

1. "I will increase my salt intake and double up on my fluid intake."
2. "I will take my diuretic pill every other day."
3. "I will weigh myself daily and notify my healthcare provider if I develop a fever or diarrhea."
4. "I will drink only one glass of water a day so I can eventually stop taking my pill."

8 A female client with type B, Rh-negative blood has been exposed to Rh-positive blood in the past. The nurse will evaluate that instruction regarding blood compatibility has been effective when the client verbalizes it is safe to receive which types of blood?

1. Type B positive and type O positive blood
2. Type B negative and type O negative blood
3. Type AB negative and type O negative blood
4. Type A positive and type O positive blood

9 Which intervention should the nurse include in a daily care plan for a client receiving intravenous (IV) crystalloid solutions?

1. Check hemoglobin and hematocrit levels.
2. Check results of serum electrolytes, BUN, and creatinine.
3. Restrict intake of oral fluids.
4. Report all intake and output (I&O) totals to the healthcare provider.

10 Which blood product should the nurse anticipate the healthcare provider will prescribe for a client diagnosed with hemophilia?

1. Whole blood
2. Packed red blood cells (PRBCs)
3. Fresh frozen plasma (FFP)
4. Albumin

➤ *See pages 180–182 for Answers and Rationales.*

I. FLUID THERAPIES

A. **Crystalloids**: intravenous solutions that contain small molecules and can pass through semipermeable membranes (flowing readily from vascular space to interstitial space and cells); have varying tonicity (isotonic, hypotonic, hypertonic); see Box 8-1
1. Isotonic solutions
   a. Have approximately same concentration (osmolality) as extracellular fluid (ECF), thereby remaining within ECF space
   b. Given to expand ECF volume
   c. Have no net effect on cellular dynamics because of equal osmolarity
   d. Examples: normal saline (NS; or 0.9% NaCl), Lactated Ringer's (LR)
   e. Note that 5% dextrose in water is isotonic in bag and during infusion, but after dextrose is metabolized it exerts a hypotonic effect by providing free water to circulating volume and cells

Box 8-1	**Isotonic Solutions**
Tonicity of Common Intravenous Solutions	0.9% sodium chloride (NaCl); also called normal saline (NS)
	5% dextrose in water (D_5W)
	Lactated Ringer's (LR)
	Hypotonic Solutions
	0.45% sodium chloride (NaCl); also called ½ NS
	0.225% sodium chloride (NaCl); also called ¼ NS
	Hypertonic Solutions
	5% dextrose in sodium chloride; also called D_5NS
	5% dextrose in 0.45% sodium chloride ($D_5\frac{1}{2}NS$)
	5% dextrose in Lactated Ringer's (D_5LR)
	10% dextrose in water ($D_{10}W$)
	3% or 5% sodium chloride (3% NaCl or 5% NaCl)
	Total parenteral nutrition (TPN) solutions

2. Hypotonic solutions
   a. Osmolality is lower than that of serum plasma
   b. Are given to reverse dehydration; provide hydration to cells
   c. With regard to cellular dynamics, cause cells to swell and possibly burst
   d. Fluid shifting occurs with administration because fluids shift out of blood vessels into interstitial spaces, causing intravascular volume depletion
   e. Due to fluid-shifting effects, hypotonic fluids should be administered cautiously
   f. Examples: ½ NS (0.45% NaCl) and ¼ NS (0.225% NaCl)
3. Hypertonic solutions
   a. Osmolality is higher than that of serum plasma
   b. Are given to increase ECF volume and decrease cellular swelling
   c. With regard to cellular dynamics, cause cells to shrink and contribute to ECF volume overload
   d. Should be administered cautiously because of fluid shifting and potential for vein irritation due to high osmolar concentration
   e. Examples: 5% dextrose in 0.9% NaCl (D_5NS), 10% dextrose in water ($D_{10}W$), 3% or 5% NaCl, and 5% dextrose in Lactated Ringer's (D_5LR)
   f. Note that total parenteral nutrition solutions need to be administered via a central line because of the high tonicity of that fluid
B. **Colloids**: solutions containing high-molecular-weight proteins or starch that do not cross capillary semipermeable membrane and remain in intravascular space (pulling fluid from intracellular and interstitial spaces) for several days, assuming client has an intact capillary membrane; although colloids contain no clotting factors, they can affect coagulation process, which must be considered with certain treatment therapies
   1. Albumin
      a. Major plasma protein available in two forms: 5% (isotonic—equivalent to 12.5 grams or 250 mL) and 25% (hypertonic—equivalent to 25 grams or 50 mL)
      b. Normal human serum albumin is derived from donor plasma and is heat-treated for viral inactivation (free from hepatitis; no known risk for human immunodeficiency virus [HIV])
      c. Changes in albumin concentration affect cellular dynamics

Practice to Pass

The healthcare provider has prescribed 0.9% NaCl IV at 250 mL per hour for a newly admitted client in diabetic ketoacidosis. How will you evaluate the effectiveness of this IV therapy for this client?

1) Increased albumin concentration results in fluid moving back into capillaries from interstitial space
2) Decreased albumin concentration results in fluid leaking through capillary walls into interstitial space (edema)
3) Clients who have underlying medical/nutritional problems (malnutrition, cirrhosis, or nephritic syndrome) can have chronically low albumin levels

 d. Comparison with crystalloid solutions
1) Remain in vascular space longer than crystalloids
2) More expensive than crystalloids
3) May cause febrile reactions
4) More likely to cause circulatory overload than crystalloid solutions (because they remain in intravascular space for a longer period of time)

 e. Indications and contraindications
1) Primary clinical use is as a volume expander when treating hypovolemic shock from trauma or surgery, raising blood pressure and cardiac output
2) Given as a volume expander in a client who needs whole blood while cross match is being completed
3) Used to support blood pressure during a hypotensive episode, create diuresis in fluid volume excess, and facilitate remobilization of fluid from third-space fluid shifts
4) Also used to treat burns, trauma, acute liver failure, hypoproteinemia, and overzealous diuresis in clients with cirrhosis or nephrotic syndrome, and to prevent and treat cerebral edema
5) Contraindicated in severe anemia and avoided in clients who are dehydrated
6) Given cautiously to clients with cardiac and pulmonary problems or in clinical situations where there is increased capillary leakage (permeability), such as with sepsis, trauma, or burns

 f. Administration and nursing actions
1) Use glass bottle with administration set and filter with vented tubing (vented tubing is required when using glass bottle)
2) Should be used within a 4-hour time frame, as there are no preservatives
3) Requires dedicated line for infusion
4) Dose and rate of infusion are based on client's blood volume and underlying condition; infuse as rapidly as tolerated in clients with hypovolemic shock to replace vascular volume; in a client with normal blood volume, infuse 5% albumin at 2–4 mL/minute and 25% albumin at 1 mL/minute
5) Assess for urticaria, fever, and manifestations of fluid volume overload; monitor vital signs (VS) and breath sounds of all clients regardless of underlying condition and rate of administration

 2. Dextran
  a. A glucose solution with colloidal activity similar to albumin that expands the plasma volume by pulling fluid from interstitial space to intravascular space, thereby promoting fluid removal from tissues
  b. Can double plasma volume within a few minutes, but this effect is limited to about 12 hours
  c. No risk of transfusion-related illnesses (not extracted from human plasma)
  d. Increased likelihood of hypersensitivity reactions during early minutes of administration because of presence of polysaccharide-reacting antibody
  e. Available in two strengths: Dextran 40 (low-molecular-weight dextran) and Dextran 70 (high-molecular-weight dextran); see Box 8-2 for additional information for Dextran 40
  f. Alterations of diagnostic tests

Practice to Pass

The healthcare provider has just prescribed 25% albumin for a 75-year-old female client in hypovolemic shock. Detail your priority assessments, interventions, and expected outcomes for the client.

Box 8-2

**Specific Information
Related to Dextran 40**

- Acts as a hypertonic colloidal solution that rapidly expands the plasma volume
- Stays in the vascular space for up to 6 hours, depending on renal clearance
- Appropriate for all types of shock states and acts as an adjunct to restore volume
- Parenteral infusion is given via dedicated line because it has a high incompatibility profile
- Will alter clotting factors because it has antiplatelet activity (decreases the adhesiveness of RBCs and improves peripheral blood flow)
- Can lead to false elevations in some laboratory tests and interfere with blood typing
- Used prophylactically during surgical procedures that present a high risk for clotting to prevent DVT and PE and can be used for pump priming in extracorporeal circulation
- Contraindicated in clients who have defined hypersensitivities, renal failure, cardiac failure, severe anemia, pregnancy, and clients receiving anticoagulant therapy
- Clients with chronic liver disease, severe dehydration, or at risk for developing renal or cardiac failure require cautious use and monitoring if therapy is indicated by the healthcare provider

1) Can affect **type and cross match** (process by which compatibility between donor and recipient blood is determined) due to presence of Rouleaux formation (RBCs stacked together in long chains)
2) Can result in *false increases* in blood glucose, total protein, total bilirubin, and urine specific gravity
3) Can increase liver enzymes, such as AST and ALT levels
4) Can alter coagulation indices and increase bleeding times by inhibiting platelet aggregation

g. Administration and nursing actions
1) Draw blood for type and cross match (especially) and other labs as needed prior to beginning dextran infusion, if possible; at minimum, notify laboratory personnel that client is receiving dextran
2) Obtain baseline hematocrit prior to dextran infusion and maintain Hct >30% during course of therapy or notify healthcare provider of decreased volume
3) Assess for signs and symptoms of **anaphylaxis** (tightness in chest, wheezing, bronchospasm, and urticaria)
4) Dextran 1 is usually given IV prior to infusion of dextran to prevent formation of immune complexes by site binding on antibody
5) Maintain hydration of client with supplemental IV fluids
6) Observe for signs and symptoms of bleeding
7) Monitor pertinent labs including Hct, serum chemistries, and serum protein levels on a frequent basis

3. Hetastarch
a. Synthetic colloid made from cornstarch and available in a 6% solution that is diluted in 500 mL of NS (approximates albumin and dextran in terms of colloidal activity)
b. Expands plasma and is used in shock precipitated by hemorrhage, trauma, burns, and sepsis; will stay in vascular space up to 36 hours, but plasma volume expansion begins to decrease at about 24 hours; causes osmotic diuresis
c. Alterations of diagnostic tests: will not interfere with blood typing or cross matching but can dilute clotting factors; prothrombin time (PT), partial thromboplastin time (PTT), and clotting times may be transiently prolonged

d. Excretion is both renal and hepatic; do not administer to clients in renal failure with oliguria or anuria; use caution in clients with liver disease

e. Use caution in clients with CHF or bleeding disorders; contraindicated in severe bleeding disorders

f. Administration and nursing actions

    1) Use opened containers immediately; contains no preservatives

    2) Monitor client for signs of hypervolemia (increased blood pressure, dyspnea, and bounding pulse)

    3) Monitor for transient changes in PT and PTT; check serum amylase level prior to beginning the infusion

    4) Assess for adequate tissue perfusion; expect an increased urine output (UO) because of osmotic diuresis; an increased UO is not an indicator of adequate blood volume

    5) Be alert to signs and symptoms of anaphylaxis and intervene accordingly (stop infusion; provide oxygen; hydrate with NS; administer epinephrine, steroids, antihistamines as prescribed; be prepared to intubate and maintain circulatory support)

    6) Clients with diabetes mellitus or clients with acid–base imbalances due to increased lactate levels should not receive this medication because it can contribute to lactic acidosis

4. Plasma protein fraction (PPF)

    a. Major component is albumin with immunoglobulins and sodium; used to expand intravascular volume

    b. Indicated for emergency treatment of hypovolemic shock, burns, and low protein states; functions as a blood-product volume expander

    c. Monitoring parameters include VS (hemodynamic—central venous pressure [CVP], if possible) and UO every 5 to 15 minutes during first hour of treatment

    d. Monitor clients closely for potential fluid volume overload, pulmonary edema, or heart failure

    e. Monitor serum protein, electrolytes, and hemoglobin and hematocrit during therapy

    f. Contraindicated in clients with CHF, history of bypass surgery, allergic reactions to albumin, and severe anemia

C. Blood and blood products

1. Packed red blood cells (PRBCs)

    a. Prepared from whole blood with each unit having approximate volume of 250 mL (some plasma, leukocytes, and platelets from whole blood are still present); usually takes six donors to make one unit PRBCs

    b. Platelets and leukocytes are not viable but can cause problems for recipient because they contain human leukocyte antigens (HLAs); recipient can form antibodies against these antigens (**HLA alloimmunization**); this can create problems with future transfusions, especially when receiving platelets

    c. Typically, PRBCs are **leukocyte depleted** (blood is filtered to remove leukocytes) to minimize risk of HLA alloimmunization

    d. Contain same red blood cell concentration as whole blood from which unit is derived; client receives same increase in oxygen-carrying capacity with less risk of fluid volume overload from whole blood

    e. Increase colloidal oncotic pressure; pull fluids from extravascular space to intravascular space to increase circulating volume

    f. Identification methods used for transfusion therapy

        1) Recipient's blood must be typed to determine **ABO blood typing** and Rh factor to ensure that client receives compatible blood

Practice to Pass

A client receiving hetastarch for hypovolemia related to hemorrhage becomes very pale and diaphoretic, complains of chest tightness, and begins wheezing. Physical examination reveals hives covering the client's chest. What nursing actions should be taken immediately?

2) Recipient must not have antibodies to major antigens on donor's RBCs (refer to Table 8-1)

3) Cross matching: to detect presence of recipient antibodies to donor's minor antigens

    a) Recipient's serum is mixed with donor's RBCs; if antibodies to donor's antigens are present, agglutination will occur (no match)

    b) If no antibodies to donor's RBCs are present, agglutination will not occur (desired)

    c) Takes approximately 20 minutes to perform; type and cross match is good for 48 hours only; must be repeated if client needs blood after time expires; blood is physically held for a specific client

4) A **type and screen** can be used to identify blood type, surface antigens, and Rh factor but blood is not physically held; useful in nonemergency situations when blood transfusion might be needed in near future

5) In an emergency, type O negative blood (universal donor) can be administered to a client, foregoing type and cross-matching procedure

6) May transmit viruses; additional tests for donated blood: hepatitis A, B, C, HIV, syphilis, ALT level (increased may be suspicious for hepatitis)

g. Specific treatments related to blood processing

1) **Irradiated blood**: blood is treated with radiation to kill donor cells that could attack an immunocompromised client (bone marrow transplant recipients; clients with Hodgkin's disease or leukemia; intrauterine neonatal transfusion recipients; or in clients being aggressively treated with chemotherapy)

    a) Goal is to prevent transmission of **transfusion graft versus host disease (TGVHD)**—donor lymphocytes attack recipient, cause liver dysfunction and bone marrow suppression, and can be fatal

    b) Leukocyte-depleted blood will not prevent TGVHD

2) Cytomegalovirus (CMV)–negative blood: for immunocompromised clients including those with HIV; CMV remains in a latent state in donor's leukocytes if previously infected with virus; transfer of leukocytes to immunocompromised recipients could cause severe illness; leukodepletion may eliminate CMV

h. One unit of PRBCs should raise hemoglobin one gram and hematocrit by 3% (assuming there is no ongoing blood loss if bleeding was either a cause or a contributing factor)

Table 8-1   **ABO Compatibility System and Safe Transfusion**

Client Blood Type (Recipient)	Donor Blood That Can Be Safely Administered	Rationale
Type A	Type A	Client has no anti-A antibodies
	Type O	*Universal donor;* donor has no antigens to which the recipient can react
Type B	Type B	Client has no anti-B antibodies
	Type O	*Universal donor;* donor has no antigens to which the recipient can react
Type AB	Type A, B, or AB	*Universal recipient;* client has no anti-A or anti-B antibodies
	Type O	*Universal donor;* donor has no antigens to which the recipient can react
Type O	Type O	*Universal donor;* donor has no antigens to which the recipient can react

Note: Rh status must also be determined as part of the blood-typing procedure. Rh-positive clients can receive Rh-positive and Rh-negative blood. Rh-negative clients can only receive Rh-negative blood.

    i. Expensive as compared to other colloids and crystalloids (collecting, testing, and screening blood and special processing contribute to this expense)

    j. Indications

        1) To improve oxygen-carrying capacity in clients with symptomatic anemia

        2) To restore blood loss caused by hemorrhage (gastrointestinal or trauma related) or surgical blood loss

    k. Transfusion options

        1) **Autologous transfusion** (to self) may be planned prior to surgical procedure (preoperative donation) or blood may also be collected and reinfused during or after surgery (perioperative, intraoperative, or postoperative blood salvage)

        2) **Homologous transfusion** (or allogenic) represents blood collected from clients for use for other clients (volunteer) or for themselves (designated)

        3) Blood collected for homologous transfusion undergoes testing for antibodies, pathologic organisms (HIV, CMV, hepatitis variants, HTLV, and syphilis)

        4) Minimum standards are set by American Association of Blood Banks (AABB) regarding criteria for donor requirements, citing age, baseline hemoglobin and hematocrit, VS, weight, no evidence of transmittable disease or drug use, and frequency of blood donation

    l. Administration (refer to Box 8-3)

        1) Pretransfusion: verify prescription and follow hospital policy and procedure for any type of transfusion therapy; ensure that client has received and signed informed consent form

        2) Start an IV if one not already in place; use an 18- to 20-gauge angiocath, which is preferred

        3) Note that if the client is an older adult with small fragile veins, a 22- to 24-gauge angiocath may be used without an infusion pump (force created by pump through a small-gauge catheter may cause cells to lyse); blood will infuse more slowly but RBCs will remain intact; blood bank may be able to divide unit into two bags (one bag can infuse while other remains properly refrigerated in blood bank); check hospital policy for managing older clients with fragile veins

        4) Administer blood with normal saline only to prevent cell lysis; obtain 500 mL of NS and Y tubing and prime Y tubing that contains blood filter; additional filters may be required, such as Pall filter, depending on blood product used and/or general health condition of client; may connect to client and run at KVO (to keep vein open) rate if blood will arrive soon

Box 8-3	• Obtain informed consent for transfusion therapy.
Principles of Transfusion Therapy	• Ensure patent IV access prior to retrieving blood from the blood bank using appropriate tubing with NS as the priming solution.
	• Follow hospital policy and procedure regarding blood typing, acquisition of unit from blood bank, and verification of prescription with two registered nurses.
	• Identify client at the bedside confirming client name and identification (ID) number, blood bank identification band (if used), unit number, blood type and Rh factor, and expiration date.
	• Remain at client's bedside during the first 15 minutes of transfusion therapy and monitor VS per protocol.
	• Obtain follow-up bloodwork to determine response to transfusion therapy.

Box 8-4

Timing Issues Relevant to Transfusion Therapy

- Transfusion should be started within 30 minutes of the time that the unit is checked out of the blood bank.
- Remain with the client during the first 15 minutes of the transfusion and monitor accordingly for signs and symptoms of possible transfusion reaction.
- Stop blood if any signs or symptoms of a transfusion reaction occur and notify the healthcare provider.
- Infuse each unit over 2 hours unless otherwise prescribed by the healthcare provider.
- Blood cannot hang more than 4 hours at room temperature because this can lead to cellular breakdown of the blood product.

5) Once blood bank indicates that blood is ready, premedicate client if prescribed; common premedications are diphenhydramine, acetaminophen, and occasionally a corticosteroid or H_2 receptor blocker; premedication may be indicated to minimize allergic potential and symptoms; furosemide can be given either as premedication or between units to minimize risk of fluid volume overload

6) Obtain blood from blood bank following hospital procedure and record baseline VS

7) Two RNs must verify identification of pertinent blood unit information (type, Rh factor, unit number, expiration date, matching with client's blood identification bracelet and original healthcare provider prescription); RNs must also identify client using two unique identifiers (such as stating name and date of birth)

8) Prior to hanging any blood product, inspect for discoloration and/or bubbling that could indicate bacterial contamination; if there is any suspicion, return blood unit to blood bank

9) Don gloves and hang blood, keeping spike and blood bag opening sterile; prime filter and tubing with blood; follow hospital policy regarding use of infusion pump for blood administration

10) Remain with client for first 15 minutes of therapy and monitor VS as per policy (refer to Box 8-4)

11) If client will receive another unit of blood, check to see if healthcare provider has prescribed a diuretic between units if client is at risk for fluid volume overload

12) Labwork (hemoglobin and hematocrit) should be prescribed 2 hours post-transfusion to assess client's response to therapy

m. Clients who undergo multiple transfusions are at risk for developing additional electrolyte problems; these may include hyperkalemia or increased ammonia levels (because of cellular release from stored blood products) and hypocalcemia (because of chelation of calcium with citrate anticoagulant used as a blood preservative)

n. Clients may still experience a transfusion reaction, regardless of all precautions used to prevent such an occurrence (refer to Box 8-5 for treatment)

2. Platelets

a. Require ABO typing only but Rh matching preferred; if no ABO-compatible platelets are available, mismatched platelets may be given, which can lead to potential allergic reactions; HLA-matched platelets are recommended to decrease risk of allergic reactions

b. Can be single donor or random donor (pooled platelets from 6 to 10 donors)

c. Stored at room temperature for up to 5 days with frequent gentle agitation of bag to keep platelets viable; half-life of platelets is 3–4 days; platelet transfusion may be repeated every 1–3 days

Box 8-5	• Stop blood immediately if you suspect client is exhibiting a significant reaction.
Transfusion Reaction Principles	• Monitor client's VS, keep IV access with NS (switch tubing), and insert indwelling urinary catheter, if needed.
	• Give old tubing and remaining blood product to lab for investigation.
	• Notify healthcare provider and lab for follow-up blood draws and report client's condition.
	• Keep client warm and provide supplemental oxygen at low flow rates.
	• Medicate as prescribed following hospital policy and procedure and new healthcare provider prescriptions.

Practice to Pass

A client being aggressively treated with chemotherapy for acute leukemia will receive two units of irradiated CMV-negative PRBCs. The client wants to know why the blood needs special treatment. What will you tell this client?

!➤

d. If platelet count $<20,000/mm^3$ and client is experiencing major bleeding, platelets may be needed; one platelet concentrate (one unit) should increase recipient platelet count by approximately $5,000–10,000/mm^3$; usual dose is 6–10 units of concentrate

e. Clients receiving platelets over a long period of time develop antibodies to HLA antigens on surface of circulating platelets (causing antigen–antibody reaction, febrile reaction, and platelet destruction); over time, client's platelet count becomes less responsive to platelet transfusions (platelet count shows little or no rise after transfusion) because alloimmunization is occurring; actions to decrease likelihood of reaction include:
  1) Use single-donor platelet transfusions from onset of therapy
  2) Use WBC filters to minimize infusion of WBCs because this will help to decrease antibody production
  3) Try to find HLA-matched donor platelets for recipient
  4) Premedicate with diphenhydramine, acetaminophen, or hydrocortisone to decrease possibility of a reaction
  5) Fever, infection, and active bleeding can modify effectiveness of transfusion

f. Indications
  1) Thrombocytopenia resulting from decreased platelet production (aplastic anemia, leukemia), increased platelet loss (bleeding), increased platelet destruction (hypersplenism in cirrhosis, transfusion reaction), and increased use or consumption as in disseminated intravascular coagulopathy (DIC)
  2) Clients undergoing needed surgery with a platelet count less than $100,0000/mm^3$ or experiencing platelet dysfunction and/or coexisting coagulation disorders

g. Contraindications
  1) Not indicated for idiopathic thrombocytopenic purpura (ITP) unless client is actively bleeding because administered platelets will also be destroyed
  2) Avoid administering platelets when client is febrile

h. Administration and nursing actions
  1) Premedicate as prescribed, especially if client has a history of platelet transfusion reaction

!➤
  2) Obtain IV access with 20- to 22-gauge angiocath, Y tubing, and NS to prime tubing

!➤
  3) Begin platelet transfusion slowly and observe for signs of a reaction; adjust rate to 1–2 mL/minute and infuse each unit over 5–10 minutes as tolerated (platelets tend to clump, which is why they should be infused quickly)
  4) A poor 15-minute platelet count means HLA antibodies are present, indicating need to use HLA-matched platelets; if there is a good 15-minute count but

poor 24-hour count, this suggests consumption (fever, sepsis), but client does not need HLA-matched platelets

5) Administer single-donor platelets whenever possible for all clients; if client will receive multiple transfusions, use single-donor platelets and use a leukodepletion filter (some platelets may be prepared as leukodepleted; check bag label); if client will receive aggressive chemotherapy or a transplant, check for anti-HLA antibodies first so that blood product administration can be carefully planned

3. Whole blood

a. One unit of donated whole blood can be broken down into one unit of packed cells, one unit of platelets, and one unit of fresh frozen plasma to replace whichever component(s) client may need

b. Not routinely used; indicated for treatment of acute massive hemorrhage and loss of >25–30% of blood volume; may also be used with cardiac surgeries, trauma situations, or major burns

c. Must be ABO and Rh compatible

d. Increases colloidal oncotic pressure and plasma volume, increases red cell mass, and improves tissue oxygenation; however, it can result in fluid volume overload

e. Should not be administered to clients with chronic anemia who only need RBCs and should have a normal blood volume

f. Stored whole blood is high in potassium

g. Administration and nursing actions

1) One unit equals approximately 500 mL; use an 18- to 20-gauge angiocath and Y tubing; use only NS as primer; infuse over 2–4 hours

2) Observe for signs and symptoms of a transfusion reaction, such as **hemolytic transfusion reaction** (refer to Table 8-2), fluid volume overload, hypothermia, electrolyte disturbances, citrate toxicity (citrate is a preservative used in blood), and infection

3) Expect a one-gram increase in hemoglobin and a 3–4% rise in hematocrit for each unit of whole blood infused, assuming no further bleeding

4. **Fresh frozen plasma (FFP)**

a. Derived from one unit of donated whole blood whereby plasma is separated from RBCs and then frozen; contains clotting factors and fibrinogen, but no platelets; volume of each unit is approximately 225 mL

b. Must know client's ABO group to ensure client's RBCs are compatible with antibodies that may be present in plasma; group AB FFP may be administered if client's blood type is unknown; Rh matching (although not required) is preferred

c. Increases colloidal oncotic pressure and moves fluid into vascular space

d. May cause fluid volume overload, hypersensitivity reaction, or hemolytic reactions

e. Indications

1) Replaces plasma volume in hemorrhage and/or hypovolemic shock

2) Replaces plasma proteins lost from burn injuries

3) Replaces clotting factors for client with a known (specific clotting factor may not be available) or unknown deficiency

4) Indicated for these clinical conditions: liver disease with significantly impaired clotting factor synthesis, DIC with active bleeding, prolonged prothrombin time/international normalized ratio (PT/INR) with active bleeding or when immediate surgery is needed, and dilutional coagulopathy (substantial volume overload)

f. Administration and nursing actions

Table 8-2	Transfusion Reactions			
Type	**Etiology**	**Clinical Presentation**	**Nursing Actions**	**Prevention**
Hemolytic	ABO or Rh incompatibility Most severe and potentially life-threatening, but accounts for a very small percentage Severe antigen–antibody reaction due to clumping of cells	Chills, low back pain, headache, chest pain, tachycardia, dyspnea, hypotension, nausea and vomiting, restlessness, anxiety, shock, flank pain, and oliguria Symptoms occur during first 30 minutes of infusion or in response to 100–200 mL of incompatible blood	*Stop transfusion immediately* Keep IV line open with NS and new tubing Follow ABCs Notify appropriate personnel (blood bank, healthcare provider, and lab) Follow hospital protocol Medicate per protocol	Follow established protocol Verify prescriptions Monitor client during therapy
Blood contamination (bacterial)	Organisms that survive the cold such as *pseudomonas* or *staphylococcus*	Sudden chills, fever, dry flushed skin, headache, abdominal pain, lumbar pain, nausea and vomiting, diarrhea, hypotension, and/or signs of renal failure	*Stop transfusion immediately* Keep IV line open with NS and new tubing Follow ABCs Notify appropriate personnel (blood bank, healthcare provider, and lab) Follow hospital protocol Medicate per protocol	Change administration set and filter per protocol (per unit) Infuse unit over prescribed time period Do not run blood unit >4 hours Maintain sterile technique
Febrile (nonhemolytic)	Most common transfusion reaction Sensitizations to HLA antibodies or plasma occur	Mild reaction—chills and fever Severe reaction—high fever, chills, headache, tightness in chest, palpitations, tachycardia, facial flushing, or flank pain Symptoms can occur within 30 minutes but may start as late as 1–2 hours post transfusion	Healthcare provider may note parameters to run blood even if the client presents with slight temperature elevation Validate prescription prior to hanging to be aware of parameters With a severe reaction, *stop the transfusion* and proceed with hospital protocol for a hemolytic reaction	Keep client warm For clients with prior history of this reaction, premedicate with acetaminophen or diphenhydramine, administer leukocyte-poor blood products, HLA-compatible products, or washed RBCs
Allergic	Sensitivity reaction, antigen-antibody reaction to plasma proteins IgE molecules on mast cells react to form histamine release	Mild reaction involves urticaria and hives Severe reaction involves chills, fever, facial and airway swelling, SOB, wheezing, loss of consciousness, shock, or possible cardiac arrest	Mild reaction—follow hospital policy and procedure, slow down transfusion, notify the healthcare provider, medicate as prescribed Severe reaction—*stop transfusion* Follow hospital policy and protocol. Medicate as prescribed. With critical situations, client may need to be intubated and managed by in-house healthcare provider	Premedication for clients who have history of allergic reactions or multiple transfusions Washed RBCs, leukocyte-depleted products, and additional filters may be needed on a routine basis for transfusion therapy

Note: It is critical to follow agency policy and procedure for *all* transfusion therapies. Many reactions can be prevented or minimized with correct administration techniques and close assessment and monitoring of client. Remain at client's bedside during first 15 minutes of any transfusion. Have all necessary equipment readily available should client experience a reaction (additional tubing and oxygen setup).

!

1) Use as soon as possible after it is thawed or within 6 hours (takes about 30 minutes to thaw)

2) Use a 20- to 22-gauge angiocath, NS not required (no RBCs present)

3) Administer as rapidly as possible, suggested rate is 4–10 mL/minute; most units are completed in 1–2 hours

4) Observe for signs and symptoms of allergic or febrile reaction and fluid volume overload; there is also a risk for hepatitis transmission

!

5) Clients receiving large amounts of FFP may become hypocalcemic due to citric acid binding with calcium in plasma; observe for signs of hypocalcemia; may need calcium gluconate intravenously

5. Cryoprecipitate

Practice to Pass

A client with disseminated intravascular coagulopathy (DIC) is receiving platelets, fresh frozen plasma, and packed red blood cells. What laboratory results will you review in evaluating the effectiveness of the transfusions? How does the disease process complicate the clinical picture?

a. Derived from one unit of FFP and contains Factor VIII (antihemophilia factor), Factor XIII (Von Willebrand factor), and Factor IX (fibrinogen)

b. ABO compatibility testing is not required; however, may cause ABO incompatibility; donor plasma and recipient RBCs should be ABO compatible (because some donor plasma is present and plasma contains the antibodies); if client's (recipient) blood group is unknown, type AB cryoprecipitate is preferred; Rh matching is not required (Rh factor is on the RBC and RBCs are not being transfused)

c. Used to treat hemophilia A, Von Willebrand disease, hypofibrinogenemia, DIC (will quickly raise fibrinogen level), and massive transfusion with hemodilution; used in uremic clients to control bleeding

d. Possibility of hepatitis or HIV transmission exists

e. Administration and nursing actions

1) Use within 6 hours once thawed; usual dose is 6–10 units

2) Use 20- to 22-gauge angiocath and standard blood filter

3) Administer as rapidly as tolerated (10 mL/min)

6. Granulocytes

a. Harvested by **leukopheresis** from a single donor; must be transfused within 24 hours after obtaining from donor

b. Each unit consists of granulocytes, lymphocytes, platelets, and RBCs in plasma

c. Donor must be ABO and Rh compatible (RBCs present in unit); it is preferable to be HLA compatible as well

Practice to Pass

A neutropenic client undergoing aggressive chemotherapy is febrile with positive blood cultures. The healthcare provider prescribes granulocytes for this client. How would you safely administer this product to the client?

d. Granulocytes are not FDA approved at the current time and are being used in clinical research trials to support febrile neutropenic clients who are not responding to other methods (antibiotic therapy or filgrastim injections) to improve white blood cell (WBC) count

e. Infusion can cause fever, allergic reaction, severe chills, mild hypertension, disorientation, and hallucinations; premedicate with diphenhydramine, steroids, and antipyretics as prescribed

f. Use an 18- to 20-gauge angiocath and Y tubing with standard inline filter; no microaggregate filter is used because it would trap the WBCs; administer slowly, generally 50 mL/hour within 4 hours

g. Treat chills with antipyretics or blankets; treat hypertension, if needed; only discontinue transfusion if client has severe respiratory distress

h. Generally one unit per day is transfused for at least 4–5 days or until infection resolves

II. DIAGNOSTIC AND LABORATORY FINDINGS

A. Serum or plasma osmolality (275–295 mOsm/kg)

1. Hydration status affects serum/plasma osmolality, and specific parenteral therapies can affect osmolality due to nature of solution (tonicity of fluid) and crystalloid or colloid status

2. Increases are seen in dehydration, hyperglycemia, and in conditions where BUN is also increased; decreases are seen in clinical states resulting in overhydration
3. Allows nurse to assess client's baseline hydration status and evaluate response to replacement therapy

B. Serum chemistries

1. Blood urea nitrogen (BUN) (8–22 mg/dL) and creatinine (0.8–1.6 mg/dL) are indicators of renal function; BUN is also affected by hydration status
   a. Increased levels seen in dehydration (BUN only), renal disease, and gastrointestinal bleeding, due to retention of urea; decreased levels are seen in clinical states that result in overhydration
   b. Creatinine is a more accurate indicator of renal function than BUN because it is a constant metabolic end product of muscle metabolism and reflects glomerular filtration rate; increased levels reflect renal dysfunction
   c. Creatinine is generally unaffected by fluid intake; however, marked fluid volume deficit can decrease glomerular filtration and slightly increase the creatinine level
   d. Determine adequate renal function before beginning fluid and electrolyte replacement (except when a fluid challenge is done to check kidneys' responsiveness); abnormal renal function can put client at risk for fluid volume overload and electrolyte disturbances
2. Electrolytes
   a. Sodium (Na^+) and chloride (Cl^-) concentration should be considered in replacement therapies because they are components in many crystalloid fluids; specific parenteral solutions (hypotonic or hypertonic) can result in fluid shifting and impact serum and urinary levels; see also Chapter 2
   b. Potassium (K^+) is usually considered in replacement therapies as an additive being used to restore normal serum levels; it is important to know client's baseline, trend pertinent laboratory values, and administer replacement according to protocol; see also Chapter 3
   c. Critical laboratory values exist for both hypokalemic and hyperkalemic states with resultant effects on cardiac system
   d. Acid–base imbalances can arise from alterations in potassium and chloride levels, and client should be properly monitored using serial arterial blood gases (ABGs); see Chapter 7
   e. Calcium levels can be affected by replacement therapies, such as multiple blood unit administration (citrate anticoagulant resulting in hypocalcemia), that require calcium administration; correlate calcium levels with serum albumin levels because binding occurs that could affect results
   f. Specific therapies such as diuretic administration, prolonged infusion of hypotonic fluids, dehydration states (malnutrition), overhydration, and underlying disease states can further impact serum electrolyte levels and response to replacement therapies
3. Serum glucose (70–110 mg/dL)
   a. Regulation of serum glucose levels is necessary to maintain normal cognitive function and prevent adverse health conditions that result in coma
   b. Because many IV solutions contain dextrose, client must be monitored closely for possible effects on blood glucose; in addition, other medications (such as dextran, diuretics, and steroids) and parenteral therapies (such as TPN) can lead to increases in blood glucose
4. Serum albumin (3.5–5.0 mg/dL)
   a. Major protein in plasma that regulates colloidal oncotic pressure and maintains intravascular integrity

     b. Hydration status affects albumin level with dehydration leading to increased albumin levels; decreased albumin from volume excess leads to fluid shifting and third spacing of fluids

     c. It is important to know the albumin level when evaluating serum calcium level because calcium is present in both ionized and nonionized forms and ionized form is bound to protein; a low albumin level can therefore be accompanied by hypocalcemia

C. Blood counts and clotting studies

  1. RBC count

     a. Normal range: male 4.5–5.3 million/mm^3, female 4.1–5.1 million/mm^3

     b. Hydration states can affect RBC count; dehydration falsely elevates RBC count (hemoconcentration) and overhydration decreases RBC count (hemodilution)

     c. CBC with differential and a peripheral smear will provide pertinent information about RBC indices and morphology

  2. Hematocrit

     a. Packed cell volume with normal range for males 37–49%; females 36–46%, which is usually three times the hemoglobin value

     b. Hydration status can affect serum values, such as hemoconcentration (with dehydration) and hemodilution (with overhydration)

     c. Serial hematocrit levels are drawn for a client with ongoing bleeding

     d. In a healthy client, transfusion is generally not needed if hemoglobin is >8 grams/dL and hematocrit is above 24% (variation depends on age and any underlying clinical condition)

     e. Each unit of PRBCs will increase hematocrit by 3%; a unit of whole blood will increase hematocrit by 3–4%

  3. Hemoglobin

     a. Normal range for males is 13–18 grams/dL and for females is 12–16 grams/dL

     b. Serial hemoglobin levels are drawn in client with ongoing blood loss

     c. Hydration can affect serum values (dehydration causes false high and overhydration decreases concentration, causing a lower value)

     d. Each unit of PRBCs or whole blood will increase hemoglobin by one gram

  4. Platelets

     a. Normal range is 150,000–400,000/mm^3

     b. Increased levels are seen with iron-deficiency anemia and decreased levels are seen with hemorrhage or coagulation disorders

     c. Each unit of platelets should increase platelet count by approximately 5000–10,000/mm^3 unless alloimmunization has occurred

     d. Dextran has antiplatelet activity

  5. Prothrombin time (PT)

     a. Used to evaluate competence of extrinsic coagulation pathway and final common coagulation pathway

     b. If clotting factors making up pathway are inadequate, PT is prolonged

     c. Normal range is 9.5–12.0 seconds

     d. Vitamin K is necessary to make prothrombin; drug interaction is seen with sodium warfarin anticoagulant therapy because it interferes with production of vitamin K–dependent clotting factors, thus prolonging PT or INR and increasing risk for bleeding; assess client for signs and symptoms of bleeding

     e. Inadequate clotting may require transfusion of FFP, cryoprecipitate, or administration of vitamin K depending on cause and urgency of situation

     f. Hetastarch can transiently prolong PT or lead to other coagulopathy in rare cases

6. Partial thromboplastin time

    a. Used to evaluate intrinsic clotting system and final common pathway

    b. Normal range for PTT is 60–70 seconds and for activated PTT (aPTT) 20–39 seconds

    c. Used to monitor heparin therapy; therapeutic range for heparin is 1.5–2.5 times the control in seconds; PTT >100 seconds or aPTT >70 seconds greatly increases risk of bleeding

    d. PTT may be abnormally prolonged due to hemophilia A or B, DIC, liver disease, or biliary obstruction

    e. Assess for signs and symptoms of bleeding

    f. FFP or cryoprecipitate may be indicated to restore missing clotting factors and vitamin K in the case of biliary obstruction

    g. Hetastarch can transiently prolong PTT or lead to other coagulopathy in rare cases

7. Antibody and immunoglobulin testing

    a. Direct antiglobulin test (direct Coomb's) detects immunoglobulins on RBC surfaces and can be used to investigate hemolytic transfusion reactions, aid in differential diagnosis of hemolytic anemia, and test for hemolytic disease of newborn

    b. Antibody screening (indirect Coomb's) determines Rh-positive antibodies in maternal blood and assists with identification of ABO incompatibility in newborns

    c. HLA antigens are identified on surface of circulating platelets, WBCs, and most tissue cells; can be used to match blood products to minimize reactions (such as HLA alloimmunization) and identify disease processes

D. Daily weights and body surface area (BSA)

1. Clients receiving IV fluids should be weighed daily (before breakfast and after voiding on same scale; have client wear similar clothing each time—i.e., hospital gown)

2. One kg (2.2 lb) of body weight is approximately equal to one liter of IV fluid; abrupt changes in weight are an important clue to changes in fluid status

3. Despite a weight gain, a client may have a significant circulating (intravascular) fluid volume deficit if there is third spacing of fluid; thorough client system assessment is critical; a weight loss is generally expected during diuretic therapy and a weight gain is expected when a client is being rehydrated for a fluid volume deficit

4. Calculation of BSA provides a more accurate determination of fluid needs for a client with critical needs; a nomogram is used to assist in calculating BSA from height and weight data

III. SELECTION OF FLUID AND ELECTROLYTE THERAPIES

A. Replacement therapies

1. Oral

    a. May be indicated if fluid loss is not excessive and if client is not vomiting, has intact gag and swallowing reflexes, has adequate GI absorption, has intact thirst mechanism and is able to drink

    b. Healthcare provider may prescribe to encourage "push" fluids for clients with actual or potential fluid volume deficits (fever, mild diarrhea)

    c. In choosing oral fluid replacement, consider client preferences, offer fluids frequently, and assist clients who have impaired swallowing by proper positioning (upright with head and neck flexed forward slightly) and providing thickened liquids or semisolid foods such as gelatin, pudding, or milkshakes

    d. It is critical to keep an accurate record of intake and output (I&O), trend results, and notify healthcare provider if imbalances occur

Practice to Pass

An older adult client with a history of CVA was admitted with dehydration because of inadequate intake and fever. What instructions should you include in discharge teaching for the client and the home health aide assigned to the client's care?

  2. Parenteral
   a. Indicated when client cannot take PO fluids because of clinical condition, when client is NPO and requires maintenance to replace insensible losses, to provide nutrients and electrolytes when GI tract is not functional, or to replace abnormal losses (GI suction, vomiting, diarrhea, fever, hemorrhage)
   b. Infusion rate is affected by maintenance and/or replacement need and underlying condition of client (administer cautiously in clients with congestive heart failure and renal failure)
   c. Refer to Table 8-3 for information about use of crystalloid fluid therapy
   d. The healthcare provider prescribes specific blood component therapy based on client's underlying health status, current medical status, and client's own personal decision (i.e., religious beliefs) to allow transfusion therapy

B. **Monitoring parameters**
  1. Daily weights
  2. I&O
   a. Maintain fluid restriction or follow prescriptions to increase fluids
   b. Properly label and time all IV solutions; run and maintain at prescribed rate
   c. Measure client's entire I&O from all sources
    1) Intake—by mouth, all IV fluids (includes IV meds), tube feedings
    2) Output—urine (urinal, bedpan, indwelling catheter, incontinence—approximate amount), nasogastric drainage, wounds, diarrhea, and emesis
   d. Accurately record findings and review 24-hour totals for several days to determine trends in fluid balance
   e. Use trended I&Os in conjunction with daily weights, labs, and knowledge of underlying pathophysiology to determine if client's response to IV therapy is sufficient
   f. Assess also for overcorrection of problem (client would experience signs of opposite fluid imbalance, such as overload with excessive fluid volume replacement or dehydration with excessive diuresis)
   g. Correlate I&O trend with changes in client's weight; generally, weight gain occurs when intake exceeds output and weight loss occurs when output exceeds intake
   h. Notify healthcare provider of any significant imbalance

Table 8-3	Crystalloid Fluid Replacement Therapy	
Hypotonic Fluids	**Isotonic Fluids**	**Hypertonic Fluids**
Indicated for cellular dehydration, hyperosmolar states (due to severe hyperglycemia), and to treat hypernatremia; hypotonic fluids provide free water that dilutes plasma and assists with renal excretion of wastes Do not give to clients with increased ICP (can increase cerebral edema), abnormal fluid shifts (third spacing), hypotension (can lower BP further), or during code situations (can worsen neurologic outcome)	Indicated for hypovolemia (ECF volume deficit) and postoperative fluid management; isotonic fluids expand vascular compartment and lower hemoglobin and hematocrit concentrations Do not give lactated solutions to clients with liver disease; monitor client for signs and symptoms of FVE; cautious use in clients with CHF or RF because they are already prone to developing FVE	Indicated for electrolyte replacement, hyponatremia, and correction of fluid shifting because this leads to cellular dehydration Do not give to clients who are already at risk for cellular dehydration (hyperosmolar serum); cautious use in clients with cardiac or renal failure

        i. In general, high UO indicates intravascular fluid volume excess (e.g., nocturia with heart failure); low UO with high specific gravity indicates intravascular fluid volume deficit (e.g., dehydration); low UO with low specific gravity indicates renal disease

    3. Trending of pertinent labs

        a. Review pertinent laboratory and diagnostic test results for improvement after use of specific replacement therapies

        b. Look also for assessment findings indicating improvement of underlying condition

        c. In general, a client being appropriately treated for an isotonic fluid volume deficit should exhibit the following:

           1) An increase in urinary output

           2) A decrease in urine specific gravity

           3) An increase in body weight

           4) An increase in blood pressure (if client was hypotensive)

           5) A decreased pulse rate

           6) Improved skin turgor and moist mucous membranes

           7) Decreased BUN, serum osmolality, and hematocrit

        d. A client being appropriately treated for a fluid volume excess should exhibit the following:

           1) Improvement in breath sounds

           2) Increase in UO (in response to diuretics), hematocrit, BUN, and serum osmolality

           3) Decreased weight

           4) Decrease in blood pressure if client's BP was elevated

           5) Decrease in or resolution of edema

C. Priority nursing concerns

    1. Fluid deficit (dehydration)

    2. Fluid overload

    3. Possible respiratory effects of fluid overload

    4. Possible reduction in cardiac output because of dehydration

D. Therapeutic management

    1. Carefully evaluate client's individualized fluid and electrolyte needs

    2. Give appropriate IV fluid(s) as maintenance and/or replacement therapy

    3. Monitor client responses to therapy daily or more often in unstable clients with review of pertinent labs, daily weights, I&O, and comprehensive client physical assessments

    4. Prevent complications (fluid overload, dehydration)

E. Client-centered nursing care

    1. Assist client to maintain and/or restore adequate plasma, cellular, or intracellular volume

        a. Encourage oral fluid intake if client able to ingest liquids

        b. Place fluids that client enjoys at bedside

        c. Infuse appropriate IV solution at prescribed rate

        d. Assess client each shift or at least daily for evidence of adequate hydration (moist mucous membranes, elastic skin turgor, no reports of thirst, VS within normal limits, adequate UO, level of consciousness within normal limits)

        e. Monitor VS frequently

        f. Carefully record I&O from all sources and weigh client daily

        g. Review pertinent laboratory results daily; closely follow any trends and interpret their significance

      h. Administer fluid challenge if needed to help determine volume status and renal status for clients with underlying clinical conditions; note that some clients may be at risk for developing fluid overload because of inability to handle fluids, such as those with heart failure

  2. Support client in achieving adequate oxygen-carrying capacity and coagulation status as needed

      a. Administer compatible blood and blood products, carefully applying knowledge of transfusion principles and following agency procedure

      b. Assess for signs of improved oxygenation: nonlabored respirations, increased tissue perfusion, improved capillary refill, increased activity tolerance, improved oxygen saturation, and possibly increased alertness

      c. Assess for signs of improved coagulation status: decreased bleeding, decreased petechiae, ecchymosis, no gingival oozing, guiac-negative stool

  3. Prevent potential complications of IV therapy

      a. Maintain a sterile IV system when priming tubings and administering IV fluids

      b. Observe IV insertion site regularly for signs of infection or phlebitis

      c. Be alert to signs and symptoms of fluid overload (pulmonary congestion, shortness of breath, elevated pulse and blood pressure, edema, and weight gain)

      d. Infuse hypertonic solutions (selected crystalloids and colloids) slowly

      e. Be alert to evidence of fluid volume deficit (dry mucous membranes, thirst, weight loss, increased heart rate, decreased blood pressure, poor perfusion, orthostatic hypotension)

      f. Do not infuse hypotonic solutions (D_5W, ½NS) in clients at risk for increased intracranial pressure or third-space fluid shifts

      g. Premedicate clients as prescribed prior to transfusions of blood or blood products; carefully assess for signs or symptoms of transfusion reaction and intervene accordingly

F. Client education

  1. Explain need for increased oral intake, if appropriate

  2. Teach client how to follow sodium and fluid restriction, if appropriate

  3. Teach client to weigh self daily

  4. Review signs and symptoms of dehydration and/or overhydration with client

  5. Instruct client to change positions slowly if dizziness or lightheadedness occurs

  6. Instruct client to report to nurse any pain, swelling, leaking, redness, or hardness (induration) at IV site

  7. Explain rationale for blood/blood product transfusion and procedure

  8. Verify that client has given informed consent prior to transfusing blood

  9. Teach client to inform nurse immediately if experiencing signs or symptoms of transfusion reaction (chills, fever, nausea, abdominal cramps)

G. Evaluation

  1. Client exhibits adequate hydration status demonstrated by warm dry skin, moist mucous membranes, no reports of excessive thirst, capillary refill <3 seconds, regular strong peripheral pulses, stable weight, VS and UO within normal limits, no edema, and clear lung sounds

  2. Client exhibits adequate oxygenation and coagulation status as demonstrated by no bleeding; VS within normal limits; adequate perfusion with improved capillary refill; hemoglobin, hematocrit, platelets, PT, and PTT within normal limits for client; and improved activity tolerance

  3. Client experiences no significant adverse effects from transfusion of blood or blood products

Case Study

A 35-year-old female client with severe anemia, tachycardia, and shortness of breath is admitted to your unit. The healthcare provider has prescribed two units of PRBCs.

1. What assessments will you make before transfusing the blood?

2. What are priority nursing concerns for this client?

3. What will you teach this client about the transfusion prior to beginning it?

4. What steps will you follow to administer the transfusion safely?

5. How will you evaluate the effectiveness of the transfusion for this client?

For suggested responses, see page 193.

POSTTEST

1 A client with dry skin and mucous membranes is weak, has orthostatic blood pressure changes, and has decreased urine output. The client's serum osmolality, however, is normal. Which type of IV fluid should the nurse anticipate being prescribed for this client? Select all that apply.

1. 5% dextrose in water
2. 0.45% sodium chloride
3. 10% dextrose in water
4. 0.9% sodium chloride
5. Lactated Ringer's

2 A client receiving a transfusion of packed RBCs suddenly sounds hoarse, begins wheezing, is diaphoretic and short of breath, and reports palpitations. Blood pressure is 76/52. What should be the nurse's priority action?

1. Stop the transfusion.
2. Infuse normal saline (NS) rapidly to maintain intravascular volume.
3. Administer epinephrine and a corticosteroid.
4. Maintain the client's airway and ask a staff member to notify the healthcare provider.

3 Which client outcome should the nurse anticipate after infusion of 25% albumin to a client in hypovolemic shock?

1. Increase in heart rate
2. Decrease in temperature
3. Decrease in peripheral perfusion
4. Increase in blood pressure

4 Which action should the nurse take when a client is receiving a granulocyte transfusion? Select all that apply.

1. Administer the granulocytes rapidly.
2. Premedicate with an antihistamine, a steroid, and an antipyretic.
3. Attach a microaggregate filter to the IV tubing.
4. Check lymphocyte count following the transfusion.
5. Administer the granulocytes slowly because of allergenicity.

5 Which laboratory test should the nurse monitor closely in an older adult client with congestive heart failure (CHF) who is receiving IV albumin?

1. Platelet count
2. Hematocrit
3. Serum bilirubin
4. Prothrombin time (PT)

6 The nurse is conducting a class for clients with cancer who frequently receive blood products. The nurse explains that if a client becomes alloimmunized, what would be the most effective way to increase the platelet count?

1. Transfuse single-donor platelet units.
2. Transfuse HLA-matched donor platelets.
3. Use a WBC filter to minimize infusion of WBCs.
4. Premedicate the client with diphenhydramine and acetaminophen.

7 A client being treated for dehydration is gaining weight as expected but remains orthostatic and tachycardic with dry mucous membranes. The nurse should assess the client for which of the following to help determine a possible etiology?

1. Jugular venous distention (JVD)
2. A third heart sound
3. Third spacing of body fluids
4. Elastic skin turgor

8 Which intervention should the nurse include in developing a plan of care for a client receiving hetastarch?

1. Draw a specimen for type and cross match prior to beginning hetastarch infusion.
2. Monitor client for signs of hypovolemia.
3. Expect decreased urine output as body begins conserving plasma volume.
4. Monitor for transient changes in PT, PTT, and clotting times.

9 A client will receive two units of packed red blood cells (PRBCs). The nurse should place highest priority on teaching the client which information related to transfusion therapy?

1. The rationale for the transfusion
2. Overview of the procedure so the client will know what to expect
3. Signs and symptoms to report to the nurse if they should occur
4. Frequency with which vital signs will be taken so as not to alarm the client

10 To promote adequate hydration in a client with impaired swallowing, which instruction for the family caregiver needs to be modified?

1. Offer fluids frequently.
2. Provide clear liquids of the client's choosing.
3. Assist the client to an upright position with head and neck flexed slightly forward.
4. Inform healthcare provider of any unusual losses (i.e., fever or diarrhea).

➤ *See pages 182–184 for Answers and Rationales.*

POSTTEST *(margin tab)*

ANSWERS & RATIONALES

Pretest

1 **Answer: 3, 5 Rationale:** A client who is hemorrhaging and in shock requires immediate restoration of oxygen-carrying capacity. With no time available for cross matching, universal donor blood (type O, Rh-negative) is administered. Establishing an intravenous site should be done prior to transfusing blood products. Type AB, Rh-positive blood can only be given to type AB, Rh-positive recipients. Albumin has no oxygen-carrying capacity, which is essential for a trauma client. Platelets may be administered if needed, but they are not oxygen-carrying cells, which is the first priority. **Cognitive Level:** Analyzing **Client Need:** Pharmacological and Parenteral Therapies **Integrated Process:** Nursing Process: Implementation **Content Area:** Adult Health **Strategy:** Recognize that the need for the client to receive a blood replacement is secondary to the type of fluid losses and to have an IV access and receive transfusions from a universal donor. **Reference:** LeMone, P., Burke, K., Bauldoff, G., & Gubrud, P. (2015). *Medical surgical nursing: Clinical reasoning in patient care* (6th ed.). New York, NY: Pearson, p. 240.

ANSWERS & RATIONALES *(margin tab)*

2 **Answer: 2 Rationale:** Normal saline is an isotonic solution that will replace lost vascular volume and promote perfusion. In addition, when blood is available, it can be hung with the normal saline. D_5W is hypotonic in the bloodstream once dextrose is metabolized, providing free water that moves into the interstitial space and cells. Administration can cause further fluid shifting, which will not help to replace lost volume or promote perfusion. A solution of 0.45% sodium chloride is hypotonic, and an isotonic solution or a volume expander would be a better choice in order to prevent fluid from moving into the interstitium. Dextrose will cause lysis of red blood cells. **Cognitive Level:** Analyzing **Client Need:** Pharmacological and Parenteral Therapies **Integrated Process:** Nursing Process: Diagnosis **Content Area:** Adult Health **Strategy:** Recognize the need for replacement with an isotonic fluid to direct you to the correct option. **Reference:** LeMone, P., Burke, K., Bauldoff, G., & Gubrud, P. (2015). *Medical surgical nursing: Clinical reasoning in patient care* (6th ed.). New York, NY: Pearson, pp. 185–187.

3 **Answer: 1 Rationale:** Each unit of PRBCs should raise the hemoglobin by 1 gram and hematocrit by 3%, making the expected changes after two transfused units to be 11 grams and 33%, respectively. A rise to 12 grams and 36% is too high. A rise to 13 grams is too high, while a rise to 30% would be expected after 1 unit is transfused. A rise to 15 grams and 39% is too high. The nurse should be aware of expected responses to therapy in order to validate that treatment has been effective. **Cognitive Level:** Applying **Client Need:** Reduction of Risk Potential **Integrated Process:** Nursing Process: Evaluation **Content Area:** Adult Health **Strategy:** Recall the expected changes that would be effected by a transfusion of PRBCs and multiply that by 2. **Reference:** LeMone, P., Burke, K., Bauldoff, G., & Gubrud, P. (2015). *Medical surgical nursing: Clinical reasoning in patient care* (6th ed.). New York, NY: Pearson, p. 240.

4 **Answer: 2 Rationale:** The client's symptoms clearly indicate fluid volume overload. A colloid solution of 25% albumin is hypertonic and pulls fluids into the intravascular space and may cause circulatory overload. The symptoms described do not demonstrate dehydration, which would be those consistent with insufficient circulating volume. Hypoalbuminemia causes fluid shifting that manifests usually as third spacing, not intravascular overload. The symptoms described do not demonstrate impaired peripheral tissue perfusion, which would include pale cool skin, delayed capillary refill, and possibly reduced peripheral pulses. **Cognitive Level:** Applying **Client Need:** Pharmacological and Parenteral Therapies **Integrated Process:** Diagnosis **Content Area:** Adult Health **Strategy:** Recognize that 25% albumin is a colloid that will draw fluid into the vascular space. Recognize the symptoms that reflect increased workload on the cardiovascular system to be directed to the correct

option. **Reference:** LeMone, P., Burke, K., Bauldoff, G., & Gubrud, P. (2015). *Medical surgical nursing: Clinical reasoning in patient care* (6th ed.). New York, NY: Pearson, p. 254.

5 **Answer: 1 Rationale:** Albumin is given to facilitate remobilization of third-space fluids. In the case of ascites, it would pull fluid from the abdomen into the intravascular space, resulting in a decrease in abdominal girth. The increase in intravascular fluid would lead to an increase in blood pressure. The pulse may increase in compensation to the increased blood volume, but this does not reflect effectiveness of the albumin treatment. A decrease in weight would most likely be seen as the reabsorbed abdominal fluid is excreted by the kidneys. **Cognitive Level:** Applying **Client Need:** Pharmacological and Parenteral Therapies **Integrated Process:** Nursing Process: Evaluation **Content Area:** Adult Health **Strategy:** Critical words are *ascites* and *albumin*. Recall the physiology of ascites and recognize the purpose of the albumin in treatment of ascites to direct you to the correct option. **Reference:** LeMone, P., Burke, K., Bauldoff, G., & Gubrud, P. (2015). *Medical surgical nursing: Clinical reasoning in patient care* (6th ed.). New York, NY: Pearson, p. 254.

6 **Answer: 2 Rationale:** The client's plasma is hypertonic (very concentrated) to begin with and thus serum osmolality, BUN, and hematocrit would be elevated from hemoconcentration. Once isotonic fluids are administered, the plasma concentration should decrease and all three laboratory test results should show a corresponding decrease. BUN and serum osmolality should not remain increased. An increase in all three parameters would be expected in a client who has not yet been treated for hypertonic dehydration. A decrease in hematocrit should occur with the administration of isotonic fluid therapy. **Cognitive Level:** Analyzing **Client Need:** Reduction of Risk Potential **Integrated Process:** Nursing Process: Evaluation **Content Area:** Adult Health **Strategy:** Critical words are *isotonic fluids* and *hypertonic dehydration*. Recall the effect of isotonic fluids on serum osmolarity to choose correctly. **Reference:** LeMone, P., Burke, K., Bauldoff, G., & Gubrud, P. (2015). *Medical surgical nursing: Clinical reasoning in patient care* (6th ed.). New York, NY: Pearson, pp. 185–187.

7 **Answer: 3 Rationale:** Abrupt changes in weight are an important clue to changes in fluid status. Unusual losses (i.e., fever or diarrhea) are significant; they need to be reported and may help the client prevent dehydration in the future, especially because the client is taking a diuretic. Increasing salt and fluids may put the client at significant risk for fluid overload considering the history of CHF. Taking a diuretic on alternate days only may put the client at risk for fluid volume excess. Drinking one glass of water a day only is grossly insufficient and can put the client at risk for fluid volume deficit. **Cognitive Level:** Analyzing **Client Need:** Physiological Adaptation

ANSWERS & RATIONALES

Integrated Process: Teaching and Learning **Content Area:** Adult Health **Strategy:** Critical words are *CHF* and *isotonic dehydration*. Eliminate incorrect options because they reflect unsafe behaviors. **Reference:** LeMone, P., Burke, K., Bauldoff, G., & Gubrud, P. (2015). *Medical surgical nursing: Clinical reasoning in patient care* (6th ed.). New York, NY: Pearson, pp. 185–187.

8 Answer: 2 Rationale: A client with type B blood can only receive type B (client/recipient has no anti-B antibodies) and type O (contains no antigens for recipient to react to). Because the client is Rh-negative and has been previously exposed to Rh-positive blood, the client may have antibodies to Rh-positive blood. Therefore only Rh-negative blood should be administered. The client cannot receive type O positive blood due to the identified negative Rh factor. The client has incompatibility with type AB negative blood because of the type A antigens. The client cannot receive type A blood or Rh-positive blood. **Cognitive Level:** Analyzing **Client Need:** Pharmacological and Parenteral Therapies **Integrated Process:** Teaching and Learning **Content Area:** Adult Health **Strategy:** Recognize the risk for Rh incompatibility existing in the client to direct you to the correct option. **Reference:** LeMone, P., Burke, K., Bauldoff, G., & Gubrud, P. (2015). *Medical surgical nursing: Clinical reasoning in patient care* (6th ed.). New York, NY: Pearson, p. 240.

9 Answer: 2 Rationale: It is important to monitor serum electrolytes, BUN, and creatinine for electrolyte imbalances and fluid balance in order to evaluate response to the infusion. Hemoglobin and hematocrit are checked if there is a concern or with transfusion of blood and blood products. Restriction of oral fluids would not be necessary unless the client is NPO. Reporting all I&O measurements would not be indicated unless significant problems are identified. **Cognitive Level:** Applying **Client Need:** Pharmacological and Parenteral Therapies **Integrated Process:** Implementation **Content Area:** Adult Health **Strategy:** The critical word is *crystalloid*. Recognize these solutions contain dextrose or electrolytes dissolved in water. Associate electrolytes in the correct option to the content of crystalloid solutions. **Reference:** LeMone, P., Burke, K., Bauldoff, G., & Gubrud, P. (2015). *Medical surgical nursing: Clinical reasoning in patient care* (6th ed.). New York, NY: Pearson, pp. 185–187.

10 Answer: 3 Rationale: FFP is derived from one unit of whole blood and contains the clotting factors that the client needs plus fibrinogen. Even though whole blood contains some clotting factors, it is deficient in others and is indicated for significant acute blood loss (which is not the client's problem). Improved oxygen-carrying capacity (rendered by the infusion of packed red cells) is something the client does not need. Hemophilia is a clotting disorder that requires clotting factor replacement. Albumin contains no clotting factors. **Cognitive Level:** Applying **Client Need:** Pharmacological and Parenteral Therapies **Integrated Process:** Nursing Process:

Assessment **Content Area:** Adult Health **Strategy:** The critical word is *hemophilia*. Recall the deficiency of clotting factors associated with this illness to choose correctly. **Reference:** LeMone, P., Burke, K., Bauldoff, G., & Gubrud, P. (2015). *Medical surgical nursing: Clinical reasoning in patient care* (6th ed.). New York, NY: Pearson, p. 254.

Posttest

1 Answer: 4,5 Rationale: The client is manifesting signs and symptoms of dehydration. Because the serum remains isotonic, this is isotonic dehydration or hypovolemia. Appropriate treatment is with an isotonic fluid to replace fluid volume. Normal saline is an isotonic solution. Lactated Ringer's is a balanced salt solution that is isotonic. Once the dextrose is metabolized, 5% dextrose in water is a hypotonic solution that would cause fluid shifting leading to cellular edema because the client's cells are normal size and free water is not needed by them. A solution of 0.45% sodium chloride is hypotonic; because the client has an isotonic dehydration, this would cause fluid shifting leading to cellular edema. A solution of 10% dextrose in water is hypertonic and could cause fluid shifting into the vascular compartment from the cells, leading to cellular dehydration. **Cognitive Level:** Analyzing **Client Need:** Pharmacological and Parenteral Therapies **Integrated Process:** Nursing Process: Diagnosis **Content Area:** Adult Health **Strategy:** Critical words are *normal osmolality*, indicating the fluid replacement will need to maintain the normal osmolality. Recognize the need to restore fluid balance with use of an isotonic solution to direct you to the correct options. **Reference:** LeMone, P., Burke, K., Bauldoff, G., & Gubrud, P. (2015). *Medical surgical nursing: Clinical reasoning in patient care* (6th ed.). New York, NY: Pearson, pp. 185–187.

2 Answer: 1 Rationale: The client is experiencing a severe allergic/anaphylactic reaction. The nurse should first stop the infusion of any more blood. The nurse should maintain IV access by infusing NS through a clean IV tubing (one not contaminated with blood) to maintain the intravascular volume and prevent vascular collapse once the transfusion is stopped. Hospital protocol may include the administration of epinephrine and corticosteroids, but it is not the first action by the nurse. The nurse should maintain the client's airway, administer oxygen, and have another staff member notify the healthcare provider immediately after the cause of the reaction (the transfusion) has been stopped. **Cognitive Level:** Analyzing **Client Need:** Pharmacological and Parenteral Therapies **Integrated Process:** Nursing Process: Implementation **Content Area:** Adult Health **Strategy:** The critical word is *priority*, indicating all or some of the options are correct and may be done almost simultaneously, but one takes highest precedence. Recognize the client's symptoms represent an anaphylactic response to direct you to the correct option. **Reference:** LeMone, P., Burke, K., Bauldoff, G., & Gubrud, P. (2015). *Medical surgical nursing: Clinical reasoning in patient care* (6th ed.). New York, NY: Pearson, p. 240.

3 **Answer: 4 Rationale:** A solution of 25% albumin is a hypertonic colloid solution that will expand the plasma volume. This increase in plasma volume should increase blood pressure. Because the albumin should increase the blood volume and blood pressure, the strain on the heart should be reduced, thus decreasing the heart rate. The increase in volume should not affect temperature. The increase in volume will not decrease peripheral perfusion; rather, it will have the opposite effect. **Cognitive Level:** Applying **Client Need:** Pharmacological and Parenteral Therapies **Integrated Process:** Nursing Process: Evaluation **Content Area:** Adult Health **Strategy:** Recognize that albumin is a plasma expander to direct you to the correct option. **Reference:** LeMone, P., Burke, K., Bauldoff, G., & Gubrud, P. (2015). *Medical surgical nursing: Clinical reasoning in patient care* (6th ed.). New York, NY: Pearson, p. 254.

4 **Answer: 2,5 Rationale:** A client receiving granulocytes is expected to experience fever and chills due to high potential for development of allergic reactions. The client should be premedicated with antihistamines, corticosteroids, and an antipyretic. Granulocytes should be administered not rapidly, but slowly. A microaggregate filter would trap the granulocytes and nullify the transfusion. Although lymphocytes are present in the transfusion, they are granulocytes and the neutrophil count is the appropriate laboratory value to trend. **Cognitive Level:** Analyzing **Client Need:** Pharmacological and Parenteral Therapies **Integrated Process:** Nursing Process: Implementation **Content Area:** Adult Health **Strategy:** The critical word is *granulocyte*. Recall the increased risk for reactions with this type of transfusion to direct you to the correct options. The wording of the question indicates that more than one option is correct. **Reference:** LeMone, P., Burke, K., Bauldoff, G., & Gubrud, P. (2015). *Medical surgical nursing: Clinical reasoning in patient care* (6th ed.). New York, NY: Pearson, p. 254.

5 **Answer: 2 Rationale:** A client with CHF has a compromised cardiac pump and therefore already has an increased risk for fluid volume excess or overload. Albumin is a hypertonic colloid solution that can cause circulatory overload. This represents a double risk, then, for a client with CHF. The hematocrit would decrease as the plasma volume increases (hemodilution). The platelet count would increase if the client had a transfusion of platelets. Serum bilirubin will be unaffected by albumin administration. The PT would not change because of an infusion of albumin. **Cognitive Level:** Analyzing **Client Need:** Pharmacological and Parenteral Therapies **Integrated Process:** Nursing Process: Assessment **Content Area:** Adult Health **Strategy:** Critical words are *older adult*, *CHF*, and

albumin. Recall the effect of albumin on fluid balance and the underlying pathophysiology of CHF to direct you to the correct option. **Reference:** LeMone, P., Burke, K., Bauldoff, G., & Gubrud, P. (2015). *Medical surgical nursing: Clinical reasoning in patient care* (6th ed.). New York, NY: Pearson, p. 254.

6 **Answer: 2 Rationale:** Clients may develop HLA antibodies in response to previous transfusions of blood that are not leukodepleted. Because platelets carry class 1 HLA antigens, the HLA antibodies will quickly destroy them. Therefore, attempting to match the donor's platelet antigens with the recipient's and then transfusing these platelets should increase the platelet count. Transfusing single-donor platelets does not ensure the platelets do not have the HLA antibodies to which the client is sensitive. Using a WBC filter does not eliminate the HLA antibodies. Premedicating the client will treat symptoms but will not reverse the process of alloimmunization. **Cognitive Level:** Analyzing **Client Need:** Pharmacological and Parenteral Therapies **Integrated Process:** Teaching and Learning **Content Area:** Adult Health **Strategy:** The critical word is *alloimmunized*. Recall the physiology of this process to direct you to the correct option. **Reference:** LeMone, P., Burke, K., Bauldoff, G., & Gubrud, P. (2015). *Medical surgical nursing: Clinical reasoning in patient care* (6th ed.). New York, NY: Pearson, p. 240.

7 **Answer: 3 Rationale:** The client's weight gain indicates retention of volume but the symptoms of extracellular fluid volume deficit (tachycardia, orthostatic, and dry mucous membranes) indicate that the fluid is moving into a third space. The presence of JVD would indicate fluid volume overload, and the client clearly has an extracellular fluid volume deficit. The presence of an S3 heart sound would indicate fluid volume overload, and the client clearly has an extracellular fluid volume deficit. The presence of elastic skin turgor indicates adequate hydration. **Client Need:** Physiological Adaptation **Cognitive Level:** Analyzing **Integrated Process:** Assessment **Content Area:** Adult Health **Strategy:** Recognize that the symptoms of hypotension and tachycardia indicate vascular volume is still depleted. **Reference:** LeMone, P., Burke, K., Bauldoff, G., & Gubrud, P. (2015). *Medical surgical nursing: Clinical reasoning in patient care* (6th ed.). New York, NY: Pearson, pp. 185–187.

8 **Answer: 4 Rationale:** Hetastarch can dilute clotting factors and therefore create transient changes in PT, PTT, and clotting times. Hetastarch will not interfere with blood typing and cross matching. Hetastarch expands the plasma volume and thus can cause hypervolemia. Urine output will be increased because hetastarch causes osmotic diuresis. **Cognitive Level:** Analyzing **Client Need:** Pharmacological and Parenteral Therapies **Integrated Process:** Nursing Process: Planning **Content Area:** Adult Health **Strategy:** Review the purpose of using hetastarch to expand intravascular fluid volume.

Recall the possible effect of hetastarch on clotting factors to choose correctly. **Reference:** LeMone, P., Burke, K., Bauldoff, G., & Gubrud, P. (2015). *Medical surgical nursing: Clinical reasoning in patient care* (6th ed.). New York, NY: Pearson, p. 254.

9 **Answer: 3 Rationale:** The nurse's highest priority is client safety; therefore, it is imperative that the client know what to report to the nurse should a reaction occur (i.e., chills, fever, itching, shortness of breath, or back pain). Providing a rationale for the procedure is appropriate but is not of higher priority than client safety. Providing an overview of the procedure is appropriate but is not of higher priority than client safety. Explaining the frequency of vital signs may help to prevent client anxiety about their frequency but does not have higher priority than client safety. **Cognitive Level:** Analyzing **Client Need:** Pharmacological and Parenteral Therapies **Integrated Process:** Nursing Process: Implementation **Content Area:** Adult Health **Strategy:** The critical words are *highest priority*, indicating all or some of the options are correct, but one takes more precedence. Choose the option that addresses safety. **Reference:** LeMone, P., Burke, K., Bauldoff, G., & Gubrud, P. (2015). *Medical surgical nursing: Clinical reasoning in patient care* (6th ed.). New York, NY: Pearson, p. 240.

10 **Answer: 2 Rationale:** Because the client has impaired swallowing, thickened liquids should be offered such as milkshakes, pudding, and gelatin because they decrease the risk of aspiration. Offering fluids frequently is an appropriate instruction and does not need to be modified. Assisting to an upright position is an appropriate instruction and does not need to be modified. Notification about unusual losses is an appropriate instruction and does not need to be modified. **Cognitive Level:** Applying **Client Need:** Physiological Integrity **Integrated Process:** Implementation **Content Area:** Adult Health **Strategy:** Critical words are *hydration* and *impaired swallowing*. Note one of the instructions needs to be modified, indicating three options are appropriate. Recall liquids often need to be thickened to enable safer swallowing to choose the correct option. **Reference:** LeMone, P., Burke, K., Bauldoff, G., & Gubrud, P. (2015). *Medical surgical nursing: Clinical reasoning in patient care* (6th ed.). New York, NY: Pearson, p. 185.

References

Adams, M. P., Josephson, D. C., & Holland, C. N. (2016). *Pharmacology for nurses: A pathophysiologic approach* (5th ed.). New York, NY: Pearson.

Berman, A., Snyder, S., & Frandsen, G. (2016). *Fundamentals of nursing: Concepts, process, and practice* (10th ed.). New York, NY: Pearson.

Holland, L., Adams, M., & Brice, J. (2018). *Core concepts in pharmacology* (5th ed.). New York, NY: Pearson.

Kee, J. L. (2017). *Pearson's handbook of laboratory and diagnostic tests* (8th ed.). New York, NY: Pearson.

LeMone, P., Burke, K., Bauldoff, G., & Gubrud, P. (2015). *Medical surgical nursing: Clinical reasoning in patient care* (6th ed.). New York, NY: Pearson.

Smith, S., Duell, D., Martin, B., Aebersold, M., & Gonzalez, L. (2016). *Clinical nursing skills: Basic to advanced skills* (9th ed.). New York, NY: Pearson.

Appendix A Practice to Pass and Case Study Suggested Answers

➤ Practice to Pass Suggested Answers

Chapter 1

Page 7: *Answer*—Hypotonic fluids (D_5W, ¼NS, ½NS) are contraindicated because they provide free water that is pulled into cells. Cerebral cells absorb such water more rapidly than other cells, which would worsen cerebral edema in a client who has sustained a head injury and insult to the brain. Isotonic fluids tend to remain in the vascular system, rather than shift into tissues.

Page 11: *Answer*—Three percent saline is very hypertonic with a high concentration of sodium. It will increase serum sodium levels and draw water from the cells into the vascular space, causing hypervolemia, hypernatremia, and cellular dehydration. Only limited doses in very controlled amounts should be infused. The infusion should be controlled with an infusion pump and the client should be closely monitored for the development of circulatory overload, pulmonary edema, rising serum sodium levels, and cerebral cell dehydration. Frequent monitoring should include:

- Vital signs and pulse oximetry
- Neurologic assessment
- Respiratory assessment with auscultation of lungs for crackles
- Hourly urine output
- Serum electrolyte levels

Page 16: *Answer*—This client's clinical manifestations are indicative of hypovolemia and impending shock. Hemorrhage from trauma is causing an isotonic fluid loss that is primarily ECF. Isotonic intravenous fluids remain in the ECF and are used to expand vascular volume. The client needs large volumes of isotonic fluids (normal saline, Ringer's solution, or lactated Ringer's) infused rapidly to increase vascular volume and prevent shock. If hemorrhage is massive, infusions of packed red blood cells and possibly other blood products to replace components of the plasma may be needed.

Page 18: *Answer*—This older adult client should be monitored closely for signs of hypervolemia and circulatory overload due to reduced cardiac and renal reserves consistent with the aging process. Monitoring should include (1) I&O, (2) observing for signs of venous congestion (neck vein distention, delayed hand vein emptying), (3) peripheral edema, and (4) pulmonary congestion (tachypnea, dyspnea, moist lung crackles). Daily weights should be done to detect weight gain in response to rehydration. Excessive weight gain could result from overcorrection, which a daily weight would also detect.

Page 19: *Answer*—Explain in simple terms that the child is losing water and minerals and needs both replaced. Suggest that she give the child small sips of a commercial oral rehydration solution frequently to replace the fluid and electrolytes lost through diarrhea and vomiting. Explain that this is a balanced solution that does not provide too much sugar or salt, which can make diarrhea worse. She should also be advised to continue a regular diet as soon as the child will eat food. This will help resolve the diarrhea and provide calories, protein, fluid, and electrolytes as well.

Page 21: *Answer*—The half-strength formula is a hypotonic solution that provides excess free water. If given on a regular basis, it could lead to inadequate calories, insufficient protein, hypotonic fluid volume excess, and water intoxication as the fluid is pulled into cells. This should be explained in simple terms that the mother can understand. If finances are a problem, she should be referred to a community agency that can help her obtain assistance in getting formula for the baby.

Page 24: *Answer*—The fluid should be controlled with an infusion pump to prevent accidental fluid overload in this infant. An infant's small body size and immature kidneys put him or her at higher risk for fluid volume overload if fluids are infused too rapidly. Monitoring should include (1) checking the intravenous infusion frequently, (2) I&O, (3) serial weights, and (4) vital signs in an effort to prevent accidental overinfusion of fluid and early detection of clinical signs of fluid overload.

Chapter 2

Page 34: *Answer*—Because serum sodium level is the primary determinant of plasma osmolality, it is easy to get a rough estimate of a client's plasma osmolality if the serum sodium level is known. Taking the known serum sodium level and doubling that figure gives a rough estimate of plasma osmolality. This can be helpful in the clinical setting to evaluate a client's osmolar state.

Page 35: *Answer*—The chief regulation of sodium occurs in the kidneys where it is reabsorbed along with chloride. The reabsorption of these two electrolytes plays an important role in water balance. Renal regulation of sodium is influenced as a response to different volume states.

Page 36: *Answer*—When sodium level is decreased, water will shift from the ECF (area of lower volume of solutes) to the ICF (area of higher volume of solutes) in an attempt to restore equilibrium. This results in a decreased circulating plasma volume and an increase in cellular swelling.

Page 39: *Answer*—The pathophysiological effects of hyponatremia are primarily seen in the central nervous system and result in neurologic depression. Muscular weakness is seen as neuromuscular involvement occurs. Nausea and other GI symptoms are seen as gastrointestinal involvement occurs. These effects are due to fluid shifting between the ECF and ICF as cellular swelling occurs.

Page 40: *Answer*—A client who is NPO and on NG suctioning is at risk for hyponatremia due to restricted oral replacement and the loss of gastric secretions. Clients who are on prolonged NPO status should have their hydration level maintained via parenteral routes. In addition, the loss of gastrointestinal secretions can lead to further electrolyte and fluid losses that will require adequate replacement therapies. Monitoring and recording intake and output is essential in the care of this client. Amount, color, and consistency of NG drainage should be monitored for potential electrolyte and fluid imbalances.

In addition, bowel sounds should be assessed on this client to see if there is resumption of normal peristalsis. Client should be in a safe position with the NG tube secure so as to prevent further complications related to potential aspiration. The suction equipment should be monitored for the correct setting and the canister changed as needed. NG tube placement should be verified at least once a shift (if not more often, such as before medication administration).

Page 46: *Answer*—The following safety measures should be instituted in taking care of a client with hypernatremia:

- Monitor neurologic status and level of consciousness (LOC) and observe for potential seizures.
- Keep the bed in the low position, side-rails up, and the call bell in place.
- Assist with ambulation and mobility as needed.
- Make sure that environment is safe so as to prevent risk of falls and injury to client.

Page 51: *Answer*—In metabolic alkalosis, chloride is decreased because the kidneys retain bicarbonate and excrete chloride. Increased bicarbonate in the body leads to potassium and sodium depletion, which affects extracellular volume depletion, resulting in accompanying chloride loss.

Page 52: *Answer*—Hypochloremia reflects a decrease in serum chloride, <95 mEq/L. Chloride levels do not usually change independently but instead are seen in conjunction with other electrolyte and acid–base imbalances. It is important to check serum sodium and potassium levels and assess

the client's acid–base status to help establish the etiology of the chloride deficit. In addition, it is important to ascertain clinical factors that would lead to chloride deficit such as disease states, GI loss, endocrine disturbance, and volume expansion in order to explain the hypochloremic state more clearly. Depending on the serum value, the following strategies can be used for correction: (1) increase intake of foods high in chloride or (2) administer sodium chloride intravenously, or potassium chloride if potassium level is also low.

Page 53: *Answer*—Methylprednisolone is a corticosteroid that causes sodium and chloride retention and fluid volume excess. Furosemide is a loop diuretic that promotes sodium, chloride, potassium, and water excretion. The methylprednisolone would be most likely to cause an increase in serum chloride levels.

Page 53: *Answer*—The nurse should assess the client with hyperchloremia for deep, rapid, vigorous respirations. In addition to respiratory manifestations, the client may also experience headache, drowsiness, and confusion. Depending on the state of acidosis, signs and symptoms will vary as the client attempts to return to normal acid–base balance by using compensatory mechanisms. The client can progress into shock states with accompanying dysrhythmias, so careful monitoring is critical to maintain client safety and establish favorable clinical outcomes.

Chapter 3

Page 62: *Answer*—Potassium (K^+) in the intracellular fluid (ICF) is important for conduction of electrical impulses, which make the muscles in the body work. Too much or too little potassium can be detrimental to health by affecting neuromuscular excitability, acid–base balance, and cardiac contractility. Elevated or decreased levels can lead to the development of cardiac dysrhythmias, which can be life-threatening. It is very important to have a K^+ level in the normal therapeutic range so as to avoid compromise.

Page 64: *Answer*—Because potassium never leaves the body in relative hypokalemia, it is important to monitor the client closely to ensure that rebound hyperkalemia does not occur with treatment. Remember, a serum potassium level that is low secondary to shifting does not indicate where the potassium loss has occurred. Clients who have relative hypokalemia may be at risk of developing hyperkalemia due to overaggressive treatment. It is important to adequately assess clients who may be exhibiting hypokalemia as a result of water intoxication, alkalosis states, and increased insulin secretion.

Page 65: *Answer*—Clients who are hypokalemic may be weak and have muscle cramps. Assist the client when ambulating to provide support and maintain balance. Have a call bell in reach and use partial side-rails when the client is in bed.

Assist the client to change position slowly to minimize the risk of orthostatic hypotension. Monitor the client's level of consciousness as well as respiratory, cardiac, and GI status. Administer medications as prescribed to restore normal serum levels. Monitor the client's labs accordingly to evaluate response to treatment.

Page 69: *Answer*—When KCl is administered intravenously, it should be diluted in enough solution so that the concentration is equal to or less than 10 mEq/mL. No more than 40 mEq should be added to a liter of solution when using a peripheral line. If a solution would deliver more than 20 mEq/hr, the client should be on continuous ECG monitoring with serum levels checked every 4–6 hours. Potassium should be infused using an infusion pump to ensure accurate rate of administration. Close monitoring of the IV site should be done because KCl is very irritating to veins. If the site is red or infiltrated, the IV must be discontinued and restarted in a new location to prevent damage to the vessel.

Page 70: *Answer*—Foods that are high in potassium include potatoes, bananas, watermelon, yogurt, and acorn squash. These are considered good sources because they contain the most K^+ per kilocalorie. Potassium is found in whole grains, meats, milk, fruits, vegetables, grains, and legumes and is present in most foods in the Western diet. In addition, it is important to note if the client is using salt substitutes because they are usually high in K^+. It is also important to assess the client for use of dietary (nutritional) supplements for their potential effects on K^+ levels. The client should avoid ingesting large amounts of licorice because this can lead to hypokalemia. Collaboration with a dietitian is essential in the management of significant hypokalemia.

Page 71: *Answer*—During massive tissue destruction, potassium is released from damaged and dying cells into the extracellular spaces. Potassium enters the vascular space and hyperkalemia develops. Because of this, all clients with injuries leading to significant cellular trauma should be monitored closely for potential problems as a result of hyperkalemia.

Chapter 4

Page 84: *Answer*—The parathyroid hormone, activated vitamin D, and calcitonin tightly control serum calcium levels. When there are alterations in any of these systems, disturbances in calcium levels can occur, leading to hypo- or hypercalcemia.

Page 86: *Answer*—Predisposing clinical conditions that can lead to calcium imbalances are related to inadequate intestinal absorption, deposition of ionized calcium into bone or soft tissue, or decreases in PTH and vitamin D levels. All of these factors can lead to decreased physiologic availability of calcium.

Page 88: *Answer*—Calcium plays an important role in determining the speed of ion fluxes through nerve and muscle membranes. The effects of too little calcium lead to an increase in nervous system irritability. This irritability is exhibited by tetany, as well as in Chvostek and Trousseau signs, and may develop into seizures if the level drops significantly.

Page 93: *Answer*—The therapeutic response to calcium gluconate therapy can be evaluated by noting resolution of dysrhythmias, tingling and paresthesias, and signs of tetany, and by noting a rise in serum calcium to within the normal range of 8.5–10.5 mg/dL. Appropriate nursing interventions for a client receiving this type of therapy should include evaluating the IV site for signs of extravasation that occur with calcium gluconate or calcium chloride, close titration of dose, and continuous ECG monitoring.

Page 93: *Answer*—CNS manifestations of hypocalcemia include depression, anxiety, irritability, delusions, hallucinations, and seizures (because of excitatory effect on CNS). Hypercalcemia produces CNS clinical manifestations such as lethargy, subtle personality changes, or acute changes such as psychosis, stupor, and possibly coma (because of CNS depression effect). Similarities in the CNS as a result of altered calcium levels (hypo- and hypercalcemia) result in clinical manifestations such as memory impairment and confusion.

Page 97: *Answer*—Foods to avoid are cheeses, milk, and other dairy products; canned salmon and sardines; rhubarb; spinach and other dark green leafy vegetables; and tofu. Calcium supplements and antacids containing calcium should be avoided. During the nursing assessment, the nurse should question the client about food likes and dislikes and for any history of peptic ulcer disease or gastric distress (which might increase the likelihood of using calcium-containing antacids and calcium-rich foods).

Chapter 5

Page 108: *Answer*—Because potassium and magnesium function together to help run the sodium-potassium pump, a change in one effects a change in the other. For this reason hypokalemia can occur with hypomagnesemia, and vice versa.

Page 110: *Answer*—Maalox, Mylanta, Riopan, Gaviscon, Gelusil, and Di-Gel are common brand-name antacids that are high in magnesium.

Page 111: *Answer*—Good sources of magnesium include dark green leafy vegetables, nuts, legumes, seafood, whole grains, bananas, oranges, cocoa, and chocolate.

Page 112: *Answer*—Cardiovascular symptoms that can occur with hypermagnesemia include hypotension, flushing and sweating, cardiac dysrhythmias, and possibly cardiac arrest.

Page 112: *Answer*—Calcium gluconate is an antagonist of magnesium and is given as an emergency treatment for severe hypermagnesemia.

Chapter 6

Page 122: *Answer*—Phosphorus is abundant in fish, poultry, eggs, red meat, and organ meats, such as brain, liver, and kidney. It is also found in dairy products such as milk. Legumes, whole grains, and nuts are other rich sources of phosphorus.

Page 125: *Answer*—The nurse should assess for subjective neurologic manifestations of hypophosphatemia such as circumoral and fingertip/extremity numbness and tingling. The client may also exhibit muscle weakness, parasthesias, tremors, spasms, and signs of tetany.

Page 127: *Answer*—When administering potassium phosphate added to IV fluids, use an infusion pump and do not exceed a rate of infusion greater than 10 mEq/hr; give the dose slowly over 2–6 hours as prescribed. Monitor for complications of IV administration, including tetany from hypocalcemia, hypotension from too rapid an infusion rate, and formation of calcium and phosphorus deposits in the tissues. Monitor infusion site for signs of infiltration, which may lead to tissue necrosis or sloughing.

Page 128: *Answer*—A client with hyperphosphatemia may exhibit any of the following manifestations:

- Metastatic calcification, including oliguria, corneal haziness, conjunctivitis, and irregular heart rate
- EKG changes and conduction disturbance, tachycardia, deposits of calcium phosphate in the cardiac tissues
- Numbness and tingling around the mouth and in the fingertips, muscle spasms, and tetany
- Decreased calcium
- Anorexia and nausea and vomiting
- Muscle weakness, hyperreflexia, and tetany

Page 129: *Answer*—Phosphate-binding medications contain either aluminum, magnesium, or calcium as the cation that binds to the phosphate anion. Products that bind phosphate will have one of these or may have aluminum and magnesium together because they have opposing effects on the GI tract (aluminum tends to cause constipation while magnesium tends to cause diarrhea).

Chapter 7

Page 142: *Answer*—The nurse would examine the client's ABG results. With uncompensated respiratory acidosis, the pH is less than 7.35, $PaCO_2$ is greater than 45 mm Hg, and the HCO_3^- is normal (22–26 mEq/L). In a client with respiratory acidosis, compensation would involve the kidneys retaining bicarbonate and returning it to the ECF. Compensation would reflect an increase in the bicarbonate level.

Page 143: *Answer*—As acidosis occurs, H^+ ions move into the cell and potassium moves into the ECF, elevating the serum potassium level. Hyperkalemia can cause serious cardiac conduction defects and can be fatal. When someone is acidotic, the potassium level must be monitored closely. Transcellular shifting of potassium is affected by acid–base balance. With acidosis, H^+ is excreted and K^+ is retained leading to hyperkalemia. With alkalosis (the opposite disorder), K^+ is excreted and H^+ is retained, leading to hypokalemia.

Page 145: *Answer*—Clients with type 1 diabetes require insulin to control glucose levels. When there is insufficient insulin, fats are metabolized and free fatty acids accumulate, which can result in the development of diabetic ketoacidosis (which is of metabolic origin, not respiratory origin). Control of glucose levels with adequate insulin is the best prevention.

Page 147: *Answer*—Monitoring the amount of NG drainage and replacing the amount lost with an equal amount of an electrolyte solution can prevent excessive H^+ ion loss. It is important for the nurse to calculate intake and output and correlate the net fluid balance with serum electrolyte levels. If fluids and electrolytes are being removed via suction, then the client may be at risk to develop further electrolyte imbalance, which could be complicated by acid–base disturbances. The nurse should consult with the healthcare provider for electrolyte replacement therapy as needed.

Page 149: *Answer*—Conditions leading to the development of metabolic alkalosis result in depleted potassium levels, which can significantly affect cardiac function. Clients who are alkalotic have decreased serum potassium levels because of transcellular shifting of potassium. Hypokalemia affects cardiac conduction, leading to the development of dysrhythmias that can become life-threatening. These clients must be monitored closely so prompt management and intervention can be implemented.

Chapter 8

Page 162: *Answer*—The client in diabetic ketoacidosis has a very hyperosmolar serum and is experiencing osmotic diuresis and dehydration. A solution of 0.9% NaCl (normal saline) will begin to replace fluid volume lost because of osmotic diuresis. It also expands plasma volume to increase the glomerular filtration rate, which will protect the kidneys from the complication of acute kidney injury. Serum osmolality should begin to decrease with rehydration (insulin is also needed, of course, to correct the causative factor). Although one might expect serum sodium to be high in this dehydrated client, a good amount of sodium is lost in the urine because of osmotic diuresis. Therefore, the serum sodium is low to begin with and should increase with 0.9% NaCl IV replacement. Blood pressure should increase, heart rate should decrease, and perfusion should improve.

Page 163: *Answer*—Priority assessments include obtaining baseline and frequent vital signs and determining adequacy of organ perfusion by assessing level of consciousness (LOC), urine output, and skin color. Be aware that the client may develop either dehydration or fluid overload because of the cellular dynamic effects of the hypertonic albumin. It is equally important to monitor the client for the possibility of a febrile reaction. Priority interventions include maintaining a patent airway and providing adequate oxygenation. Albumin should be infused as rapidly as the client will tolerate, while paying close attention to lung sounds for possible pulmonary edema and other indicators of fluid volume excess (FVE). The client may be at higher risk for fluid volume excess if there is a significant cardiac history. Even without a cardiac history, given the client's age, there may be some cardiac insufficiency associated with the normal aging process. It is important to place the client in a supine position with legs elevated (modified Trendelenburg or antishock position) to maximize organ perfusion. If the client cannot tolerate this position due to respiratory compromise, then elevate the head of bed to no higher than 30–45 degrees. If the client is at risk for increased intracranial pressure (if head injury present), elevate the head of bed to 30 degrees. Keep the client warm. If trauma occurred or may have occurred, observe for increased bleeding, especially as the blood pressure rises. Monitor hemoglobin, hematocrit, electrolytes, and serum albumin. Expected outcomes for this client include improved organ perfusion with a corresponding increase in cardiac output, blood pressure, and urine output, and a decrease in heart rate, respiratory rate, and hematocrit (if shock was not caused by hemorrhage).

Page 165: *Answer*—Stop the infusion because the client may be experiencing an anaphylactic reaction. Maintain the client's airway and provide high-flow oxygen. Enlist assistance and have one colleague bring the crash cart and another notify the healthcare provider. Administer epinephrine per hospital protocol. Quickly change the IV line at the hub and infuse 0.9% normal saline (NS) to help maintain blood volume. Place the client on a cardiac monitor and initiate pulse oximetry. Monitor heart rate, respiratory rate, and oxygen saturation continuously and measure blood pressure frequently. Additional medications such as diphenhydramine, methylprednisolone sodium succinate, and aminophylline may be prescribed. The client may need to be intubated. The healthcare provider may prescribe additional IV fluids. A vasopressor (i.e., dopamine) may be prescribed if the client is unable to maintain an adequate blood pressure. Once the client has stabilized, continue to observe the client for several hours. Once it has been determined that the client is allergic to hetastarch, the client should be advised to wear a medical alert bracelet indicating the allergy.

Page 169: *Answer*—An example of an appropriate response to a client's question about the rationale for irradiated CMV-negative blood would be, "The chemotherapy that you are receiving to treat the leukemia puts you at increased risk for infection. Specially treating the blood you will receive helps to ensure that it will not be a source of infection for you while you are at increased risk."

Page 172: *Answer*—Laboratory results to review in evaluating the effectiveness of transfusion therapy for a client with DIC include hemoglobin, hematocrit, RBC count, platelet count, partial thromboplastin time (PTT), prothrombin time (PT) or International Normalized Ratio (INR), and fibrinogen level. While transfusions of PRBCs, platelets, fresh frozen plasma (FFP), and possibly cryoprecipitate will help to replenish blood components, additional blood loss may occur because of this coagulopathy. The presence of DIC complicates the clinical picture because unless the underlying mechanism is identified and treated, replacement therapies are aimed at supportive management and are not curative. Therefore, lab values are likely to plunge again and again until the underlying cause is identified and treated.

Page 172: *Answer*—First explain to the client what the granulocyte transfusion is for, what to expect during the transfusion (chilling, fever, and allergic reaction), and answer any client questions. To safely administer granulocytes, begin by premedicating the client as prescribed, generally with diphenhydramine, corticosteroids, and an antipyretic. When hanging the unit, verify that it is ABO and Rh compatible because it contains RBCs (note it is preferable for the unit to be HLA compatible as well). Granulocytes must be administered within 24 hours after being collected and are maximally effective when given as soon as possible after collection. Use a standard inline filter (not a microaggregate filter, which will trap the WBCs) and administer the transfusion slowly, generally at a rate of 50 mL per hour for 4 hours. Monitor the client for expected side effects. Cover the client with a warm blanket to prevent chilling. Monitor the client for hypertension and treat it if needed. Only discontinue the transfusion if the client develops severe respiratory distress. Be aware that granulocytes are generally administered for at least 4–5 days, one unit a day or until the infection resolves.

Page 175: *Answer*—If the client has any difficulty swallowing as a result of a prior stroke, it is important that the home health aide assists the client to an upright position with the head and neck flexed slightly forward. Liquids should be thickened if prescribed based on results of a swallowing evaluation. The home health aide should offer the client fluid frequently and consider preferences when purchasing and preparing the fluids. It is also important that cold fluids are served cold and warm fluids are served warm. The client and home health aide must be aware of and maintain any prescribed fluid restriction if there is underlying CHF and/or renal insufficiency. The home health aide should keep a record of the client's intake and output and, if appropriate, note the characteristics of urine output. It is important that daily weights be obtained. The aide should be instructed to report to the nurse if the client's skin and mucous membranes become dry. The client should be instructed to report any excess thirst to the aide. All abnormal losses from fever, diaphoresis, or diarrhea, for example, should be reported to the healthcare provider. Finally, the client and aide should be instructed about proper hand hygiene techniques and other measures to protect against infection.

Case Study Suggested Answers

Chapter 1

1. Questions to ask the mother include:
   - How high has the fever been, how many times has the infant vomited, how many stools has the infant had today?
   - Has the infant been able to keep any food or fluids down?
   - When did the infant last urinate?
   - Is the infant acting "normal"? Are there any changes in behavior or activity?
   - Has there been any weight lost in the past 2 days?
   - Have you used any treatments or medicines at home? If so, which ones and how often? What effect did they have?
2. Serious fluid imbalance is indicated by these assessments and related findings:
   - Level of alertness, activity, interaction and response to others (lethargy, listlessness, and/or reduced activity/interaction are signs of serious dehydration).
   - Heart rate (tachycardia is an early sign of fluid volume deficit in infants).
   - Skin and mucous membranes (dry oral mucosa and tongue, furrowed tongue, and no tears when crying are all signs of fluid volume loss).
   - Palpation of fontanels (sunken fontanels are a sign of significant fluid volume loss).
3. Control the fluid rate with an infusion pump to prevent infusing a volume too large for the child's size. Explain all procedures to the parents and provide emotional support. Monitor the child for signs of improvement as well as fluid overload as a complication of overcorrection.
4. Give the child small, frequent sips of a commercial oral rehydration solution recommended by provider to replace both fluid and electrolyte losses without giving excess sugar or salt, which can make diarrhea worse. Resume regular foods as soon as the infant will eat them. Once the infant is eating and the diarrhea is resolving, add a variety of fluids the infant likes, avoiding those with high sugar or salt content.
5. The BRAT diet is a transition diet that might be recommended when clients have gastrointestinal tract alterations (nausea and vomiting or diarrhea). It is not meant for long-term use as it does not provide adequate amounts of required nutrients and calories. Once the infant is able to keep food and fluids down, it is important to progress the diet back to the original pattern.

Chapter 2

1. Client's past medical history (PMH) reveals hypertension diagnosed 6 weeks ago with a prescription of hydrochlorothiazide and a low-sodium diet. Current findings related to history of present illness (HPI) or chief complaint reveals dizziness, nausea, weakness, abdominal cramps, and headache. Onset of symptoms 3 days ago with worsening by today indicates that the client's condition is becoming more acute. These findings suggest that the client might be experiencing a sodium deficit. The use of a thiazide diuretic can lead to a sodium deficit, and the increase in neurologic symptoms of dizziness, weakness, and headache are consistent with hyponatremia.
2. Questions that should be asked prior to performing a physical examination should include:
   - Are you taking your diuretic as prescribed? Clarify information relative to dosage, frequency, and compliance with treatment regimen.
   - Have you ever experienced these kinds of symptoms before?
   - Are there any contributory health problems that could affect your overall condition? Have you been diagnosed with any acute or chronic disease process?
   - Are you taking any other medications, either prescription or OTC or herbal supplements?
   - Have you been experiencing thirst?
   - Have you had excessive perspiration or sweating in the last few days?
   - You stated that you have been dizzy. Can you explain what that means to you? Are you having blurred vision? Are you having difficulty concentrating?
   - Can you tell me where you feel your headache and describe the type of discomfort that you experience (obtain pain characteristics)?
   - Have you taken any medication today to relieve any of your symptoms?
   - Obtain an accurate intake and output record from the client for the past 24 hours.
3. Clinical findings consistent with hyponatremia should be expected. These physical examination findings include tachycardia, hypotension, dry mucous membranes, muscular weakness, and flat neck veins.
4. Based on the data obtained thus far and knowledge of fluid and electrolytes, the nurse should expect a Na^+ level <135 mEq/L (which would indicate hyponatremia), a serum osmolality <275 mOsm/kg (which would indicate decreased plasma osmolality), a serum chloride level <95 mEq/L (which would indicate hypochloremia), and a specific gravity of <1.008 (which would indicate a decreased ability to concentrate urine).
5. Discharge teaching that would be important for this client includes:
   - Signs and symptoms of hyponatremia (such as abdominal cramps, nausea, muscle weakness) so that he will be able to identify and report potential problems to the healthcare provider.
   - Importance of drinking liquids containing sodium during periods of heavy sweating and/or high environmental temperatures, especially since the client's occupation requires him to be outdoors.

- Comply with regularly scheduled lab/diagnostic tests to monitor sodium and other electrolyte levels while taking hydrochlorothiazide, a diuretic.
- Adherence to low-sodium diet instructions (also verify that the client is meeting dietary goals). Refer to a dietitian for follow-up if needed.
- Safety measures to use when ambulating while on diuretic therapy (fluid volume loss can potentially lead to dizziness and orthostasis—a drop in blood pressure when arising from a lying or sitting position). Discuss slow change of positioning and monitor BP during therapy.
- Keep all regularly scheduled health care appointments and report findings immediately to healthcare provider so that prompt recognition and treatment of symptoms can be started.

Chapter 3

1. The nurse should question this client closely about any medications that the client is taking (prescription, over-the-counter, and dietary or herbal supplements). Particular attention should be given if the client is taking potassium supplements and/or digitalis preparations. The nurse should question this client about any acute or chronic disease process that could increase the risk for developing hypokalemia. In addition, any recent medical or surgical treatment should be explored. The nurse should obtain diet history. Finally, the nurse should ask the client about any signs and symptoms of hypokalemia being experienced.
2. The client could manifest many other signs and symptoms, such as fatigue, muscle weakness, leg cramps, nausea and vomiting, paralytic ileus, paresthesias, polyuria, weak and irregular pulse, hyperglycemia, and ECG changes consistent with hypokalemia.
3. A serum chemistry panel should be drawn because episodes of diarrhea are associated with potential fluid and electrolyte depletion. Magnesium levels and calcium levels should be reviewed because hypokalemia often occurs in conjunction with losses of these two electrolytes. Arterial blood gases might be drawn to determine acid–base status because GI fluids are lost in diarrhea (including pancreatic juices that are rich in bicarbonate), leading to the development of metabolic acidosis. ECG monitoring is indicated for this client because the client is reporting cardiac effects (feeling of heart racing). Depending on ECG baseline, additional labs, such as cardiac enzymes, might be prescribed if further cardiac compromise was suspected. If the client continues to have diarrhea, then a stool sample should be obtained for culture and sensitivity.
4. The client would be given either oral or parenteral potassium supplements depending on the baseline potassium level. If the level was low (below 3.0 mEq/L), then IV potassium would be the treatment of choice until the level reached 3.0 mEq/L; then oral supplements would be sufficient. Even at higher levels, some clients are unable to consume sufficient potassium to raise serum levels. These clients might have to remain on IV therapy with KCl in addition to oral supplements. If the diarrhea continues and the stool sample identifies a specific pathogen, then further medical treatment may be warranted by using antibiotic therapy to treat the organism; otherwise, antidiarrheal agents may be prescribed to prevent excess fluid loss.
5. The client should be given information about signs and symptoms of hypokalemia and to report them to the healthcare provider if they occur. If relevant, client teaching should include specific information about the client's diet and/or current medications that contribute to potassium balance. Because the client will most likely be started on K^+ supplementation, the client should be aware of potential interactions and adequate sources of dietary potassium to maintain normal serum levels. Regarding the most effective teaching methods for the client, it is important to individualize so that the client can have both verbal and written information. Including significant family members may be warranted in order to reinforce information and help others participate in the client's healthcare upon discharge.

Chapter 4

1. These signs and symptoms are caused by hypercalcemia from bone osteoclastic activity associated with malignancy of multiple myeloma.
2. The pathophysiological mechanism appears to be osteoclastic bone resorption, mediated by PTH or other substances secreted by the tumor. The result is that more calcium is released from the bone into the ECF.
3. Isotonic saline diuresis will lead rapidly to increased renal excretion, depending on renal function. Bisphosphonate drugs (such as pamidronate) are used with saline diuresis because they inhibit osteoclasts from resorbing bone. Plicamycin is extraordinarily effective in clients who have hypercalcemia that results from skeletal metastasis.
4. Priority nursing interventions include:
   - Monitor for signs of continuing hypercalcemia.
   - Monitor for signs of impending hypocalcemia from overcorrection secondary to treatment.
   - Monitor client carefully for signs of heart failure from saline diuresis.
   - Monitor for side effects of bisphosphonate therapy.
   - Monitor for side effects of plicamycin.
   - Move the client with great care to avoid pain or fractures.
   - Pain management therapy should be an integral part of the treatment plan.
5. If therapy is effective, there should be an absence of the presenting clinical manifestations. Calcium and phosphorus levels should normalize. Serum creatinine should

indicate effectively functioning kidneys and a urine output of 2–3 L/day. The client should experience minimal side effects of medication therapy and no signs of heart failure. Fluid volume should be stable with no signs of overload. The client should state a reduction in pain, with no increase in pain during moving or ambulation.

Chapter 5

1. The client has low weight for height. This leads to questions about starvation, dietary habits, anorexia, and bulimia. Any of these could lead to a state of hypomagnesemia.

2. Subjective data should also be gathered about alcohol use and over-the-counter medications or supplements, including those with diuretic or laxative effects, enemas, and diet aids.

3. Diagnostic evaluation should include electrolytes, including potassium, magnesium, and calcium levels, and an electrocardiogram (ECG).

4. Depending on the findings, dietary evaluation, mental health counseling, and endocrinology evaluation could be indicated.

5. Instructions that would help to prevent fluctuating magnesium levels include avoiding foods high in magnesium, antacids, laxatives, enemas, and magnesium supplements if there are high magnesium levels. Instructions would further include avoiding alcohol, diuretics, hyperglycemia, and treating unresolved vomiting or diarrhea if there were low magnesium levels.

Chapter 6

1. The client is expected to have hyperphosphatemia because the chronic renal failure inhibits the ability of the kidneys to eliminate excess phosphates.

2. As the kidneys fail, the nephrons (the functional units of the kidney) are not able to perform their intended functions adequately. Because the kidneys ordinarily eliminate excess phosphorus, this substance is retained in the bloodstream, leading to high phosphorus levels.

3. Many foods are naturally rich in phosphorus, making dietary management somewhat difficult. The client should avoid foods that are especially rich in phosphorus, such as fish, poultry, eggs, red meat, organ meats, dairy products, legumes, whole grains, and nuts.

4. Hemodialysis will compensate for the lack of kidney function and will help to remove excess phosphates from the bloodstream.

5. The client will likely receive a phosphate-binding agent as part of his medication therapy. The active ingredient in the prescribed medication will be aluminum, magnesium, or calcium. Currently, calcium-based products (with calcium carbonate as an example) are popular for use in clients with renal failure because they often have concurrent hypocalcemia (recall the reciprocal effect between calcium and phosphorus). The client should also be taught to read the labels of over-the-counter medications and products and avoid using those that are high in phosphorus or phosphate content.

Chapter 7

1. Due to the chronic nature of COPD, this client would most likely have ABG values consistent with chronic respiratory acidosis. Compensation would be expected because of the chronic nature of COPD, but because of the acute onset of URI, decompensation could occur depending on the client's baseline status and nature of acute exacerbation. Due to retention of acids, the pH would be low and the $PaCO_2$ would be elevated, with the HCO_3^- elevated to compensate. The presence of mild renal insufficiency should not lead to concurrent metabolic acidosis.

2. To help improve respiratory status, the nurse should administer medications on time and position the client upright as appropriate to enhance respirations. The nurse should reinforce information about how to manage COPD, including purse-lipped breathing to eliminate CO_2, the importance of taking bronchodilators as prescribed, signs and symptoms of infection to report to healthcare provider, and the benefits of getting pneumonia and flu vaccines per recommended schedules (because these two conditions could exacerbate the respiratory condition).

3. Because of chronic lung disease, this client's alveoli have difficulty eliminating excess CO_2, which leads to chronically high CO_2 levels on ABG results. This is considered an abnormal but expected finding in clients with chronic COPD. A client who does not have COPD retains the normal response stimulus of CO_2 for ventilatory drive. Clients without airway disease are able to ventilate and perform gas exchange using normal mechanisms. They are able to maintain CO_2 balance by breathing patterns and are not subject to CO_2 retention.

4. Clients with COPD frequently develop cardiac problems along with their lung disease. The chronic hypoxemia leads to pulmonary vasoconstriction, which can lead to development of right heart failure. Potassium-wasting diuretics are used to treat both conditions. When potassium is lost, hydrogen ions tend to move out of cells into the blood, creating an alkalotic state. The client should learn the signs and symptoms of hypokalemia and metabolic alkalosis and to report potential problems to the healthcare provider. The client should eat foods high in potassium, if not already on a potassium supplement. The client should be taught to notify the healthcare provider immediately if severe diarrhea develops, as this might increase risk of metabolic alkalosis.

5. If the client's kidney function deteriorates further over time from renal insufficiency due to chronic renal failure, the client would be at risk for metabolic acidosis.

Because of ongoing respiratory acidosis, the client would then be more at risk for general signs and symptoms associated with acidosis.

Chapter 8

1. Check baseline vital signs, heart rhythm, and lung sounds as well as assess for other signs and symptoms of anemia. Be aware of the type of anemia the client has, its cause, and the client's current hematocrit and hemoglobin (as well as total RBC count and RBC indices if available). Ask the client whether she's ever had a transfusion of blood or a blood product before, when that was, and whether she had a reaction (including signs and symptoms experienced). Ensure that the client has given informed consent after speaking with the healthcare provider and that all transfusion-related questions have been answered.

2. The following are priority nursing concerns: inadequate gas exchange, adverse changes in breathing pattern, reduced tissue perfusion, and reduced activity tolerance. While the blood is transfusing, the client may also have a potential risk for transfusion reaction. The client may have insufficient understanding of the reason for the transfusion (to improve the oxygen-carrying capacity of the blood), procedures that will be done during the transfusion process (identification of blood product, frequent vital signs, length of transfusion therapy, and signs and symptoms of transfusion reactions), and posttransfusion procedures (follow-up bloodwork and continued observation).

3. Prior to beginning the transfusion, it is important to determine that the client has informed consent and has signed the consent form. It is important to answer all questions regarding the administration of this blood product. If the client has additional questions or concerns that are beyond the scope of nursing practice, the healthcare provider should be notified. If there are no questions or if the client's questions have been answered to satisfaction, then the nurse should inform the client of the steps that will be taken during the blood transfusion procedure. Once the type and cross-match has been completed, an IV site will be established for the transfusion if the client does not already have IV access. Once the blood unit is brought to the floor, the nurse will verify the original order with another licensed nurse and (at the bedside) check the client's blood bank band with the blood unit in order to verify client name, date of birth, blood bank client identifier number and blood unit number, ABO type and Rh, and expiration date. The client will be monitored throughout the course of therapy with frequent vital signs and observation. If any additional medication is prescribed either as a premedication or in between units, the nurse will administer it per the healthcare provider's prescription. Following completion of the transfusion of the units, labwork will be drawn to see how the client responded to the therapy.

4. To administer the transfusion safely, follow hospital policy and procedure, which will reduce the likelihood of a transfusion action. Verify the prescription for the transfusion and ensure the client has been typed and cross-matched for two units of PRBCs by the lab. Hang the first unit of blood after performing the appropriate verifications for the blood unit; use only normal saline as a priming solution. Remain with the client during the first 15 minutes of any transfusion therapy to assess for potential transfusion reactions. If the client should develop any signs or symptoms of a transfusion reaction, stop or slow the transfusion depending on type of reaction and hospital policy, attend to the client, and notify the healthcare provider and the blood bank according to established agency procedure. Using proper equipment, monitoring parameters, and assessing the client (not merely the equipment) will promote transfusion safety in the clinical setting.

5. Effective transfusion therapy for anemia should lead to a decrease in heart rate, respiratory rate, improvement of clinical symptoms (decrease in shortness of breath and increased tissue perfusion), and increased activity tolerance. After transfusion of two units of packed red blood cells, diagnostic results should reflect an increase of 2 grams in hemoglobin and a 6% increase in hematocrit, which is the equivalent of a 1-gram increase in hemoglobin per unit and a 3% increase in hematocrit per unit.

Preparing for the NCLEX-RN® Exam

SAFE AND EFFECTIVE CARE ENVIRONMENT: MANAGEMENT OF CARE

Management of Care makes up 17–23% of the questions on the NCLEX-RN® exam.

Key Testing Strategies:

- Recognize questions that require priority setting through words in the question such as first, initial, best, most important, essential, and most therapeutic.
- When answering questions related to delegation to caregivers, such as float registered nurses from other clinical specialties, LPNs/LVNs, and unlicensed assistive personnel (UAPs), recall that the task being delegated needs to be part of that caregiver's skill set and that the other rights of delegation must be upheld.
- Immediately eliminate distracters that violate client rights or ethical principles.

Areas of Focus for Management of Care Questions		
	Ethical and legal concepts for nursing practice	Performance or quality improvement
	Maintaining client rights, including confidentiality and informed consent	Communication with interdisciplinary team (collaboration, client advocacy, case management, making referrals, and maintaining continuity of care)
	Assisting client with self-determination (such as with life planning, advance directives, and organ donation)	
	Nursing management concepts	Skills involving clinical reasoning, such as priority setting, assignment-making, delegation, and supervision
	Using information technology in clinical care	

Essential Rights of Delegation

1. **Right Task:** Nurses determine those activities team members may perform. For each situation, the nurse must consider the client's condition, the complexity of the activity, the UAP's capabilities, and the amount of supervision the nurse will be able to provide.
2. **Right Circumstances:** The nurse evaluates the individual clients and the individual UAPs and matches the two. The nurse assesses the client's needs, looks at the care plan, and considers the setting, ensuring that UAPs have the proper resources, equipment, and supervision to work safely.
3. **Right Person:** The nurse follows organizational policies, which are congruent with state law, in determining the appropriate staff to which to delegate a nursing activity.
4. **Right Direction and Communication:** The nurse needs to communicate the acceptable tasks and activities. The nurse needs to clearly understand the organization's policies and procedures to carry out effective delegation. In turn, staff nurses need to direct UAPs' actions and communicate clearly about each delegated task. Nurses must be specific about how and when UAPs should report back to them. Nurses should feel comfortable asking, Do you know how to do this? Where did you learn? How many times have you done it in the past? Where is your experience documented?
5. **Right Supervision and Evaluation:** Nurse managers must ensure that each unit has adequate staffing and time, identify the task inherent to each staff role, and evaluate the impact of the organization's nursing service on the community. The delegating nurse then must supervise, guide, and evaluate the UAPs' task implementation. The nurse must ensure that UAPs meet expectations and must intervene if they aren't performing well.

© 2018 Pearson Education, Inc.

*Based on the April 2016 Test Plan

Strategies for Setting Priorities in Clinical Practice	**Guiding Principles**	**First Priority**	**Second Priority**
	Physiology	**Airway, breathing, and circulation**	
	Maslow's Hierarchy of Needs theory	Physiological (primary) needs: air, breathing, circulation, water, food (oxygen therapy, circulatory support, IV hydration, nutrition, critical lab values, treatment of pain)	Safety and security (primary) needs: prevention of falls, reorientation to surroundings, abnormally high or low values that are not critical, may include some client teaching (e.g. insulin administration)
	Policies and Procedures	Activities governed by agency policy or procedure that involves strict timelines (e.g., restraints, falls, stat medications)	Activities governed by policy or procedure that directly affect client care (e.g., non-stat, regularly scheduled medications, dressings)
	Care activities related to clinical condition of client	Life-threatening or potentially life-threatening occurrences (adverse changes in VS, change in LOC, potential for respiratory or circulatory collapse); often unanticipated	Activities essential to safety: life-saving medications and equipment that protect clients from infections or falls
	Medication or IV therapy priorities	Medications that prevent or treat physiological distress (e.g., analgesics, updrafts or inhalers); medications ordered more frequently (e.g., every 4 hours) because late medication delivery could affect next dose; IV therapy for hydration in clients who are NPO because of nonfunctional GI tract	Medications that prevent reoccurrences of symptoms of disease processes (such as digoxin or antibiotics); medications ordered once per shift, routine maintenance of IV therapy or heparin/saline lock care

Ethical Principles and Decision-making		
	Autonomy	Beneficence
	Accountability	Justice
	Fidelity	Veracity
	Confidentiality	Nonmaleficence

Informed Consent

- Requirements of client: has mental capacity to consent; it is voluntarily done; and client understands treatment and information presented
- Requirements of healthcare provider (performing treatment, procedure, or surgery): shares information about planned treatment, procedure or surgery, its associated risks and benefits, and alternatives to treatment; gives client opportunity to ask questions and have them answered
- If a client waives right to informed consent, document this in the medical record
- If client is deemed incompetent to make informed decisions about healthcare in court of law, a court-appointed guardian makes these decisions
- Informed consent for minors is obtained from parent or legal guardian, except in emergency situations, when minor is married or emancipated from parents, or has special care needs, such as with sexually transmitted infection or pregnancy

Upholding HIPAA (Health Information Portability and Accountability Act)

- Protect personal identifying information (such as name, social security number, date of birth) and information about diagnosis or treatment
- Share information only with individuals involved directly in client's care, payment for care, and/or management of client's care
- Verify identify of persons asking for client information
- Dispose of confidential documents in accord with agency policy (such as shredder, locked recycle bin)

- Keep contents of medical record out of public view by placing in a secure area and turning computer screens displaying client data away from general view
- Discuss client's care only in areas where cannot be overheard

SAFE AND EFFECTIVE CARE ENVIRONMENT: SAFETY AND INFECTION CONTROL

Safety and Infection Control makes up 9–15% of the questions on the NCLEX-RN® exam.

Key Testing Strategies

- Questions that focus on assessing the home environment of a client may be seeking to determine knowledge of risks to safety in the home, such as risk of falls (e.g., throw rugs, no night lights, handrails, or bathroom safety bars) or risk of fire (e.g., oxygen in the home, frayed electrical cords, lack of smoke detectors).
- When answering a question that addresses an infectious disease, consider that the question may be determining knowledge of precautions to prevent disease transmission, and discriminate the need to use contact, airborne, or droplet precautions.
- When answering a question that addresses a client with a compromised immune system or who is receiving chemotherapy, consider that the question may be determining whether the client has a need for neutropenic precautions (for low white blood cell count) or thrombocytopenic precautions (for low platelet count).

Areas of Focus for Safety and Infection Control Questions	Using ergonomic principles	Preventing accidents, errors, and injuries
	Using equipment safely	Implementing infection control practices such as standard precautions, transmission-based precautions, and surgical asepsis
	Using equipment for client safety (such as restraints or safety devices) correctly	
	Workplace safety measures such as security plan/emergency response plan and reporting adverse events using incident/irregular occurrence/variance reports	Safe handling of hazardous materials or infectious materials
		Assessing and assisting with home safety

4 Steps to Maintain Client Safety During a Fire	Remove clients from danger	Contain the fire
	Activate the fire alarm	Evacuate the area (do horizontal evacuation if possible before vertical evacuation)

Fall Risk Factors in Older Adults	Intrinsic Age-Related Changes	Intrinsic Disease Related Changes	Extrinsic Risk Factors
	Gait (step length and height)	Orthostatic hypotension	Floor surface; waxed, scatter rugs, tears in carpeting
	Gait (symmetry and path)	Dehydration	Steps uneven, without hand rails
	Balance when sitting	Cardiac arrhythmias and anemias	Edges and curbing without contrasting colors
	Balance when standing	Urinary tract and other infections	Dim lighting, bright lights that cause glare
	Balance when turning	Osteoporosis and fractures	Bathrooms without grab bars and tub or shower seats
	Stability	Hypoglycemia	High-heeled shoes
	Cognition	Seizures, TIA, CVA, adverse effects of medication, delirium	Clutter

Principles of Surgical Asepsis

- All objects used in a sterile field must be sterile.
- Sterile objects that touch unsterile objects become unsterile.
- Sterile items that are out of vision or below waist level are considered unsterile.
- Sterile objects can become unsterile by prolonged exposure to airborne microorganisms.
- Fluids flow in the direction of gravity.
- Moisture that passes through a sterile object exerts capillary action to draw microorganisms from unsterile surfaces above or below to the sterile surface.
- The edges of a sterile field are considered unsterile.
- The skin is unsterile and cannot be sterilized.
- Conscientiousness, alertness, and honesty are essential qualities in maintaining surgical asepsis.

Centers for Disease Control and Prevention (CDC) Precautions	**Tier 1: Standard Precautions** Hand hygiene Gloves Face protection (mask, goggles, face shield) Gowns and other protective apparel Others **Tier 2: Transmission Based Precautions** **Airborne Precautions:** Use when small ($<5\ \mu$m) pathogen-infected droplet nuclei may remain suspended in air over time and travel distances greater than 3 feet. *Examples: varicella, measles, tuberculosis* **Droplet Precautions:** Use with large ($>5\ \mu$m) pathogen-infected droplets that travel 3 feet or less via coughing, sneezing, etc. or during procedures (suctioning). *Examples: Haemophilus influenzae, Neisseria meningitides, others* **Contact Precautions:** Use with known or suspected microorganisms transmitted by direct hand-to-skin client contact or indirect contact with surfaces or care items in the environment. *Examples: Clostridium difficile, diphtheria (cutaneous), herpes simplex (mucocutaneous or neonatal), impetigo, pediculosis, scabies, zoster (disseminated, immunocompromised host), viral/hemorrhagic infections (Ebola, Lassa, Marburg), others*

HEALTH PROMOTION AND MAINTENANCE

Health Promotion and Maintenance makes up 6–12% of the questions on the NCLEX-RN® exam.

Key Testing Strategies

- Make note of whether the client's age is identified in the question. If so, the question may be determining ability to apply concepts of normal growth and development.
- Because health promotion often involves client education, be prepared to apply principles of teaching and learning to questions in this area.
- When determining interventions to enhance a client's wellness, consider options that promote healthy nutrition, regular exercise, proper weight maintenance, proper rest, and avoidance of harmful chemicals, such as nicotine, and risk-taking behaviors, such as not wearing a seat belt.

Areas of Focus for Health Promotion and Maintenance Questions	Growth and development concepts, including the aging process, developmental stages, and assisting clients with transitions Assisting clients with self-care Activities to promote health and prevent disease, including health screenings	Client lifestyle choices and high-risk behaviors Maternal-newborn concepts such as antepartum, intrapartum, postpartum, and newborn care Physical assessment techniques

Health Screening for Cancer	*Use common sense when monitoring for signs of cancer in clients or yourself:*

Use common sense when monitoring for signs of cancer in clients or yourself:

Pay attention to body changes:

- Unexplained weight loss
- Changes in the characteristics or timing of bowel movements
- Alterations in tissue (moles, thicknesses, lumps)
- Hoarseness, cough, difficulty swallowing

Follow recommended guidelines (USPSTF, ACS, other) for screening recommendations at different ages

Ensure family history of cancer is reviewed as part of record

---

ABCDE Rule for Evaluating a Suspicious Skin Lesion

A = Asymmetry (one half of lesion does not match the other half)

B = Border irregularity (edges are blurred, jagged, or have a notched appearance)

C = Color variation is present or has a dark black color change

D = Diameter is greater than 6 millimeters in size

E = Evolving (color, size, or shape is changing)

Techniques of Physical Assessment

- Inspection: utilizes observation to obtain important information about a client's state of health; have adequate lighting to visually inspect the body without distortions or shadows; lighting can be sunlight or artificial
- Palpation: uses the sensation of touch and pressure of the hands and fingers to determine masses, elevations, temperature, organ position, and any abnormal findings; can be light or deep depending on the area of the body being examined
  - Light palpation is 1 cm in depth
  - Deep palpation is about 4 cm in depth
  - Deep palpation should occur after light palpation
- Percussion: a skill in which the finger of one hand touches or taps a finger of the other hand to generate vibration, which in turn produces a specific, diagnostic sound; the sound changes as the practitioner moves from one area to the next
- Auscultation: uses the sense of hearing to identify sounds produced by the body; some sounds can be heard and identified without a stethoscope; others can only be identified in a quiet environment with a stethoscope

Basic Teaching Principles

- Set priorities for client's learning needs.
- Use appropriate timing.
- Organize materials so that learning proceeds from simple to complex.
- Promote and maintain learner attention and participation.
- Build on the client's existing knowledge.
- Select appropriate teaching methods, including discussion, question and answer, role-play, or discovery, or computerized instruction.
- Use appropriate teaching aids: visual aids (drawings, charts, models, printed materials), audiotapes, films or videotapes, programmed instruction, games, and others.
- Provide teaching related to developmental level.

Age-Related Changes

Skin: Subcutaneous tissue loss and dermal thinning, leading to wrinkling; increase in lentigines (brown age spots); hair thins and loses pigment; nail growth slows and nails may become thicker; skin tissue is more fragile

Sensory/perceptual: Visual acuity changes; ocular changes lead to near vision problems (presbyopia), increased sensitivity to glare, decreased ability to adjust to darkness; cataracts may develop; eyelids lose elasticity; ear canal narrows with calcification of ossicles and increased cerumen, resulting in progressive hearing loss (presbycusis); reduced ability to smell and discriminate odors; sense of taste decreases (especially to sense sweet taste); touch sensation changes with reduced ability to sense heat and cold

Neurologic: Conduction speeds of neuron firing and transmission decrease; memory retrieval is slower; sleep stages 2–4 shorten, leading to a decrease in deep sleep; proprioception decreases

Musculoskeletal: Muscles atrophy; joint cartilage deteriorates; intervertebral disks atrophy, resulting in a loss of height of 1–3 inches

Pulmonary: Chest wall becomes rigid; thoracic muscles weaken; ciliary activity decreases; delivery and diffusion of O_2 to tissues decreases

Cardiovascular: Cardiac output and stroke volume decrease; valves stiffen; conductivity is altered; blood vessels are less elastic, leading to increasing blood pressure

Renal: Decreased glomerular filtration rate and creatinine clearance; possible residual urine or nocturia

Gastrointestinal: Thirst decreases; swallowing time is delayed; possible loss of teeth; decreased saliva; decreased gastric enzymes; weaker intestinal walls

Endocrine: Slowed basal metabolism; insulin levels increase but insulin sensitivity decreases

Genital: Males: prostate enlarges (often benign); decreased sperm protection. Females: vaginal dryness and atrophy

Immune: First sign of infection in an older adult may be a fall; temperature pattern may be lower than younger adult with the same infection

PSYCHOSOCIAL INTEGRITY
Psychosocial Integrity makes up 6–12% of the questions on the NCLEX-RN® exam.

Key Testing Strategies

- For communication questions, select answers that use therapeutic communication techniques and eliminate options that represent communication blocks.
- If a question suggests that a client is at risk for abuse, assess the client without caregivers present and be aware of mandatory reporting laws.
- When responding to a client's communication, look for options that address the client's concern or issue.
- When answering questions of a psychosocial nature when all options seem of equal importance, follow the SEAs: **s**afety, **e**xpressing feelings, and **a**ssisting with problem solving.

Areas of Focus for Psychosocial Integrity Questions	
	Cultural and spiritual/religious influences on health
	Therapeutic communication and environment
	Coping mechanisms, stress management, support systems, and crisis intervention
	Mental health concepts
	Supporting client who has sensory-perceptual alterations
	Assisting clients with grief and loss; end-of-life care
	Family dynamics
	Recognizing and intervening with client abuse or neglect
	Working with clients who have chemical or other dependencies or substance use disorders
	Using behavioral interventions

Components of a Mental Status Exam

General Appearance	Appears stated age? Hygiene? Body odors? Dressed to season? Layered? Cleanliness?
Orientation	Person, place, time, and situation?
Thought Process	Clear, coherent, appropriate to topic? Concentration? Hallucinations or delusions?
Memory	Short-term (What did you have for breakfast?), long-term (Who is the president, and the president before that?)
Judgment	Appropriate? Safe? Impaired? Poor?

Communication Techniques to Avoid	Self-disclosure	Giving personal opinions or advice
	Inattentive listening	Prying to satisfy personal curiosity
	Overuse of medical jargon	Changing the subject

Suicide Precautions

When a client is acutely or actively suicidal, the following precautions should be taken:

- If not already hospitalized, someone should stay with the client until he or she can be admitted to prevent self-harm and maintain the safety of the client.
- Remove all sharp or dangerous objects from the client and the immediate vicinity, including knives or forks, scissors, mirrors, glass, and other objects that could be used for self-harm.
- Remove clothing that could be used as a tourniquet to cause self-harm, including belts of all kinds, neckties, stockings, handbags with long straps, etc.
- Remove all substances that could be ingested to toxic levels, including alcohol, recreational drugs, and medications. Keep client's medications locked.
- Ensure that the client swallows all pills, tablets, or other oral forms of medication, so that they are not kept in the cheek and then stored for later overdose.
- Keep the client in seclusion under one-to-one supervision while actively suicidal; explain in a gentle manner that this is for the client's safety until he or she is able to resist suicidal urges.
- Monitor a client who is not under one-to-one supervision with a nursing unit staff member every 10 to 15 minutes on an irregular schedule of observation.

Ensuring Your Safety on the Psychiatric Unit

1. Never be with a client by yourself. Alert staff to your whereabouts at all times.
2. Always have the ability to exit; do not put yourself in a position where your back is toward a closed-in area without an escape route.
3. Dress in casual clothes. Avoid sexually provocative clothing. Avoid having too much skin exposed.
4. Psychotic clients generally experience three delusional themes: 1) sexual, 2) political, and 3) religious. Avoid these topics unless you are experienced in managing them.
5. Remember that staff members are trained in managing client behavioral problems. Obtain the assistance of more experienced staff members when encountering unsafe situations early in practice.
6. Avoid wearing necklaces or other items that can be used as a weapon to strangle. Wear closed-toe shoes. Do not wear loop earrings (or rings).
7. Remember safety first. Always listen to your primary or gut instinct. Enlist the aid of other staff to help in maintaining control.

Therapeutic Communication Techniques		
	Acknowledging:	Gives nonjudgmental recognition to a client for a certain behavior or contribution, or indicates attention to and care of the client
	Clarifying:	Asks for additional information to ensure understanding of the message sent; a statement like "Would you tell me more about what you have just said?" indicates that understanding the client's message is important to the nurse
	Focusing:	Focuses the client on information that is pertinent and helps the client expand on that information; this technique directs the client towards information that is important
	Giving information:	Provides specific information to a client either with or without the client's request
	Offering self:	Offers the nurse's presence without attaching any expectations or conditions about the client's behavior during that time
	Restating or paraphrasing:	Ensures the nurse understands the message sent; utilizing this technique the nurse repeats the main thought of the message sent
	Reflecting:	Redirects the content of a client's message back to the client for further thought or consideration
	Summarizing:	May be used at the end of an interaction to identify material discussed; it helps to sort out relevant information from irrelevant
	Using silence:	Allows for quiet time without conversation for several seconds or minutes to allow for reflection about the discussion that just occurred, to reduce tension, or to gather thoughts about how to proceed

PHYSIOLOGICAL INTEGRITY: BASIC CARE AND COMFORT

Basic Care and Comfort makes up 6–12% of the questions on the NCLEX-RN® exam.

Key Testing Strategies

- Use principles of administering basic physiological care to clients when answering questions in this part of the test plan.

- When questions address a client's mobility, select answers that will preserve muscle tone and joint function and prevent contractures or skin breakdown.

- Keep principles of safety in mind when answering questions about the use of assistive devices, such as canes, walkers, and crutches.

- Promote good nutrition by selecting meal choices that are balanced and that address any diet restrictions, such as low sodium or reduced fat.

- Use principles of gravity when considering how to position the clients or when working with clients who have drainage or wound tubes.

Areas of focus for Basic Care and Comfort Questions	
	Assisting with or supporting client self-care needs for hygiene, elimination, rest and sleep, and nutrition and oral hydration
	Assisting client with mobility, including use of assistive devices, and caring for clients who are immobile
	Maintaining client comfort using nonpharmacological interventions

Safety Precautions During Oxygen Therapy

- Instruct the client and visitors about the danger of smoking when oxygen is in use. If necessary, remove matches, lighters, and ashtrays.

- If oxygen therapy is used at home, instruct family members or caregivers to smoke only outside. If smoking is permitted, teach visitors to use smoking room.

- Avoid materials that generate static electricity such as woolen blankets and synthetic fabrics; instead use cotton fabrics.
- Avoid use of volatile, flammable substances such as acetone in nail polish removers, alcohol, ether, and oils near clients using oxygen.
- Remove any friction type or battery operated gadgets, devices, or toys.
- Make sure electric devices such as radios, razors, and televisions are in good working order to prevent short-circuit sparks.
- Ensure that electric monitoring equipment and suction machines are properly grounded. Disconnect any ungrounded equipment.
- Personnel need to be aware of the location of fire extinguishers and be able to use them properly.
- Know location of oxygen meter turn-off value.

Therapeutic Diets

Regular diet	High-residue/high-fiber diet
Clear liquids	Low-residue/low-fiber
Full liquids	Carbohydrate controlled
Pureed diet	Fat controlled
Dysphagia diet	Protein controlled
Soft diet	Gastric bypass diet
Mechanical soft diet	Restricted diets (gluten, tyramine, others)
Bland diet	

Types of Dressings

Dressing Type	Description
Gauze	Plain or impregnated with an antimicrobial • Packs and fills wound • Absorbs drainage • Used for full- and partial-thickness wounds with drainage • May be apply dry, wet-to-moist, and wet-to-wet
Transparent film	Adhesive plastic semipermeable membrane that allows oxygen into wound but is occlusive to liquids and bacteria • Protects wound from contamination and friction
Impregnated nonadherent	Cotton or synthetic material impregnated with saline, zinc-saline, antimicrobials, petrolatum or others • Protects nonexudative partial- and full-thickness wounds • Requires secondary dressing to keep in place, hold in moisture, and protect wound
Hydrocolloid	Adhesive made of gelatin • Is occlusive to microorganisms and liquids and promotes absorption of wound exudates • Enhances autolysis of necrotic tissue within wound bed • Duo-Derm and Tegasorb are examples
Hydrogel	Water or glycerin is primary component of jelly-like sheet, granules, or gels • Maintains moist wound bed and helps liquefy necrotic tissue or slough • Permeable to oxygen and can fill dead spaces in a wound • Secondary nonadhesive dressing is required
Alginate (exudate absorbers)	Nonadherent dressings with granules, ropes, paste or other materials; requires secondary dressing • Purpose is to absorb up to 20 times their weight in drainage
Polyurethane foam	Nonadherent dressings that absorb large amounts of exudates while keeping wound moist • Use secondary dressing or tape around edges to secure it
Clear absorbent acrylic	Absorbs exudate and allows moisture to evaporate • Aids in wound assessment and protects from bacteria and shearing forces

PHYSIOLOGICAL INTEGRITY: PHARMACOLOGIC AND PARENTERAL THERAPIES

Pharmacologic and Parenteral Therapies makes up 12–18% of the questions on the NCLEX-RN® exam.

Key Testing Strategies

- Use knowledge of drug action, intended effects and key side and adverse effects to answer a question about a specific medication.

- For questions addressing medication history, do not forget to ask about over-the-counter and herbal supplements as well as prescription medications.

- Double-check drug dosages and make sure the answer passes the common sense test (e.g., answer for a subcutaneous dose should not be more than 1 milliliter for an adult).

- Look for certain prefixes and suffixes in drug names to help identify the drug if the name is unfamiliar.

Areas of Focus for Pharmacologic and Parenteral Therapies Questions	Expected medication actions and client outcomes	Calculating drug dosages
	Unintended medication effects such as side and adverse effects, drug interactions; contraindications to specific medications	Pharmacological pain management
		Maintaining central venous access devices
		Administering blood and blood products
	Administering medications and parenteral/ intravenous therapies	Administering total parenteral nutrition

Calculating Medication Dosages

Formula 1

$$\frac{\text{dose ordered (desired)}}{\text{dose on hand (have)}} \times \text{amount available (quantity)} = \text{amount to give}$$

Formula 2 (ratio and proportion)

$$\frac{\text{dose ordered}}{\text{dose on hand}} = \frac{\times}{\text{quantity available}}$$

Formula 3 (dimensional analysis)

Rule 1: Multiplying one side of an equation by a conversion factor will not change the value of the equation.

Rule 2: Set up the problem so that all labels cancel from the numerator and denominator except the label desired in the answer.

Calculating IV Drip Rates

$$\frac{\text{volume (of fluid)}}{\text{time (in minutes)}} \times \text{drop factor} = \text{flow rate}$$

Steps for Calculating Pediatric Medication Dosages

1. Convert the child's weight from pounds (lb) to kilograms (kg); 1kg = 2.2 lb.
2. Calculate the safe total daily dose in mg/kg or in mcg/kg for a child of this weight as recommended in a standard drug reference book (mg/kg recommended × weight in kg). Then calculate the amount of one dose (total daily dose divided by the number of doses/day).
3. Compare the ordered dose to the recommended dose and determine if the dose is safe.
4. If the dose is safe, calculate the amount of one dose using one of the medication dosage formulas shown. If unsafe, consult prescriber before administering.

Reducing the Risk of Medication Errors

- Question any medication order that is not written clearly, has an unusual dose, or is not in keeping with treatment for client's known health problems.
- Prepare medications in a quiet area away from noise and distractions.
- Check client drug allergies before giving medications; if there is no notation in the allergy section(s) of the medical record, STOP and be sure to obtain allergy history prior to administration. Verify order for a medication that is questionable based on allergy history before administration.
- Be knowledgeable about medications: various names, correct dosage ranges, method of administration, and side/adverse effects.
- Have another nurse check dosage of parenteral medications (such as heparin, digoxin, and insulin) that could pose immediate harm to client if given incorrectly.
- Be aware of drug-food and drug-drug interactions to reduce risk of either ineffective treatment or toxic effects. Sometimes interactions reduce drug's effectiveness and sometimes they heighten its effect.
- Identify client correctly by asking client to state his or her name; checking identification bracelet is the next best method if client is nonverbal. Be especially careful when there are two clients or more in room. Use two unique identifiers per agency policy. If medication bar coding technology is in use, scan medication per agency policy.
- If client questions a medication or states it is different than one taken at home, STOP and recheck medication order and client history. Verify order as necessary before proceeding to administer.
- Carefully and promptly document medication administration.
- Check results of ordered therapeutic drug levels as soon as they are expected to be available and report results promptly.
- Teach clients and significant others/family members about medications well in advance of discharge so they are prepared for safe self-administration following discharge.

Memory Aid for Drugs by Generic Name Prefix, Root, or Suffix*	Syllable in Generic Name	Interpretation	Examples by Generic Name
	-ase, -plase	Thrombolytic agent (-ase usually indicates enzyme)	alteplase, anistreplase, reteplase, streptokinase, tenecteplase
	-azole	Antifungal antimicrobial	itraconazole, fluconazole, clotrimazole, miconazole
	cef-, ceph-	Cephalosporin, antibiotic; check allergy to this class and penicillins	cefazolin, cephalexin, cefotetan, ceftazidime, ceftriazone
	-cillin	Penicillin, antibiotic; check allergy	amoxicillin, penicillin, piperacillin, ticarcillin, nafcillin, oxacillin
	-cycline	Tetracycline, antibiotic	doxycycline, minocycline, tetracycline
	-dipine	Calcium channel blocker, antianginal, antihypertensive	amlodipine, nicardipine, nifedipine, felodipine
	-dronate	Bisphosphonate, bone resorption inhibitor	alendronate, etidronate, pamidronate, risedronate
	-floxacin	Fluoroquinolone, antibiotic	ciprofloxacin, levofloxacin, norfloxacin, sparfloxacin
	-micin, -mycin	Aminoglycoside, antibiotic**	gentamicin, kanamycin, netilmicin, tobramycin
	nitr-, -nitr-	Nitrate, vasodilator, antianginal	nitroglycerin, isosorbide dinitrate
	-olol, -lol	Beta adrenergic blocker, antihypertensive and/or antianginal	propranolol, atenolol, metoprolol, nadolol, labetalol, timolol

Syllable in Generic Name	Interpretation	Examples by Generic Name
-parin	Anticoagulant, heparin or heparinoid	heparin, dalteparin, enoxaparin
-phylline	Xanthine type of bronchodilator	aminophylline, theophylline
-prazole	GI proton pump inhibitor, antiulcer	omeprazole, lansoprazole
-pril	Angiotensin converting enzyme (ACE) inhibitor, antihypertensive	captopril, enalapril, fosinopril, lisinopril, quinapril
sal-, -sal-	Contains salicylate; check allergy to salicylates or aspirin	salsalate (nonopioid analgesic), sulfasalazine (GI anti-inflammatory)
-sartan	Angiotensin II receptor antagonist, antihypertensive	candesartan, eprosartan, losartan, valsartan
-sone, -lone, pred-	Corticosteroid	prednisone, betamethasone, dexa-methasone, cortisone, triamcinolone, prednisolone
-statin	HMG-Coenzyme A reductase inhibitor, lipid lowering agent	atorvastatin, fluvastatin, lovastatin, pravastatin, simvastatin
sulfa-	Sulfonamide, antibiotic; check allergy to sulfa	sulfacetamide, sulfamethoxazole
-terol	Adrenergic type of bronchodilator	albuterol, formoterol, levabuterol, pirbu-terol, salmeterol
-tidine	Histamine H2 antagonist (GI), antiulcer	cimetidine, ranitidine, famotidine, nizatidine
-triptan	Vascular headache sup-pressant, serotonin (5-HT1) agonist	almotriptan, naratriptan, sumatriptan, zolmitriptan
-vir	Antiviral antiinfective	acyclovir, cidofovir, famciclovir, gangciclo-vir, valacyclovir
-zepam, -zolam	Benzodiazepine, antianxiety, sedative/hypnotic	diazepam, lorazepam, oxazepam, alprazolam, midazolam
-zosin	Peripherally acting anti-adrenergic, antihypertensive	doxazocin, prazosin, terazosin

* This is not an exhaustive list and may not be inclusive of every drug in each category.
** This category does not include erythromycin, azithromycin, or clarithromycin, all of which are a macrolide type of antibiotic.

PHYSIOLOGICAL INTEGRITY: REDUCTION OF RISK POTENTIAL

Reduction of Risk Potential makes up 9–15% of the questions on the NCLEX-RN® exam.

Key Testing Strategies

- Memorize common laboratory values and use them to answer questions about specific laboratory test results.
- Always ask if a female client of childbearing age is pregnant before she has x-rays taken.
- Remove all metal objects before a client has an x-ray.
- Ask routinely about allergies to contrast dyes or media before a client undergoes a diagnostic test using inject-able contrast material.
- Recall that clients cannot wear or have imbedded metal (prostheses, for example) to be eligible for magnetic resonance imaging (MRI).

Key Assessments in the Immediate Post-surgical Period

- Adequacy of airway
- Adequacy of ventilation
- Cardiovascular status
- Level of consciousness
- Presence of protective reflexes (e.g., gag, cough)
- Activity, ability to move extremities
- Skin color (pink, pale, dusky, blotchy, cyanotic, jaundiced)
- Fluid status: intake and output, status of IV infusions (type of fluid, rate, amount in container, patency of tubing), signs of dehydration or fluid overload
- Condition of operative site, dressing and presence of drainage
- Patency of and character and amount of drainage from catheters, tubes, and drains
- Discomfort (i.e., pain) (type, location, and severity), nausea, vomiting
- Safety (e.g., necessity for side rails, call bell within reach)

Areas of Focus for Reduction of Risk Potential Questions	Recognizing changes and abnormal trends in vital signs Laboratory and diagnostic tests Potential for body system alterations Implementing therapeutic procedures	Potential for complications of diagnostic tests, client treatments or procedures, client health alterations, or surgery Assessments specific to one or more body systems

Vital Signs by Age

Age	Heart Rate Range & (Avg) in bpm*		Respiratory Rate Range in rpm**		Median Blood Pressure (mm Hg)***	
Newborn (NB)–1 mo	NB	110–170 (120)		30–60	NB	73/55
	1 mo	90–130 (110)			1 mo	86/52
6 months–1 year		80–130 (110)	6 mo	24–36	6 mo	90/53
			1 yr	20–40	1 yr	90/56
2 years		70–120 (100)		20–40		90/56
3–5 years		70–120 (100)		20–30		92/55
6–9 years		70–110 (90)		16–22	6 yrs	96/57
					9 yrs	100/61
10–15 years		60–100 (85)		16–20	10 yrs	100/61
					12 yrs	107/64
					15 yrs	114/65
18 years		60–100 (85)		12–20		121/70

* Beats per minute.
** Respirations per minute; higher when awake; slower during sleep.
*** Blood pressure varies by gender as well as age.

Normal Arterial Blood Gas Values

Arterial Blood Gas Parameter	Normal Value
pH	7.35–7.45
PCO_2	35–45 mm Hg
HCO_3^-	22–26 mEq/L
PO_2	80–100 mm Hg

Adult Reference Range for Common Laboratory Tests	Coagulation Studies	Prothrombin time (PT): 10–13 seconds; 1.5–2.0 times the control in seconds for anticoagulant therapy; Activated partial thromboplastin time (APTT): 20–35 seconds (1.5–2.5 times the control in anticoagulant therapy); Partial thromboplastin time (PTT): 60–70 seconds; 1.5–2.5 times the control in anticoagulant therapy; International normalized ratio (INR): 2.0–3.0 for most anticoagulation needs
	Electrolytes	Sodium (Na^+): 135–145 mEq/L; Potassium (K^+): 3.5–5.1 mEq/L Chloride (Cl^-): 95–105 mEq/L CO_2 combining power: 22–30 mEq/L; 22–30 mmol/L Calcium, total (Ca^{++}): 4.5–5.5 mEq/L, 9–11 mg/dL, 2.3–2.8 mmol/L Calcium (ionized): 4.25–5.25 mg/dL, 2.2–2.5 mEq/L, 1.1–1.24 mmol/L Magnesium (Mg^{++}): 1.5–2.5 mEq/L, 1.8–3.0 mg/dL
	Glucose	Fasting (FBS): 70–110 mg/dL (serum, plasma); 60–100 mg/dL (whole blood); 70–120 mg/dL (elderly); panic values: < 40 or > 700 mg/dL Fingerstick glucose (self-monitoring device): 60–100 mg/dL
	Hematology	White blood cells (WBC): 5000–10,000 microliter or 4500–11,500/mm^3 Neutrophils: 1935–7942 (absolute count) or 45–75% Red blood cells (RBC): 4.5–5.3 million or (10^6)/mm^3 (men), 4.1–5.1 million or (10^6)/mm^3 (women) Hemoglobin (Hgb): 13.0–18.0 grams/100 mL (men), 12–16 grams/100 mL (women) Hematocrit (Hct): 37–49 % (men), 36–46 % (women) Platelet count: 150,000–400,000/mm^3 (or microliter)
	Renal Function Studies	Blood urea nitrogen (BUN): 5–25 mg/dL Serum creatinine: 0.5–1.5 mg/dL
	Therapeutic Drug Levels	Digoxin: 0.5–2.0 ng/mL; Phenytoin: 10–20 mcg/mL Theophylline derivatives: 10–20 mcg/mL or 10–20 mg/mL

PHYSIOLOGICAL INTEGRITY: PHYSIOLOGICAL ADAPTATION

Physiological Adaptation makes up 11–17% of the questions on the NCLEX-RN® exam.

Key Testing Strategies

- Think about the underlying pathophysiology when selecting interventions to assist a client with a health problem affecting a particular body system.
- Remember when a client's status is deteriorating rapidly, follow the ABCs—airway, breathing, and circulation.
- When evaluating the condition of a client with a particular health problem, use knowledge of normal findings or the client's usual baselines as a gauge as to the effectiveness of care.

Areas of Focus for Physiological Adaptation Questions	Body system alterations and pathophysiology	Responding to medical emergencies
	Management of illness	Assessment and treatment of fluid and electrolyte imbalances
	Recognizing and providing care during unexpected response to therapies	Client hemodynamics

Symptom Analysis	O	When was the onset of symptom and what was the client doing?
	P	What was the provoking incident (aggravating factor[s]) that caused the symptom, if any? Any palliating factors?
	Q	What is the quality of the symptom? Is it burning, throbbing, aching, stabbing, other?
	R	Where is the region of symptom? Does it radiate? Does anything relieve the symptom?
	S	How severe is the symptom? (intensity, quantity)
	T	What is the timing of the symptom? When does it occur; how long does it last? (pattern, duration)

Glasgow Coma Scoring System

Type of Response Tested	Score	Indicator
Physical (Motor) Response	6	Acts out a simple command
	5	Reacts to a localized discomfort and offensive stimulus
	4	Moves purposelessly or flexes in response to pain
	3	Exhibits abnormal flexion (decorticate posture)
	2	Exhibits abnormal extension (decerebrate posture)
	1	Has no motor response
Verbal Response	5	Has full orientation (time, place, person)
	4	Shows confusion and disorientation
	3	Uses disorganized or inappropriate words; cannot sustain a conversation
	2	Uses sounds instead of words
	1	Makes no verbal response
Eye Response	4	Open when a person approaches (spontaneous response)
	3	Open when a person speaks
	2	Open only when in pain
	1	Open never, even in presence of painful stimuli

Note: Add numbers to find score from 3 (profound coma) to 15 (normal conscious state).

Neurovascular Status: Checking the "6 Ps"	**Pain:** is there pain or discomfort in the extremity? **Pallor:** is the skin color paler than normal or baseline? **Polar:** is the skin cooler to the touch than normal or baseline in the area? **Paresthesia:** are there any unusual sensations, such as numbness or tingling? **Paralysis:** is the extremity without movement or weaker than normal or baseline? **Pulse:** is the affected pulse (or pulses) diminished or absent?

Nursing Care of the Client in a Cast

- Casts made from plaster of Paris should not get wet and cast padding should not be removed; if cast becomes soiled, clean with a damp cloth. Casts made of synthetic material dry more quickly and allow mobility in less than an hour.
- Smooth rough edges to prevent skin injury; explain that no foreign objects should be inserted into the cast (sticks, food crumbs, etc.) to prevent skin breakdown.
- Avoid covering a new plaster cast with blanket or plastic for extended periods (air cannot circulate, and heat builds up in cast).
- Turn client from side to side (using palms, not fingertips) every 2 hours to facilitate drying for the first 24 to 72 hours.
- Apply ice (crushed or small cubes to avoid denting cast) for the first 24 hours over fracture site to control edema, ensuring that ice is securely contained to avoid wetting cast.
- Elevate extremity above the level of the heart to promote venous return for the first 24 hours after application.
- Encourage active range of motion (AROM) to joints above and below immobilized extremity.
- Report to healthcare provider: increasing pain in immobilized extremity, excessive swelling and discoloration of exposed limb, burning or tingling under cast, sores, or foul odor under cast.

Rule of Nines for Calculating Burn Injury

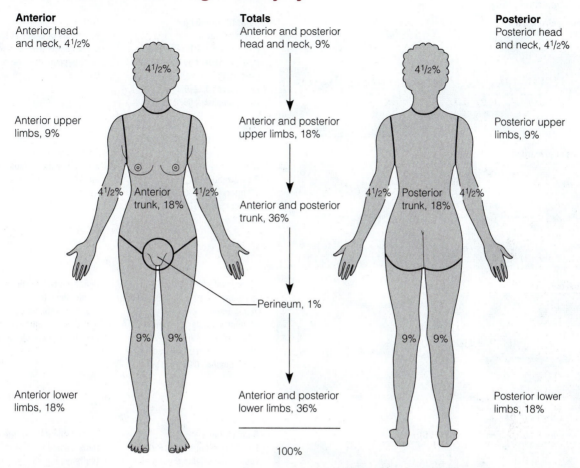

Anterior
Anterior head and neck, 4½%

Anterior upper limbs, 9%

Anterior trunk, 18%

Anterior lower limbs, 18%

Totals
Anterior and posterior head and neck, 9%

Anterior and posterior upper limbs, 18%

Anterior and posterior trunk, 36%

Perineum, 1%

Anterior and posterior lower limbs, 36%

100%

Posterior
Posterior head and neck, 4½%

Posterior upper limbs, 9%

Posterior trunk, 18%

Posterior lower limbs, 18%

Clinical Manifestations of Chronic Renal Failure

Body System	Clinical Manifestations	Cause of Manifestations
Cardiovascular	Hypervolemia, hypertension, tachycardia, arrhythmias, congestive heart failure, pericarditis	Increased fluid volume, build-up of metabolic wastes, chronic hypertension, change in renin-angiotension mechanism
Hematologic	Anemia, leukocytosis, decreased platelet function, thrombocytopenia	Decreased production of erythropoietin and RBCs, decreased survival of RBCs, decreased platelet activity; blood loss through dialysis and bleeding
Gastrointestinal	Anorexia, nausea, vomiting, abdominal distention, diarrhea, constipation, bleeding	Build-up of uremic toxins, electrolyte imbalances, changes in platelet activity, conversion of urea to ammonia by saliva
Neurologic	Lethargy, confusion, convulsions, stupor, coma, sleep disturbances, behavioral changes, muscle irritability	Uremic toxins, electrolyte imbalances, cerebral swelling caused by fluid shifts
Dermatologic	Pallor, pigmentation, pruritus, ecchymosis, excoriation, uremic frost	Anemia, decreased activity of sweat glands, dry skin, phosphate deposits on skin
Urinary	Decreased urine output, decreased specific gravity, proteinuria, casts and cells in the urine	Damage to the nephron
Skeletal	Osteoporosis, renal rickets, joint pain	Decreased calcium absorption, decreased phosphate excretion

Priority Cardiac Dysrhythmias

Rhythm/ECG Appearance	ECG Characteristics	Management

Supraventricular Rhythms

Sinus tachycardia

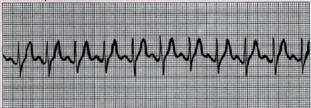

Rate: 101 to 150 bpm
Rhythm: regular
P:QRS ratio is 1:1 (with very fast rates, P wave may be hidden in preceding T wave)
PR interval: 0.12–0.20 sec
QRS complex: 0.06–0.10 sec

Treat only if client is experiencing symptoms or is at risk for myocardial damage; treat underlying cause (e.g., hypovolemia, fever, pain); beta blockers or verapamil may be used

Sinus bradycardia

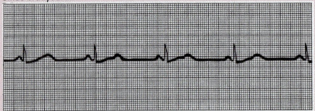

Rate: less than 60 bpm
Rhythm: regular
P:QRS ratio is 1:1
PR interval: 0.12–0.20 sec
QRS complex: 0.06–0.10 sec

Treat only if client is experiencing symptoms; intravenous atropine and/or pacemaker therapy may be used

Atrial fibrillation

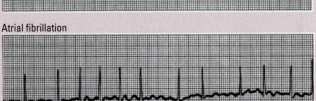

Rate: atrial 300–600 bpm (too rapid to count); ventricular 100–180 bpm in untreated clients
Rhythm: irregularly irregular
P:QRS ratio is variable
PR interval: not measured
QRS complex: 0.06–0.10 sec

Synchronized cardioversion; medications to reduce ventricular response rate: verapamil, propranolol, digoxin, anticoagulant therapy to reduce risk of clot formation and stroke

Ventricular Rhythms

Premature ventricular contractions (PVC)

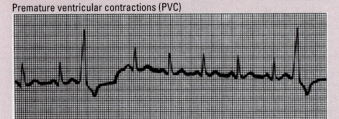

Rate: variable
Rhythm: irregular, with PVC interrupting underlying rhythm and followed by a compensatory pause
P:QRS ratio: no P wave noted before PVC
PR interval: absent with PVC
QRS complex: wide (greater 0.12 sec), bizarre in appearance; differs from normal QRS complex

Treat if client is experiencing symptoms; advise against stimulant use (caffeine, nicotine); drug therapy includes intravenous lidocaine, procainamide, quinidine, propranolol, phenytoin, amiodarone

Ventricular tachycardia (VT or V tach)

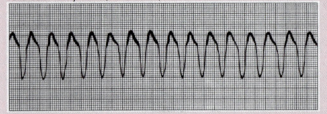

Rate: 100–250 bpm
Rhythm: regular
P:QRS ratio: P waves usually not identifiable
PR interval: not measured
QRS complex: 0.12 sec or greater; bizarre shape

Treat if VT is sustained or if client is experiencing symptoms; treatment includes intravenous procainamide or lidocaine and/or immediate defibrillation if the client is unconscious or unstable

Ventricular fibrillation (VF or V fib)

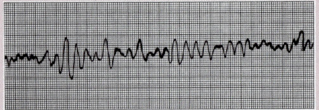

Rate: too rapid to count
Rhythm: grossly irregular
P:QRS ratio: no identifiable P waves
PR interval: none
QRS: bizarre, varying in shape and direction

Immediate defibrillation

Index

NOTE: Page numbers followed by *b* indicate box; those followed by *f* indicate figure; those followed by *t* indicate table.